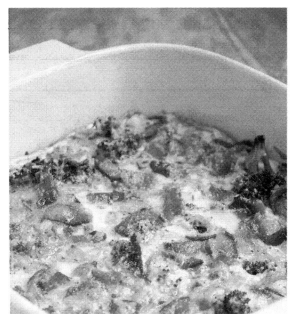
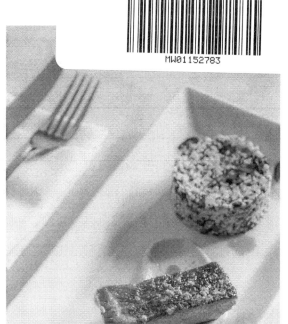

Keto for Women Over 60

500 DAYS OF TASTY RECIPES AND A STRESS-FREE 30-DAY DIET PLAN

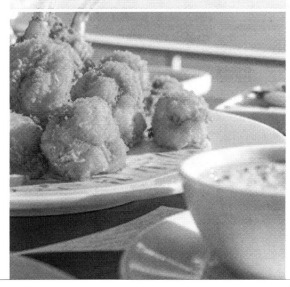
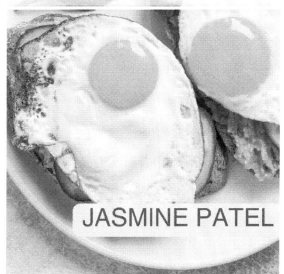

JASMINE PATEL

NOTES

INTRODUCTION

CHAPTER 1

CHAPTER 2

CHAPTER 3

BREAKFAST

- KETO BREAKFAST DAIRY-FREE SMOOTHIE BOWL 39
- CRISPY KETO CORNED BEEF & RADISH HASH 39
- COCONUT FLOUR PORRIDGE 39
- EASY SHAKSHUKA 39
- STEAK AND EGGS 40
- FARMER CHEESE PANCAKES 40
- FRENCH OMELET 40
- SOUTHWESTERN OMELET 41
- BROCCOLI & CHEESE OMELET 41
- HAM & FETA OMELET 41
- BACON AND MUSHROOM OMELETTE 42
- SCRAMBLED EGGS WITH MUSHROOMS AND COTTAGE CHEESE 42
- BACON AND EGG STUFFED ZUCCHINI BOATS 42
- BACON AND ZUCCHINI EGG MUFFINS 43
- DENVER OMELET SALAD 43
- TURKEY BREAKFAST SAUSAGE 43
- CHICKEN AVOCADO SALAD 44
- SPINACH-MUSHROOM SCRAMBLED EGGS 44
- EGGS FLORENTINE CASSEROLE 44
- TACO BREAKFAST SKILLET 45
- CHORIZO BREAKFAST BAKE 45
- SPINACH AND CHEESE EGG BAKE 46
- KETO BREAKFAST CASSEROLE 46
- AVOCADO OMELETTE 46
- BRUSCHETTA WITH AVOCADO AND EGG 46
- LEMON POPPY RICOTTA PANCAKES 47
- EGG STRATA WITH BLUEBERRIES AND CINNAMON 47
- SWEET BLUEBERRY COCONUT PORRIDGE 47
- SWEET APPLE CINNAMON COCONUT PORRIDGE 48
- LOW-CARB BREAKFAST QUICHE 48
- QUICHE WITH BOILED CHICKEN BREAST AND MUSHROOM 48
- COCONUT FLOUR PANCAKES 49
- PEPPERONI, HAM & CHEDDAR STROMBOLI 49
- EGGS AND ASPARAGUS BREAKFAST BITES 50
- CHEDDAR BISCUITS 50
- VEGETABLE TART 50
- KETO SAUSAGE BREAKFAST SANDWICH 51
- CABBAGE HASH BROWNS 51
- OMELET-STUFFED PEPPERS 51
- BACON AVOCADO BOMBS 52
- HAM & CHEESE EGG CUPS 52
- KETO PIZZA EGG WRAP 52
- GREEN EGGS 52
- MASALA FRITTATA WITH AVOCADO SALSA 53
- KETO BREAKFAST PARFAIT 53
- KETO SAUSAGE & EGG BOWLS 53
- CHEESE AND EGG STUFFED PEPPERS 54
- EGG WRAPS WITH HAM AND GREENS 54
- KETO CROQUE MADAME 55
- KETO SPINACH SHAKSHUKA 55
- KETO SAUSAGE CREAM CHEESE ROLLS 55
- KETO BISCUITS AND GRAVY 56
- PROTEIN BREAKFAST SCRAMBLE 56
- RADISH AND TURNIP HASH WITH FRIED EGGS 57
- KALE AND GOAT CHEESE FRITTATA CUPS 57
- ROASTED RADISH AND HERBED RICOTTA OMELET 58
- MIXED MUSHROOM EGG BAKES 58
- CHICKEN AND CHEESE BREAKFAST BOWLS 59
- SPICY CHICKEN BREAKFAST BOWLS 59
- KETO BREAKFAST SANDWICH 59
- POACHED EGGS MYTILENE 60
- HEALTHY BREAKFAST CHEESECAKE 60
- BLUEBERRY PANCAKES 61
- LOW CARB PUMPKIN CHEESECAKE PANCAKES 61
- TURKISH-STYLE BREAKFAST RECIPE 61
- POACHED EGG AND BACON SALAD 62
- SPINACH PANCAKES 62
- PECAN & COCONUT ' N ' OATMEAL 62
- CHEDDAR CHIVE BAKED AVOCADO EGGS 63
- KETO EGG ROLL IN A BOWL 63
- KETO PIGS IN A BLANKET 63
- KETO MEAL PREP BREAKFAST BOMBS 64
- KETO CAULIFLOWER BUNS 64
- KETO THREE CHEESE CAULIFLOWER MAC AND CHEESE CUPS 65
- KETO YOGURT PARFAIT 65
- KETO HOT POCKET 66
- KETO BREAKFAST CHILI 66
- BIG MAC BREAKFAST PIE 67
- CREAM OF WHEAT CEREAL 67
- GREEN EGGS AND HAM: AVOCADO HOLLANDAISE 67
- DUTCH BABY 68
- CARNIVORE QUICHE 68
- HUEVOS RANCHEROS WITH A PROTEIN-SPARING TWIST 69
- PROTEIN SPARING PANCAKES 69

POULTRY

- PAPRIKA CHICKEN 71
- STUFFED CHICKEN BREASTS 71
- BACON-WRAPPED CHICKEN WITH SHRIMP 71
- BACON-WRAPPED BLUE CHEESE CHICKEN 72
- GARLIC CHICKEN WITH ROASTED VEGETABLES 72
- CREAM CHEESE STUFFED CHICKEN 72
- ONE PAN KETO CHEESY JALAPEÑO CHICKEN 73
- KETO CRACK CHICKEN 73
- CHICKEN FLORENTINE 74
- HUNAN CHICKEN 74
- KETO ORANGE CHICKEN 75
- CHICKEN WITH CREAMY PEPPER SAUCE 75
- CHICKEN AND EGGPLANT CURRY WITH ALMONDS 76
- COCONUT BREADED CHICKEN 76

INDIAN-STYLE KETO CHICKEN 76
CHICKEN FRICASSEE WITH VEGETABLES 77
CHICKEN STIR-FRY WITH MUSHROOMS 77
GRILLED CHICKEN FILLET WITH CREAMY WINE SAUCE 78
CHICKEN FILLET STUFFED WITH SHRIMP 78
CHICKEN SALAD PUFFS 78
SESAME CHICKEN AVOCADO SALAD 79
EASY CASHEW CHICKEN 79
KETO PESTO STUFFED CHICKEN BREASTS 79
SMOKED CHICKEN SALAD SANDWICH 80
THAI CHICKEN LETTUCE WRAPS 80
GARLIC, LEMON & THYME ROASTED CHICKEN BREASTS 81
GRILLED CHICKEN KABOBS 81
CHICKEN ENCHILADA BOWL 81
CHICKEN PHILLY CHEESESTEAK 82
DUCK ACCORDING TO UKRAINIAN RECIPE 82
DUCK STEWED WITH PRUNES 83
DUCK WITH STEWED CABBAGE 83
DUCK AND CAULIFLOWER STIR-FRY 84
CREAMY DUCK WITH SPINACH RECIPE 84
DUCK AND SPINACH SALAD 85
CREAMY DUCK SOUP 85
KETO DUCK ROLLS 86
DUCK, BACON, GREEN BEAN, AND MUSHROOM SKILLET 86
KETO DUCK DUMPLINGS 87
DUCK AND BROCCOLI "ALFREDO" 87
DUCK A L'ORANGE RECIPE 88
DUCK BREAST WITH CHERRY PORT SAUCE 88
DUCK BREAST WITH BLUEBERRY SAUCE 89
CHICKEN EGG SALAD WRAPS 89
CHICKEN HEARTS AND LIVER IN A CREAMY TOMATO SAUCE 89
CHICKEN HEARTS IN A CREAMY SAUCE 90
KETO CHICKEN HEARTS 90
KETO THIGH PULPS WITH MUSTARD 90
KETO CHICKEN LIVER PATE 91
KETO WHITE CHICKEN CHILI 91
GARLIC PARMESAN CHICKEN WITH BROCCOLI 91
CHICKEN FILLET STUFFED WITH CHICKEN LIVER PATE 92
BUFFALO CHICKEN CANNOLI 92
CHICKEN CHORIZO CHILI 93
CHICKEN WINGETTES WITH CILANTRO DIP 93
TURKEY AND CAULIFLOWER RICE BOWL 94
FAT HEAD CHICKEN BRAID 94
CHICKEN MILANESE 94
TURKEY AND SOY SPROUTS STIR FRY 95
TURKEY STEW RECIPE 95
MUSHROOM & SAGE ROLLED TURKEY BREAST 96
WHOLE ROASTED BRINED TURKEY 96
COBB SALAD 97
JALAPENO POPPER CHICKEN 97
CHICKEN WONTONS 97
REUBEN CHICKEN 98

CRACK SLAW 98
KETO TANDOORI CHICKEN WINGS 99
YAKISOBA CHICKEN 99
KETO RICED CAULIFLOWER & CURRY CHICKEN 99
TURKEY AND ZUCCHINI FRITTERS 99
SWEET AND SOUR CHICKEN 100
BAKED CHICKEN NUGGETS 100
CURRIED CHICKEN SOUP 100
COCONUT CHICKEN TENDERS 101
TURKEY LASAGNA WITH RICOTTA 101
CREAMY TURKEY AND CAULIFLOWER SOUP 102
PINE NUT BREADED BLUE CHEESE STUFFED TURKEY POCKETS 102
SALSA CHICKEN 102
TURKEY AND SPINACH CASSEROLE 103
TURKEY AND WALNUT SALAD 103
ROASTED TURKEY BREAST WITH MUSHROOMS & BRUSSELS SPROUTS 103

BEEF AND LAMB

BLUE CHEESE BACON BURGERS 105
BACON CHEESEBURGER SKILLET 105
BACON MUSHROOM SWISS STEAK 105
BACON BEEF SKILLET WITH CHEESY GREEN BEANS 105
BEEF AND VEGETABLE SKILLET WITH YOGURT SAUCE 106
CREAMY BEEF AND SPINACH SKILLET 106
BACON-WRAPPED BEEF ROLLS 107
SESAME-CRUSTED BEEF ROLLS 107
BEEF AND VEGETABLE STIR-FRY 107
CREAMY GARLIC BEEF AND BRUSSELS SPROUTS SKILLET 108
VITELLO TONNATO 108
KETO BEEF WELLINGTON 108
AVOCADO WITH GROUND BEEF AND CHEESE 109
KETO BEEF NACHOS 109
CHINESE CABBAGE BEEF ROLLS 109
KETO EGG-STUFFED BEEF CUTLETS WITH MUSHROOMS 110
CREAMY BEEF LIVER WITH CARAMELIZED ONIONS 110
BEEF LIVER PATE 110
CREAMY BEEF LIVER AND VEGETABLES 111
BEEF LIVER WITH VEGETABLES IN TOMATO SAUCE 111
BEEF LIVER JAPANESE STYLE 111
KETO BEEF LIVER FRITTERS 112
PANCAKES STUFFED WITH BEEF LIVER 112
BEEF LIVER GOULASH 112
BEEF LIVER CASSEROLE 113
BEEF LIVER WITH ZUCCHINI PANCAKES 113
VIETNAMESE BEEF LIVER 114
BEEF LIVER WITH MIXED VEGETABLES SAUTEED 114
KETO BAKED BEEF WITH MIXED VEGETABLES 114
PARMESAN-CRUSTED BEEF LIVER CUTLETS 115

PORK AND HAM

ROASTED PORK LOIN WITH GRAINY MUSTARD SAUCE 153

FISH AND SEAFOOD

SALMON AND CREAM CHEESE SUSHI ROLLS 156
SALMON AND CAULIFLOWER RICE SUSHI ROLLS 156
KETO CRISPY SKIN SALMON IN WHITE WINE SAUCE 157
ALASKAN SALMON WITH BUTTER CREAM SAUCE AND AVOCADO 157
GRILLED SALMON WITH PESTO AND ROASTED ASPARAGUS 158
KETO ASIAN GLAZED SALMON 158
BACON-WRAPPED SALMON WITH SPINACH SALAD 158
SMOKED SALMON AND ASPARAGUS FRITTATA 159
PARMESAN CRUSTED FLOUNDER FISH 159
SIMPLE TUNA SALAD ON LETTUCE 159
FRIED TUNA AVOCADO BALLS 159
CREAMY SMOKED SALMON ZUCCHINI SPAGHETTI 160
SHRIMP AVOCADO SALAD 160
CAPRESE TUNA SALAD STUFFED TOMATOES 160
SPICY KIMCHI AHI POKE 161
PROSCIUTTO BLACKBERRY SHRIMP 161
SPICY SHRIMP TACO LETTUCE WRAPS 161
SHRIMP AND NORI ROLLS 162
CRISPY FISH STICKS WITH CAPER DILL SAUCE 162
CREAMY SHRIMP AND MUSHROOM SKILLET 162
BUTTERED COD IN SKILLET 163
BROCCOLI AND SHRIMP SAUTÉED IN BUTTER 163
KETO CALAMARI 164
LOW CARB ALMOND CRUSTED COD 164
MEXICAN FISH STEW 164
CREAMY KETO FISH CASSEROLE 165
GRILLED SALMON WITH AVOCADO SALSA 165
CREAMY CHILE SHRIMP 166
LEMON KALAMATA OLIVE SALMON 166
SEAFOOD MEDLEY STEW 166
FLAVORED OCTOPUS 167
CRUNCHY ALMOND TUNA 167
ARUGULA AND SALMON SALAD 167
GRILLED PESTO SALMON WITH ASPARAGUS 167
GRILLED SALMON AND ZUCCHINI WITH MANGO SAUCE 168
FRIED COCONUT SHRIMP WITH ASPARAGUS 168
BALSAMIC SALMON WITH GREEN BEANS 168
SHRIMP AND SAUSAGE "BAKE" 169
HERB BUTTER SCALLOPS 169
PAN-SEARED HALIBUT WITH CITRUS BUTTER SAUCE 170
FISH CURRY 170
ROASTED SALMON WITH AVOCADO SALSA 170
SOLE ASIAGO 171
BAKED COCONUT HADDOCK 171
CHEESY GARLIC SALMON 172

DESSERTS

KETO MUFFINS CLASSIC CINNAMON 174
KETO BLUEBERRY MUFFINS 174
KETO CHOCOLATE MUFFINS 175
KETO LEMON MUFFINS 175
KETO ALMOND FLOUR MUFFINS 176
1-MINUTE KETO MUFFINS RECIPE 176
KETO PUMPKIN MUFFINS 176
KETO STRAWBERRY, ALMOND AND CHOCOLATE MUFFINS 177
KETO CHOCOLATE CREAM CHEESE MUFFINS 177
TRIPLE CHOCOLATE ZUCCHINI MUFFINS 178
KETO PECAN MUFFINS 178
KETO PUMPKIN CHIA MUFFINS 179
KETO CARROT MUFFINS 179
KETO CRANBERRY ORANGE MUFFINS 180
KETO CHEESECAKE MUFFINS 180
CREAM CHEESE PUMPKIN MUFFINS 181
CHEESY CAULIFLOWER MUFFINS 181
DOUBLE CHOCOLATE MUFFINS 181
KETO CINNAMON EGG LOAF MUFFINS 182
CHOCOLATE CHIP BANANA BREAD MUFFINS 182
KETO CHEESY HERB MUFFINS 183
KETO RICOTTA LEMON POPPYSEED MUFFINS 183
CRANBERRY SOUR CREAM MUFFINS 184
KETO LEMON BLUEBERRY MUFFINS 184
KETO BANANA NUT MUFFINS 184
KETO SNICKERDOODLE MUFFINS 185
KETO COFFEE CAKE MUFFINS 185
STRAWBERRY VANILLA MUFFIN 186
FLAXSEED MUFFIN IN A MUG 186
FLOURLESS PEANUT BUTTER MUFFINS 187
KETO GINGERBREAD MUFFINS 187
KETO PEACH MUFFINS 187
KETO JELLY DONUT MUFFINS 188
KETO CAPPUCCINO MUFFINS 188
KETO PANCAKE MUFFINS 189
KETO MOCHA MUFFINS 189
BROWN BUTTER PECAN MUFFINS 190
MAPLE WALNUT MUFFINS 190
PECAN CHEESECAKE MUFFINS 190
BLUEBERRY LEMON MUFFINS 191
BUTTER PECAN COOKIES 191
KETO JAM COOKIES 192
ENGLISH TOFFEE CAPPUCCINO COOKIES 192
CRUNCHY PEANUT COOKIES 192
KETO VANILLA COOKIES 193
MAPLE CREAM SANDWICH COOKIES 193
'APPLE' PIE COOKIES 194
LOW CARB LEMON COOKIES 194
KETO FRUIT PIZZA COOKIES 194
GLAZED MAPLE WALNUT COOKIES 195
CHOCOLATE CHIP SHORTBREAD COOKIES 195
CRANBERRY COOKIES 195
KETO MAGIC COOKIES 196
SUGAR FREE LEMON BARS 196

KETO SMOOTHITES AND DRINKS

INTRODUCTION

Dear reader,

Congratulations on taking the first step toward a transformative journey that will revolutionize your life and your approach to aging. Within the pages of this book, we embark on an exhilarating and empowering exploration of the immense potential of a ketogenic diet specifically tailored for women over 60. It is a life force that knows no boundaries, as age is merely a number. Together, we will unravel the mystery of finding the fountain of youth and unlock your full potential in terms of physical and mental well-being.

Turning 60 opens the door to a remarkable new phase of life, filled with wisdom, experience, and a newfound sense of independence. However, it can also present unique challenges, particularly when it comes to maintaining a healthy weight and managing age-related health issues. The good news is that it is never too late to make significant changes and embrace a new lifestyle that will profoundly impact your well-being. For women over 60, the low-carb, high-fat ketogenic diet holds immense promise.

Before delving into the specifics of this meal plan, let us first grasp the science behind the ketogenic diet. By shifting your body's primary fuel source from glucose to ketones, you can enter a metabolic state called ketosis. Ketosis is an alternative metabolic state that sets off a chain reaction of positive outcomes, including increased energy levels, enhanced mental clarity, reduced inflammation, and decreased body fat. Moreover, studies have demonstrated that the ketogenic diet offers particular benefits to women over 60, addressing many of the challenges that older women may encounter.

The ketogenic diet serves as an alternative approach to nourishing your body with essential nutrients, as nutrition forms the foundation of any healthy lifestyle. This chapter will guide you through the fundamentals of the diet and provide helpful tips on creating a personalized meal plan that caters to both your preferences and requirements. We will explore a range of delectable and satisfying options that not only please your taste buds but also contribute to your overall well-being. These choices encompass sourcing high-quality fats and proteins and incorporating a variety of nutrient-dense vegetables into your diet.

When embracing the ketogenic diet, the goal extends beyond mere body fat reduction. In the subsequent chapter, we will delve into the myriad benefits that ketosis can bestow upon your life. You will discover how a low-carb, high-fat diet can be a game-changer in multiple aspects, such as increasing energy and mental acuity, enhancing insulin sensitivity, and reducing the likelihood of developing chronic diseases. Additionally, we will explore the impact of ketosis on hormonal balance, bone health, and cognitive function, emphasizing their direct relevance to the needs of women over 60.

Commencing any dietary modification can be challenging, and the ketogenic diet is no exception. However, you will find the necessary tools and resources to maintain commitment and motivation throughout your journey towards optimal health. These include managing cravings, navigating potential plateaus, mastering social situations, dining out, and everything in between. Remember, perseverance is absolutely crucial, and every step forward represents progress towards a brighter and healthier future.

Dear reader, you possess the power to reclaim your youth and vitality with a little effort. By embarking on this exclusive ketogenic journey designed for women over 60, you are taking a bold stride towards a healthier and more fulfilling life. Now is the time to prioritize your well-being, and through the ketogenic diet, you can unlock the potential of a vibrant and energized future under your complete control. Believe in your ability to effect positive changes in your life and explore the countless opportunities that lie ahead. Allow this book to serve as your guiding companion as you embark on this remarkable voyage.

Do you possess the determination to uncover the secret of everlasting youth? Let us embark on this life-altering adventure together and dive into the depths of possibility!

Jasmine Patel

2023

CHAPTER 1

WHY DO WE NEED KETO? REMARKABLE BENEFITS FOR WOMEN OVER 60

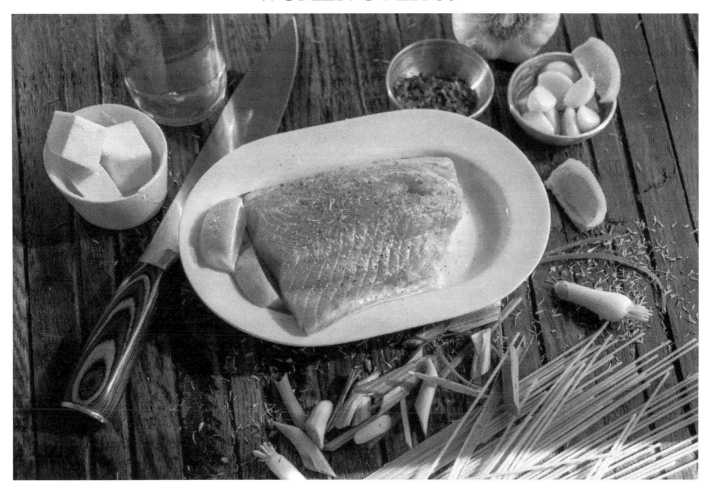

Recently, the ketogenic diet has been making waves across social media and online forums. It is frequently touted as a quick remedy for losing excess pounds, and this is one of the reasons for its popularity. Weight loss is just one of the many benefits that come along with following the keto diet, which is designed specifically for women over the age of 60. However, it is undoubtedly one of the most important ones. Let's have a look at some of the reasons why a nutritional strategy like this one is so beneficial during menopause and beyond:

An Extraordinary Method That Involves the Melting of Fat.

The ketogenic diet, in contrast to the vast majority of other diets, which mainly result in a reduction in water weight, is very effective at lowering overall body fat. This is because the ketogenic diet prioritizes fat loss over weight loss of any other kind. By using fats as the primary fuel source rather than glucose, you can improve the efficiency with which your body uses the glucose it stores and the fat it stores by switching the primary fuel source it uses, which is glucose, to fats. For many women over the age of 60, menopause is connected with an increase in abdominal fat, and the keto diet does an outstanding job of focusing on and removing this sort of resistant fat. In addition, the keto diet is associated with a reduction in overall body fat. By cutting down on the amount of excess fat in your body, you can lower your chances of developing cardiovascular conditions like heart disease, stroke, and sudden cardiac arrest.

Improving one's insulin sensitivity is absolutely necessary for continuing to enjoy good health.

Insulin resistance is becoming increasingly prevalent in those over the age of 60, particularly those who are overweight or obese. The aging of the population is exacerbating this pattern. Because of this issue, it is difficult for the body to adequately transport glucose from the bloodstream to the muscles and liver. This can lead to increased body fat as well as an increased chance of getting diabetes. On the other hand, low-carbohydrate diets such as the ketogenic diet and other programs that are very similar to it have been shown to boost insulin sensitivity in some people. If you process fewer carbohydrates, your body will make less fat from glucose, which will lower your risk of getting type 2 diabetes and keep you from gaining weight unnecessarily. If you process fewer carbohydrates, your body will produce less fat from protein, which will lower your risk of developing type 1 diabetes.

How to Regain Command of Your Thoughts and Improve Your Brain's Health.

The process of aging is linked to a natural decline in cognitive ability, which is typically accompanied by changes in mood, the inability to remember things, and diminished focus. It's possible that these challenges will become much more challenging as menopause progresses. On the other hand, the ketogenic diet offers the opportunity for a cure by providing an efficient source of fuel for the brain. This makes the ketogenic diet a potential candidate for a remedy. Glucose is the source of energy that the brain uses when everything is functioning normally; however, as estrogen levels decline, the amount of glucose that is able to reach the brain also drops. When you convert to using ketones as a fuel source when you are on the ketogenic diet, your brain receives a flow of energy that is more reliable and useful. This is because ketones are derived from fat. Both the prevention of neurological diseases and the treatment of those that already exist are helped by this.

A reduction in the amount of inflammation, in addition to providing relief from aches and pains.

If you are a woman over the age of 60, it is highly likely that you have suffered from the excruciating pain of migraine headaches, knee pain, and joint inflammation at some point in your life. Walnuts, avocados, and olive oil are a few examples of sources of anti-inflammatory fat that are prevalent in a ketogenic diet. These fats may help alleviate some of the unpleasant side effects of the ketogenic diet. In addition, it has been found that an association exists between the consumption of processed foods and sources that are high in carbs and increased levels of inflammatory markers. By limiting your consumption of these items and adopting a lifestyle that is more in line with the ketogenic diet, you can effectively reduce inflammation and find relief from chronic pain. This is accomplished by adopting a lifestyle that is more in line with the ketogenic diet.

Keeping a healthy ratio of lipids in order to promote healthy heart functioning.

Blood tests taken on women once they reach the age of 60 typically reveal an increase in LDL cholesterol, which is also known as low-density lipoprotein cholesterol, as well as triglycerides, which are commonly referred to as "bad" fats. This rise in LDL cholesterol and triglycerides is associated with an increased risk of cardiovascular disease. When there are no limitations placed on a person's diet, it is usual for the consumption of unhealthy fats to outnumber the consumption of healthy fats, such as high-density lipoprotein (HDL) and omega-3 fatty acids. This is because harmful fats tend to have a higher caloric density than omega-3 fatty acids do. Researchers have shown a link between low HDL levels and an increased likelihood of developing cardiovascular disease (CVD). If, on the other hand, you adhere to the keto diet, you will take in the necessary quantity of fat, and within that fat will be a large portion of HDL. HDL is a kind of cholesterol that has been demonstrated to lower the risk of developing cardiovascular disease.

Maintaining a Healthy Blood Pressure Level While Keeping Your Hypertension Under Control.

Beyond the age of sixty, the roles switch around: While men typically have higher blood pressure than women, women's blood pressure tends to rise beyond that age. This is in contrast to the normal situation, in which men have higher blood pressure than women. If the condition is not addressed, hypertension can become a significant risk factor for a variety of other health conditions, including kidney and heart disorders. The elimination of processed foods from your diet and the adoption of a more heart-healthy eating pattern are two major components of the ketogenic diet. Both of these factors contribute to a drop in blood pressure, which is one of the primary benefits of the ketogenic diet.

Increasing the bone density in your body is one of the most effective preventative measures you can take against osteoporosis.

After menopause, bone loss and fragility are two symptoms that frequently affect women in their 50s. These symptoms, if left untreated, can eventually develop into osteoporosis in the advanced stages of the disorder. The ingestion of an adequate amount of calcium is crucial for the preservation of bone health, and the ketogenic diet includes green leafy vegetables that are rich in calcium as part of its selection of vegetables. In addition, the diet avoids a number of foods and substances that prevent the body from properly absorbing calcium. This serves as an extra line of defense against the development of osteoporosis.

Keep your strength up and don't stop moving if you want to keep your muscles strong.

When women age, they often have a higher rate of muscle loss than men do, which can lead to decreased strength and exhaustion in addition to a general decline in physical performance. Men, on the other hand, typically experience a slower rate of muscle loss than women do. Because it promotes the consumption of protein-rich foods in moderate proportions, the ketogenic diet is beneficial for the growth, maintenance, and repair of muscle tissue. Because it contains all of the nutrients that are necessary for the proper functioning of your muscles, the ketogenic diet makes it possible for you to maintain your muscular mass as well as your strength, energy, and active lifestyle.

Remember that going on the keto diet isn't just about reducing your calorie intake or your overall weight. Women over the age of 60 who want to enhance their health and extend their lives may find that adopting a ketogenic way of life is an option that can completely transform their situation.

In the chapters that follow, we will go more into the specifics of the ketogenic diet for women over the age of 60. Our intention is to make available to you helpful guidelines, mouthwatering recipes, and strategies that will allow you to triumph over challenges that may appear along the route. Prepare to uncover your true potential and embark on the first step of your journey toward a life that is rich in vitality, energy, and satisfaction. Let's all start following the ketogenic diet and lifestyle together, and together we can rewrite the rules of getting older!

HOW DOES ONE ADHERE TO A KETOGENIC DIET?

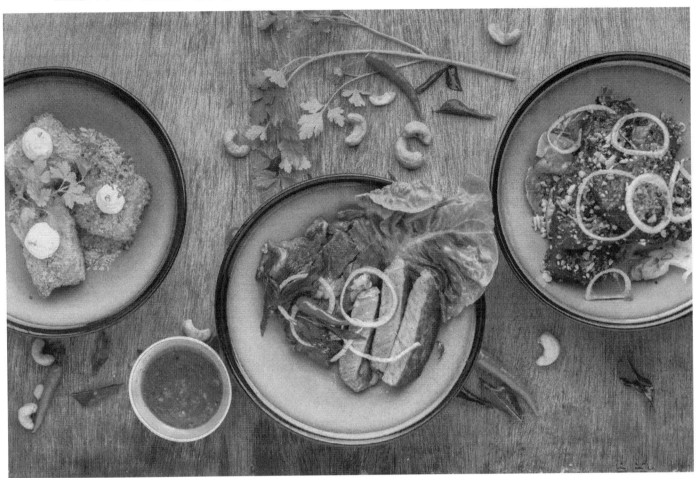

It is a type of diet that contains a restricted amount of carbs. On the other hand, you will need to reduce the amount of carbohydrates you eat to an exceptionally low level and increase the amount of fat you consume in order to achieve your goal. Because of this, your body will transition from obtaining the majority of its energy from carbohydrates, specifically glucose, to obtaining the majority of its energy from ketones instead. Ketones are produced from lipids, and just like glucose, they have the ability to supply the brain with a source of energy. Ketones are produced when lipids are broken down.

Because of this change, your body will go through a process that is referred to as "ketosis." Your body enters a state of ketosis when it switches from using carbs as its primary source of fuel to using fat as its primary fuel source.

This change will result in weight loss for you, in addition to having positive effects on your health in other areas.

Several distinct methods exist for following the ketogenic diet.

This diet can be modified in a number of different ways, some of which are described in the paragraphs that follow.

Standard Ketogenic Diet (SKD): This diet plan is typically followed by individuals who are engaged in the process of reducing their overall body mass. It has a moderate quantity of protein, an extremely low consumption of carbohydrates, and an unlimited supply of fat. The majority of the calories come from fat, which makes up about 70 to 75 percent of the total, and you are also required to consume a set quantity of vegetables that are low in carbohydrate content.

The Targeted Ketogenic Diet, also known as the TKD, is a type of ketogenic diet that has shown some promise for helping people lose weight when combined with regular physical exercise. Carbohydrates are something that may be ingested either immediately before or on the day that a workout session is planned to take place. You can get your workout energy from carbohydrates.

According to this school of thought, carbohydrates provide a greater gain in energy and performance when the focus is on exercise. This is because carbohydrates include glucose, which the body converts into energy.

The cyclic ketogenic diet, more commonly referred to as the CKD, is a form of diet that is intended to provide high-intensity athletes with additional energy. This diet allows for two days of "backloading," which means you can consume carbs for those two days, and then it transitions you into eating ketogenic for the next five days.

It is possible, with the assistance of this diet, to restore the glycogen reserves that are found in the muscles, which, in turn, helps to boost performance.

High-Protein Ketogenic Diet/High-Protein Ketogenic Diet: This diet is comparable to a typical ketogenic diet; however, it obtains a greater proportion of its daily calorie intake from protein than the traditional ketogenic diet does. In contrast to the SKD, there is a restriction on the amount of fat that can be taken in at any given time. In normal circumstances, fat makes up roughly sixty percent of the calories, whereas protein only accounts for thirty-five percent of the total.

HISTORY

The ketogenic diet may be traced back to the 1920s, when it was first used as a treatment for seizures and epileptic symptoms in children by Dr. Russell Wilder. Since that time, the ketogenic diet has become increasingly popular. A large amount of progress has been made in the ketogenic diet since that time. Since antiepileptic drugs are now more readily available, the ketogenic diet has suffered a steady decline in popularity, despite the fact that it was once quite successful in treating epilepsy.

On the other hand, the ketogenic diet wasn't brought to the attention of the general public until 1994. An episode of a television program in the United States told the story of Hollywood producer Jim Abrahams and his son, who was a patient suffering from epilepsy at the age of two. The child was just two years old at the time. Abrahams heeded the counsel of other members of his family and pleaded with the medical staff at the hospital to place his son on a ketogenic diet. Abrahams was delighted with how things turned out as a result of the fact that the child's condition significantly improved as a consequence of this. A greater interest in and comprehension of the ketogenic diet among members of the scientific community eventually led to the year 1998. Abrahams, who was impressed by the results, donated funds for additional research into the diet.

In recent years, there has been a rise in popularity of the ketogenic diet, and many Hollywood celebrities have joined the bandwagon to promote its use. Because it can boost one's energy levels, assist weight loss, and even improve certain medical conditions, the diet is becoming increasingly popular. It consists of decreasing the quantity of carbohydrates that one consumes while at the same time raising the quantity of healthy fats that are consumed.

One of the most well-known celebrities who has been seen following the ketogenic diet is the actress Halle Berry. She has been photographed doing so on multiple occasions. During the course of an interview, she disclosed this information and indicated that adopting a ketogenic diet and lifestyle had assisted her in better managing her type 2 diabetes. She believes that the diet she has been adhering to is the cause of her improved health and decreased levels of blood sugar.

One more well-known figure from the world of reality television is on board with the ketogenic diet, and she goes by the name of Kourtney Kardashian. She has been an ardent advocate of the diet, recording her progress and experiences across a variety of social media channels, including Instagram, Twitter, and Facebook. She even started a food blog and a meal delivery service in order to aid others in adopting the ketogenic diet and lifestyle. She did this so she could help others.

Jonah Hill, an actor, is yet another well-known person who says that adhering to a ketogenic diet is the secret to his smaller figure. During the course of an interview, he revealed that he had reduced his weight by forty pounds by following a stringent ketogenic diet and working out on a regular basis. As a result of adhering to the diet, he continued, he has been able to achieve his physical goals and establish a good connection with food.

The actress Vanessa Hudgens is yet another well-known person who has been successful while following the ketogenic diet. Hudgens was able to accomplish both of her health and fitness goals with the assistance of the diet. She has credited the ketogenic diet with helping her lose weight and improving her overall sense of well-being, and she has posted pictures of her astonishing transformation on a variety of social media channels.

The ketogenic diet is thought to provide additional benefits, including the promotion of mental clarity and an increase in energy levels. These advantages come on top of the diet's ability to facilitate weight loss. In addition to its benefits for weight loss, it also has several other benefits. This is one of the key reasons why a huge number of celebrities from Hollywood, such as football star Tim Tebow, DJ Khaled, and even supermodel Gisele Bundchen, have adopted this way of life. Other reasons include the fact that this style of life is healthier.

To draw a conclusion, the ketogenic diet is no longer just a trend but rather has developed into a well-liked way of life for many prominent people in Hollywood. This is a conclusion that can be drawn because the ketogenic diet has been around for a while.

CHAPTER 2

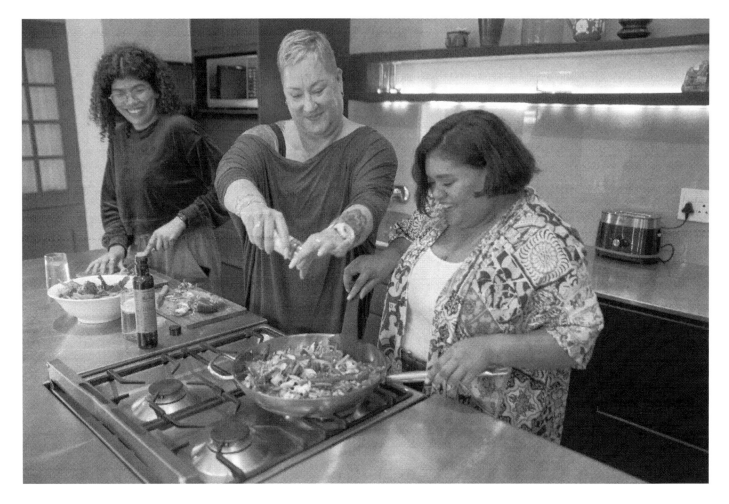

TAILORING THE KETOGENIC DIET TO FIT THE NEEDS OF WOMEN OVER THE AGE OF 60

A gradual decline in metabolism is one of the many changes associated with the natural aging process in women. It is crucial to adapt the ketogenic diet to meet the specific needs of women over 60. This chapter explores how to adjust calorie intake and macronutrient ratios to achieve optimal results and meet health goals. Additionally, it emphasizes the importance of maintaining muscle mass and the role of resistance training and adequate protein intake in overall health preservation.

Adjusting calorie intake:

To meet personal calorie requirements, it is essential to determine the optimal calorie intake based on individual goals and activity level. Women over 60 often have lower energy requirements due to a slower metabolism. However, to achieve weight loss and maintain good health, it is necessary to create a calorie deficit while still meeting nutritional needs.

Determining basal metabolic rate (BMR) is a starting point. This can be calculated using online calculators by entering age, weight, height, and activity level. Once the BMR is determined, the number of calories consumed can be adjusted according to weight loss, weight maintenance, or weight gain goals.

Remember that the quality of calories is as important as quantity. Prioritize a diet that is nutritionally dense, rich in vitamins, minerals, and antioxidants for optimal health.

Adjusting macronutrient ratios:

The ketogenic diet is characterized by high fat, moderate protein, and low carbohydrate content. However, these proportions need to be adjusted for women over 60. Recommended macronutrient ratios are as follows:

Fat: Consume sufficient healthy fats as the primary fuel source. Include a variety of sources such as avocados, nuts, seeds, olive oil, coconut oil, fatty fish, and foods high in saturated fat. Aim for 70-75% of daily calories from healthy fats.

Protein: Consume adequate protein to maintain muscle mass, support tissue regeneration, and overall health. It becomes increasingly important for women over 60 due to muscle atrophy that commonly occurs with age. Include lean meats, poultry, fish, eggs, dairy products, and plant-based proteins as part of a balanced diet. Strive for 20-25% of daily calorie intake from protein.

Carbohydrates: To achieve and maintain ketosis, limit daily carbohydrate intake to 5-10% of total calories. Focus on non-starchy vegetables like leafy greens, broccoli, cauliflower, and zucchini. These vegetables have minimal impact on blood sugar levels while providing essential minerals and fiber.

Maintaining muscle mass:

Preserving muscle mass is crucial for strength, mobility, and reducing the risk of fractures and falls. Incorporate resistance training into your workout routine to maintain and develop muscle strength. Seek guidance from a qualified fitness professional to design a safe and effective program tailored to your needs and goals.

In addition to resistance training, ensure adequate protein intake to maintain muscle mass. Protein provides the structural components for muscle development and maintenance. Aim to consume 0.6-0.8 grams of protein per pound of body weight. For example, if you weigh approximately 150 pounds, strive to consume 90-120 grams of protein per day. Distribute protein intake evenly across meals to facilitate recovery and muscle synthesis.

Promoting overall well-being:

Maintaining proper hydration is crucial, particularly for women over 60 who may experience reduced thirst sensation. Aim to drink at least eight glasses of water per day, adjusting for physical activity and temperature.

In addition to hydration, prioritize a nutrient-rich diet. Include a variety of fruits, vegetables, lean proteins, healthy fats, and whole grains within your carbohydrate limit. These choices provide essential vitamins, minerals, and antioxidants to maximize health and well-being.

Adapting the ketogenic diet to meet the specific needs of women over 60 is vital for optimal results and overall health. By adjusting calorie intake, macronutrient ratios, preserving muscle mass through resistance training and protein consumption, and prioritizing hydration and nutrient density, you can maximize the benefits of the diet.

THE KETOGENIC DIET'S POSITIVE EFFECTS ON ONE'S HEALTH

The ketogenic diet is gaining popularity among people of all ages and genders, including menopausal women over the age of 60. Contrary to some beliefs, this diet has benefits for individuals of all age groups. In this chapter, we will explore the numerous positive health effects associated with following a ketogenic diet.

Remarkable weight loss results

One of the key advantages of the keto diet is its remarkable effectiveness in promoting weight loss. Within three to six months of starting the program, significant weight loss can be observed, particularly in areas that are typically resistant to weight loss, such as the abdomen and hips. Unlike other diets, the ketogenic diet facilitates the conversion of fat into ketones, which requires more energy. This leads to increased satiety, reduced appetite, and ultimately, consuming fewer calories without feelings of deprivation or exhaustion.

Potential cancer prevention methods

Several studies suggest that following a ketogenic diet may help slow down or inhibit the growth of cancer cells. By lowering blood sugar levels and insulin production, the keto diet restricts the fuel supply that cancer cells need to survive. However, further research is required to fully understand the extent of the diet's influence on cancer prevention.

Improved heart health

Contrary to common belief, consuming a diet rich in healthy fats can contribute to maintaining a healthy heart. Research has shown that following a ketogenic diet can reduce levels of LDL, or "bad" cholesterol, while increasing levels of HDL, or "good" cholesterol. This shift in lipid profile helps reduce the risk of arterial plaque buildup, thereby lowering the risk of heart disease and high blood pressure.

Clearer skin and reduced acne

Acne can be a bothersome skin condition, and there is a correlation between carbohydrate consumption, insulin levels, and acne severity. Following a low-carbohydrate diet like keto can effectively manage acne symptoms. Additionally, the consumption of healthy fats in the diet has been shown to decrease the severity of acne. However, further research is needed to understand the specific mechanisms and duration of this impact.

Potential diabetes management

For individuals with diabetes, careful monitoring and control of carbohydrate consumption are essential for maintaining stable blood sugar levels. Those with type 2 diabetes may find it easier to manage their blood glucose by adhering to a low-carb diet like keto. However, individuals with type 1 diabetes should approach with caution due to the potential adverse effects of high levels of ketones in the body. It is always advisable to consult with a qualified medical practitioner before making significant changes to your diet.

Beneficial for epilepsy

The ketogenic diet has a long history of use in the treatment and management of epilepsy. Since the 1920s, it has been recognized for its potential to reduce the frequency and severity of seizures, even in cases where medication is ineffective. However, it is crucial to consult with a qualified medical practitioner before considering the ketogenic diet as a management strategy for epilepsy.

Management of nervous system disorders

Preliminary evidence suggests that following a ketogenic diet may lower the risk of neurodegenerative diseases such as Alzheimer's and Parkinson's. Ongoing studies are exploring its potential use in the treatment of sleep disorders and other neurological conditions. While these findings are in the early stages, the neuroprotective properties of the keto diet offer hope for individuals seeking alternative methods to maintain brain health.

PCOS treatment

Polycystic ovary syndrome (PCOS) can significantly impact a woman's life and fertility, with insulin resistance being a primary cause. Following a keto diet can help control insulin levels and reduce glucose demands, potentially aiding in the treatment of PCOS when combined with exercise.

Improved athletic performance

Although the ketogenic diet may not be specifically designed for enhancing strength and exercise performance like some other diets, it has shown promise in boosting endurance performance. The higher fat-to-muscle ratio associated with keto can benefit endurance athletes, such as cyclists and runners, by enhancing muscle endurance and reducing fatigue during prolonged exercise.

In summary, women over the age of 60 can experience various health benefits by following a ketogenic diet. This dietary approach can enhance overall well-being and vitality by aiding in the management of conditions such as epilepsy, neurological disorders, weight loss, and potential cancer prevention. Additional benefits include reduced acne and improved heart health.

In the next chapter, we will explore customizing the keto diet to meet the specific needs of women over the age of 60, considering factors such as metabolism, muscle mass maintenance, and overall health optimization. Get ready to embark on a personalized journey towards a healthier and more vibrant life.

Remember, it is crucial to consult with a healthcare professional before making significant changes to your diet, especially if you have preexisting medical conditions or are taking any medications.

Let's embrace the keto diet and lifestyle to unlock its full potential for women over the age of 60.

HOW TO RAPIDLY ACHIEVE KETOSIS ON A KETOGENIC DIET

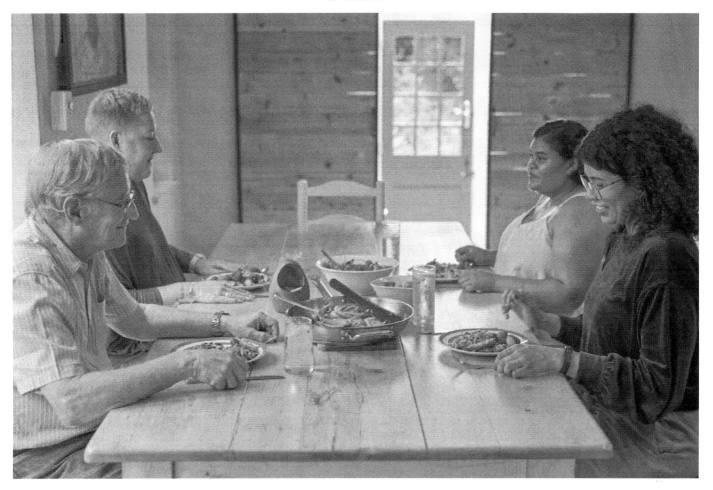

When starting a ketogenic diet, especially for women over the age of 60, it's beneficial to expedite the process of entering ketosis. In this chapter, we will discuss effective methods to quickly achieve ketosis and maximize the benefits of the ketogenic diet.

Reduce carbohydrate intake:

To initiate ketosis, it's crucial to significantly decrease your carbohydrate consumption. The lower your carb intake, the faster your body will enter ketosis. Variations of the ketogenic diet that restrict daily carbs to 20 grams or less can accelerate the process of reaching ketosis compared to the traditional ketogenic diet.

Increase physical activity:

Regular exercise can aid in your journey to ketosis. Studies have shown that exercise raises ketone levels in the blood, leading to improved physical performance, particularly in endurance activities. During the initial weeks of the diet, start with less strenuous workouts to allow your body to adapt to ketosis and achieve optimal results.

Incorporate MCTs (medium-chain triglycerides):

MCTs, a specific type of fat, play a key role in expediting ketosis. MCTs, like lauric acid, are easily converted into ketone bodies by the liver, providing a source of energy. Adding coconut oil, a rich natural source of MCTs, to your diet can hasten the process of entering ketosis. Consider using MCT oil supplements, which offer a concentrated amount of MCTs and can be added to meals or blended drinks.

Embrace healthy fats:

Since the ketogenic diet emphasizes high-fat consumption, focus on incorporating a variety of healthy fats to elevate ketone levels and expedite ketosis. Include foods such as salmon, avocados, and olive oil in each meal to ensure a diverse range of healthy fats. If weight loss is a goal, be mindful of calorie intake and practice portion control to avoid impeding progress.

Explore fasting techniques:

Fasting has been shown to be a safe and effective method for inducing ketosis. Specific fasting protocols, such as fat fasting, can hasten the process of entering ketosis. Fat fasting involves consuming at least 90 percent of daily calories from fat. While this method shows promise, further research is needed to fully understand its efficacy. Before starting any fasting regimen, consult a qualified medical professional.

Optimize protein intake:

Proper protein consumption is essential on a ketogenic diet. Both insufficient and excessive protein intake can have negative effects. Inadequate protein can lead to muscle breakdown, while protein is necessary for the production of enzymes, hormones, and overall bodily functions. Maintain a balanced protein intake to preserve muscle mass and promote overall health.

Monitor ketone levels and adjust as needed:

Since individual responses to the keto diet vary, it's important to adapt your approach based on your ketone levels. Testing methods include blood, breath, and urine tests. Blood testing is the most accurate but more expensive, while urine testing is cost-effective but less precise. Once you choose a preferred method, adjust your diet accordingly based on the results. Find the most effective strategy for your journey by keeping what works and discarding what doesn't.

By implementing these strategies, women over 60 can optimize their ketogenic diet experience, accelerate the process of entering ketosis, and improve their overall health. In the next chapter, we will delve into tailoring the keto diet specifically for women over 60, considering factors such as metabolism, muscle preservation, and overall well-being.

Always consult a qualified medical professional before making significant changes to your diet, especially if you have preexisting medical conditions or take medications.

How can you determine if you are already in ketosis?

To help you identify the signs of ketosis, we have compiled a list of common symptoms associated with it.

- Bad breath: When in full ketosis, your breath may have a fruity odor. This is due to the ketone called acetone being exhaled. To mitigate this, you can chew sugar-free gum, consume sugar-free beverages without carbs, or increase your oral hygiene routine.

- Steady weight loss: In the initial week, you may experience rapid weight loss, primarily from water and stored carbohydrates. After this initial drop, weight loss becomes more gradual as your body burns fat for fuel while maintaining a calorie deficit.

- Blood ketone test: A blood test provides the most precise measurement of ketosis. Ketone molecules such as hydroxybutyrate, acetone, and acetoacetate can be measured, indicating the level of ketosis. Test kits are available, but they can be costly.

- Ketones in breath and urine: Ketone bodies are excreted through breath and urine. Using a ketone breath analyzer or urine indicator strips can give you an indication of ketosis, but these methods may not be as accurate.

- Reduced hunger and appetite: Many people experience a decreased interest in food while in ketosis. The reasons behind this are not yet fully understood, but increased consumption of protein and fiber-rich vegetables or changes in hormone levels may play a role.

- Increased mental clarity: As your body adapts to using fat as its primary source of energy, you may initially experience symptoms like irritability, mental fog, and fatigue. However, once you transition fully, many people report improved attention and mental clarity.

- Periods of fatigue: During the adaptation phase, some individuals may experience weakness and fatigue, often referred to as the "keto flu." This is temporary and can be alleviated by taking energy supplements or electrolytes.

- Decreased physical performance: In the beginning, your physical performance may decline due to depleted glycogen stores. However, once your body becomes fat-adapted, you will be able to burn fat more efficiently during exercise.

- Stomach troubles: It is common to experience digestive issues such as constipation, bloating, or diarrhea when starting the keto diet. These symptoms are temporary and can be managed by consuming fiber-rich, low-carbohydrate vegetables and maintaining a diverse diet.

- Sleep disturbances: Some individuals may experience sleep troubles, like insomnia, when first entering ketosis. This is a transient effect and should resolve itself within a week or two.

- emember, these symptoms can vary from person to person, and it is essential to consult with a healthcare professional before making significant changes to your diet or if you have any preexisting medical conditions.

How can I optimize my ketosis levels?

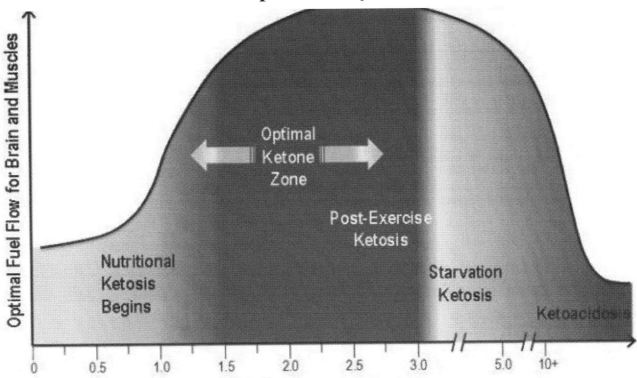

The ketogenic diet has been surrounded by a lot of misinformation lately. Here are some practical tips to maximize your experience and achieve optimal weight loss.

Focus on calorie intake: To lose weight effectively, it's essential to monitor your calorie intake and avoid high-calorie foods. Pay attention to your calorie consumption and prioritize foods that are high in protein and fiber, which promote feelings of fullness. Restrict foods that are high in calories.

Stick to ketogenic foods and drinks: To enter ketosis, it's crucial to be mindful of the food you consume. Organize your meals and recipes according to the requirements of the diet. Check restaurant menus in advance for keto-friendly options to avoid high-carb meals and prevent "cheating." There is a wide range of food options available on the ketogenic diet, including baked goods made with almond or coconut flour.

Monitor your calorie intake: Even if you're consuming keto-friendly foods, consuming fewer calories is essential for efficient weight loss. Many people underestimate their calorie intake, which can hinder progress. Consider using a keto calculator app, a calorie-counting app, or a food scale to track your calories accurately.

Make adjustments to your food environment: Be honest with yourself about your cravings and temptations. Replace high-carb foods in your kitchen with keto-friendly alternatives, such as almond flour and berries. Avoid making or buying "binge-worthy" foods that may lead to overeating.

Connect with fellow keto dieters: Joining a community of people following the ketogenic diet can provide motivation and support. You can share experiences, ask questions, and seek advice from others who understand the challenges and successes of the diet.

Prepare meals at home: When eating out, it's challenging to track the exact ingredients and quantities in your meals. To ensure accurate measurements and control over your calorie and carbohydrate intake, prioritize cooking meals at home using carefully crafted recipes.

Plan your budget: Proper budget planning is essential to sustain the ketogenic diet in the long term. Avoid overspending by buying keto-friendly ingredients in bulk and preparing meals in advance. Look for coupons and sales to save money and stick to your shopping list to prevent impulsive purchases.

Remember, transitioning to a low-carb diet may cause temporary discomfort, such as the keto flu. Stay hydrated and consider taking mineral supplements or electrolytes to support your body during this adjustment phase.

By implementing these strategies, you can optimize your ketosis levels and enhance your overall experience on the ketogenic diet.

Chapter 3

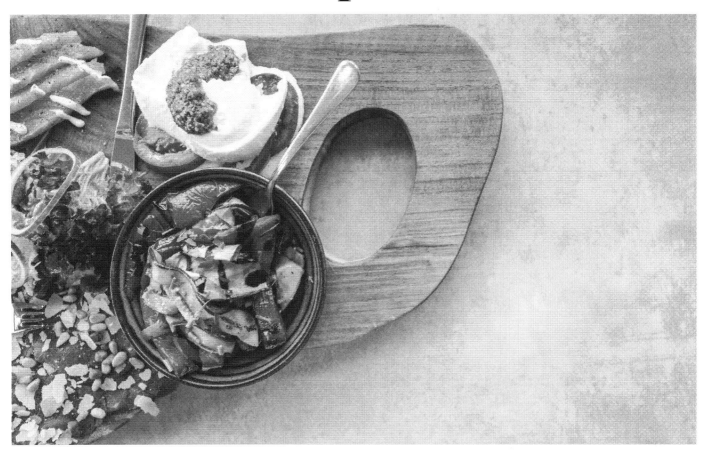

PRODUCTS FOR HEALTH

LIST OF APPROVED PRODUCTS

On the ketogenic diet, you are allowed to consume the following foods:

Free to Eat:

- Various types of fish and seafood, including mackerel, salmon, sardines, albacore tuna, etc.

- Eggs

- Avocado

- Cheese, especially cottage cheese

- Poultry, such as chicken and turkey

- Nuts like almonds, cashews, pistachios, Brazil nuts, etc.

- Seeds: chia seeds, flaxseed, sesame seeds, etc.

- Healthy oils, such as olive oil, coconut oil, etc.

- Plain Greek yogurt without added sugar

- Coffee without added sugar

- Tea without added sugar

Consume in Moderation:

While these foods are permitted, it's important to exercise moderation to avoid excessive consumption.

- Low-carb vegetables like cauliflower, green beans, spinach, broccoli, bell peppers, zucchini, etc.

- Berries with a low glycemic index, including blackberries, blueberries, raspberries, etc. (a good option for diabetics)

- Bittersweet chocolate made with unsweetened cocoa powder

- Unsweetened varieties of milk, such as almond milk, coconut milk, hempseed milk, etc.

List of Restricted Items:

On the ketogenic diet, you are not allowed to consume the following foods:

- Legumes, including beans, chickpeas, lentils, black beans, pinto beans, etc.

- Grains like cereal, rice, pasta, bread, beer, etc. This includes whole wheat and bean paste.

- Starchy and high-carb vegetables such as corn, potatoes, sweet potatoes, and beets

- Sugary fruits like bananas, dates, mangoes, pears, etc.

- Avoid all forms of sugar and sweeteners, including honey, syrups, and maple syrup.

- Gluten-free baked goods are not permitted as they still contain carbs.

- Both commercially made and natural juices

Keto Supplements:

Here are some recommended vitamins and supplements for those following a ketogenic diet. However, it's advisable to consult your primary care physician if you have any preexisting medical conditions.

- Magnesium: Since the diet restricts magnesium-rich foods that are high in carbs, a magnesium supplement of approximately 300 grams per day can help prevent deficiencies and improve sleep quality and mood.

- MCT Oil: Medium-chain triglycerides (MCTs) are popular among keto dieters as they increase fat consumption and promote the production of ketones, aiding in ketosis. MCT oil supplements provide a concentrated dose.

- Exogenous Ketones: These are ketone molecules consumed through diet rather than produced by the body. They can accelerate the process of entering ketosis, enhance satiety, and improve performance in physical activities.

- Green Powder: Since the ketogenic diet limits vegetable intake, green powder made from crushed green vegetables like broccoli can help address nutrient deficiencies and provide essential vitamins and minerals.

- Digestive Enzymes: Starting a ketogenic diet may cause digestive issues like bloating. Adding digestive enzyme supplements can help alleviate these symptoms.

- Electrolytes or Mineral Supplements: Maintaining proper levels of electrolytes like sodium and potassium is crucial on the keto diet. Consuming electrolyte fluids or mineral supplements can support various bodily processes.

- Energy Supplements: Essential for athletes, these supplements boost performance, preserve muscle mass, and reduce fatigue associated with exercise.

- Omega-3 Fatty Acids: These supplements offer additional health benefits by reducing inflammation and the risk of heart disease. They help maintain a healthy balance of omega fats.

By incorporating these supplements and vitamins, you can enhance the benefits of the ketogenic diet and support your overall well-being.

MEAL PLAN

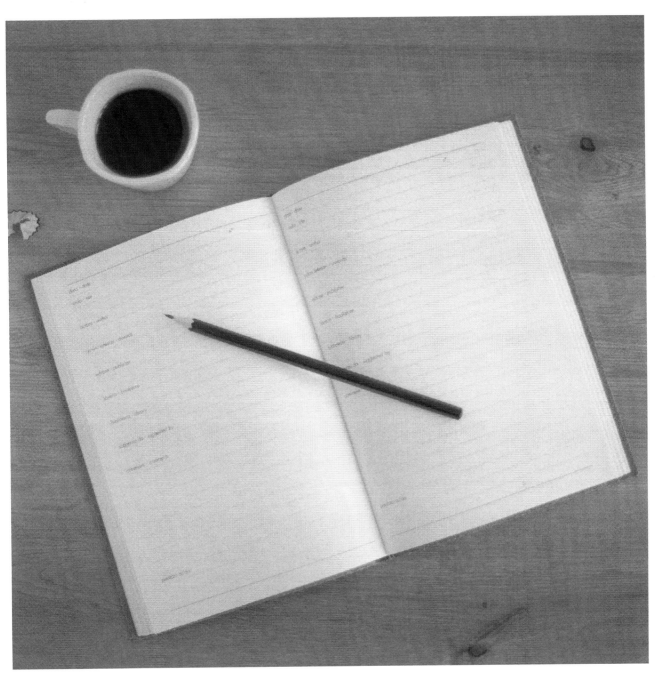

We would like to bring to your attention a meal plan that covers the next 30 days. This is a general plan that can be modified to fit your diet and the number of calories you require. In addition, many dishes are served without the accompaniment of side dishes; however, you are free to include these in your diet according to your preferences.

30 DAY Meal Plan 1

MONDAY

Breakfast	Lunch	Dinner	Snacks
COCONUT FLOUR PORRIDGE	YAKISOBA CHICKEN	HAM AND PROVOLONE SANDWICH	KETO MUFFINS CLASSIC CINNAMON

TUESDAY

Breakfast	Lunch	Dinner	Snacks
EASY SHAKSHUKA	FISH CURRY	KETO CHICKEN LIVER PATE	CREAMY CHOCOLATE MILKSHAKE

WEDNESDAY

Breakfast	Lunch	Dinner	Snacks
FARMER CHEESE PANCAKES	BACON MUSHROOM SWISS STEAK	VITELLO TONNATO	KETO LEMON MUFFINS

THURSAY

Breakfast	Lunch	Dinner	Snacks
BROCCOLI & CHEESE OMELET	JALAPENO POPPER CHICKEN	COBB SALAD	BLUEBERRY BLISS

FRIDAY

Breakfast	Lunch	Dinner	Snacks
AVOCADO OMELETTE	BALSAMIC SALMON WITH GREEN BEANS	MEATBALLS IN TOMATO SAUCE	CINNAMON ROLL SMOOTHIE

SATURDAY

Breakfast	Lunch	Dinner	Snacks
CHORIZO BREAKFAST BAKE	COCONUT CHICKEN TENDERS	KETO BEEF NACHOS	KETO CARROT MUFFINS

SUNDAY

Breakfast	Lunch	Dinner	Snacks
EGGS FLORENTINE CASSEROLE	BEEF AND PASTA CASSEROLE	CHICKEN HEARTS IN A CREAMY SAUCE	BLUEBERRY AVOCADO SMOOTHIE

30 DAY Meal Plan 2

MONDAY

Breakfast	Lunch	Dinner	Snacks
LEMON POPPY RICOTTA PANCAKES	LEMON KALAMATA OLIVE SALMON	HAM, EGG, AND CHEESE SANDWICH	ORANGE CREAMSICLE

TUESDAY

Breakfast	Lunch	Dinner	Snacks
SWEET BLUEBERRY COCONUT PORRIDGE	BEEF LIVER GOULASH	DUCK A L'ORANGE RECIPE	KETO CHEESECAKE MUFFINS

WEDNESDAY

Breakfast	Lunch	Dinner	Snacks
LOW-CARB BREAKFAST QUICHE	TURKEY STEW RECIPE	CRUNCHY ALMOND TUNA	SHAMROCK SHAKE

THURSAY

Breakfast	Lunch	Dinner	Snacks
VEGETABLE TART	PORK MEATBALLS WITH VEGETABLE MARINARA SAUCE	BEEF LIVER PATE	AVOCADO ALMOND SMOOTHIE

FRIDAY

Breakfast	Lunch	Dinner	Snacks
COCONUT FLOUR PANCAKES	CREAMY DUCK SOUP	CREAMY CHILE SHRIMP	KETO CHEESY HERB MUFFINS

SATURDAY

Breakfast	Lunch	Dinner	Snacks
KETO SAUSAGE BREAKFAST SANDWICH	GARLIC PARMESAN CHICKEN WITH BROCCOLI	DUCK AND CAULIFLOWER STIR-FRY	RASPBERRY SMOOTHIE

SUNDAY

Breakfast	Lunch	Dinner	Snacks
OMELET-STUFFED PEPPERS	MOROCCAN LAMB	MEXICAN FISH STEW	CREAMY STRAWBERRY

30 DAY Meal Plan 3

MONDAY

Breakfast	Lunch	Dinner	Snacks
HAM & CHEESE EGG CUPS	PAPRIKA CHICKEN	KETO CALAMARI	KETO BANANA NUT MUFFINS

TUESDAY

Breakfast	Lunch	Dinner	Snacks
GREEN EGGS	BUTTERED COD IN SKILLET	CHICKEN SALAD PUFFS	PEPPERMINT MOCHA

WEDNESDAY

Breakfast	Lunch	Dinner	Snacks
KETO SAUSAGE & EGG BOWLS	KETO BAKED BEEF WITH MIXED VEGETABLES	BROCCOLI AND SHRIMP SAUTÉED IN BUTTER	RED VELVET SMOOTHIE

THURSAY

Breakfast	Lunch	Dinner	Snacks
KETO CROQUE MADAME	CREAM CHEESE STUFFED CHICKEN	DUCK STEWED WITH PRUNES	KETO CAPPUCCINO MUFFINS

FRIDAY

Breakfast	Lunch	Dinner	Snacks
KETO SPINACH SHAKSHUKA	PORK MEATBALLS WITH CREAMY MUSHROOM SAUCE	SESAME CHICKEN AVOCADO SALAD	WHIPPED SHAKE

SATURDAY

Breakfast	Lunch	Dinner	Snacks
PROTEIN BREAKFAST SCRAMBLE	KETO LAMB KOFTAS	SHRIMP AVOCADO SALAD	KETO JAM COOKIES

SUNDAY

Breakfast	Lunch	Dinner	Snacks
MIXED MUSHROOM EGG BAKES	KETO CRACK CHICKEN	CAPRESE TUNA SALAD STUFFED TOMATOES	CREAMY BLACKBERRY

30 DAY Meal Plan 4

MONDAY

Breakfast	Lunch	Dinner	Snacks
SPICY CHICKEN BREAKFAST BOWLS	KETO CHICKEN HEARTS	BEEF AND PEPPER KEBABS	CRANBERRY COOKIES

TUESDAY

Breakfast	Lunch	Dinner	Snacks
KETO BREAKFAST SANDWICH	KETO LEMON-ROSEMARY BEEF BAKE	SMOKED CHICKEN SALAD SANDWICH	COCONUT CHAI SMOOTHIE

WEDNESDAY

Breakfast	Lunch	Dinner	Snacks
POACHED EGGS MYTILENE	BAKED COCONUT HADDOCK	FRIED TUNA AVOCADO BALLS	PEACH PIE SHAKE

THURSAY

Breakfast	Lunch	Dinner	Snacks
BLUEBERRY PANCAKES	HUNAN CHICKEN	KETO LAMB CURRY WITH SPINACH	KETO BROWNIE COOKIES

FRIDAY

Breakfast	Lunch	Dinner	Snacks
TURKISH-STYLE BREAKFAST	KETO BEEF AND CABBAGE SKILLET	DUCK AND SPINACH SALAD	MANGO ALMOND SMOOTHIE

SATURDAY

Breakfast	Lunch	Dinner	Snacks
PECAN & COCONUT ' N ' OATMEAL	PORK ROLS WITH WALNUT, PRUNE, AND CHEESE	BACON-WRAPPED SALMON WITH SPINACH SALAD	PIGNOLI COOKIES

SUNDAY

Breakfast	Lunch	Dinner	Snacks
SPINACH PANCAKES	COCONUT BREADED CHICKEN	BLUE CHEESE BACON BURGERS	CHOCOLATE AVOCADO CREAM SMOOTHIE

30 DAY Meal Plan 5

MONDAY

Breakfast	Lunch	Dinner	Snacks
KETO EGG ROLL IN A BOWL	KETO ASIAN GLAZED SALMON	KETO DUCK ROLLS	MOCHA KETO COFFEE SHAKE

TUESDAY

Breakfast	Lunch	Dinner	Snacks
KETO CAULIFLOWER BUNS	BRAISED LAMB SHANKS	SALMON AND CREAM CHEESE SUSHI ROLLS	SOUR CREAM CAKE

WEDNESDAY

Breakfast	Lunch	Dinner	Snacks
BIG MAC BREAKFAST PIE	CHICKEN STIR-FRY WITH MUSHROOMS	CHICKEN EGG SALAD WRAPS	GOLDEN MILK KETO SMOOTHIE

BREAKFAST

KETO BREAKFAST DAIRY-FREE SMOOTHIE BOWL

Nutrition: Cal 642;Fat 45 g;Carb 10 g;Protein 22 g
Serving 3; Cook time 10 min

Ingredients

- 1 ½ cups (350 ml) full-fat coconut milk
- 1 cup (110 g) frozen raspberries
- ¼ cup (60 ml) MCT oil or melted coconut oil, or ¼ cup (40 g) unflavored MCT oil powder
- ¼ cup (40 g) collagen peptides or protein powder
- 2 tablespoons chia seeds
- 1 tablespoon apple cider vinegar
- 1 teaspoon vanilla extract
- 1 tablespoon erythritol, or 4 drops liquid stevia

Instructions

Place all the pudding ingredients in a blender or food processor and blend until smooth. Serve in bowls with your favorite toppings, if desired.

CRISPY KETO CORNED BEEF & RADISH HASH

Nutrition: Cal 252;Fat 16 g;Carb 1,5 g;Protein 23 g
Serving 2; Cook time 10 min

Ingredients

- 2 tablespoons olive oil
- 1/2 cup diced onions
- 2 cups radishes, diced to about 1/2 inch
- 1 teaspoon kosher salt
- 1/2 teaspoon ground black pepper
- 1 teaspoon dried oregano (Mexican if you have it)
- 1/2 teaspoon garlic powder
- 2 twelve-ounce cans corned beef or 2 cups finely chopped corned beef, packed

Instructions

1. Heat the olive oil in a large saute pan and add the onions, radishes, salt, and pepper.
2. Saute the onions and radishes on medium heat for 5 minutes or until softened.
3. Add the oregano, garlic powder, and corned beef to the pan and stir well until combined.
4. Cook over low to medium heat, stirring occasionally for 10 minutes or until the radishes are soft and starting to brown.

Press the mixture into the bottom of the pan and cook on high heat for 2–3 minutes or until the bottom is crisp and brown.

COCONUT FLOUR PORRIDGE

Nutrition: Cal 345;Fat 28,5 g;Carb 11 g;Protein 13 g
Serving 1; Cook time 7 min

Ingredients

- 2 tablespoons coconut flour
- 2 tablespoons golden flax meal
- 3/4 cup water
- Pinch of salt
- 1 large egg, beaten
- 2 teaspoons butter or ghee
- 1 tablespoon heavy cream or coconut milk
- 1 tablespoon low-carb brown sugar (or your favorite sweetener)

Instructions

1. Measure the first four ingredients into a small pot over medium heat and stir. When it begins to simmer, turn it down to medium-low and whisk until it begins to thicken.
2. Remove the coconut flour porridge from heat and add the beaten egg, a half at a time, while whisking continuously. Place back on the heat and continue to whisk until the porridge thickens.Remove from the heat and continue to whisk for about 30 seconds before adding the butter, cream, and sweetener.

Garnish with your favorite toppings (4 grams net carbs).

EASY SHAKSHUKA

Nutrition: Cal 216;Fat 12 g;Carb 16 g;Protein 12 g
Serving 6; Cook time 35 min

Ingredients

- 2 tablespoons olive oil
- 1 large yellow onion, chopped
- 1 large red bell pepper or roasted red bell pepper, chopped
- 1/4 teaspoon fine sea salt

- 3 cloves garlic, pressed or minced
- 2 tablespoons tomato paste
- 1 teaspoon ground cumin
- 1/2 teaspoon smoked paprika
- 1/4 teaspoon red pepper flakes (reduce or omit if sensitive to spice)
- 1 large can (28 ounces) crushed tomatoes, preferably fire-roasted
- 2 tablespoons chopped fresh cilantro or flat-leaf parsley, plus addition cilantro or parsley leaves for garnish
- Freshly ground black pepper, to taste
- 5 to 6 large eggs

Instructions

1. Preheat the oven to 375°F. Warm the oil in a large, oven-safe skillet (preferably stainless steel) over medium heat. Once shimmering, add the onion, bell pepper, and salt. Cook, stirring often, until the onions are tender and turning translucent, about 4 to 6 minutes.
2. Add the garlic, tomato paste, cumin, paprika, and red pepper flakes. Cook, stirring constantly, until nice and fragrant, 1 to 2 minutes.
3. Pour in the crushed tomatoes with their juices and add the cilantro. Stir, and let the mixture come to a simmer. Reduce the heat as necessary to maintain a gentle simmer and cook for 5 minutes to give the flavors time to meld.
4. Turn off the heat. Taste (careful, it's hot!), and add salt and pepper as necessary. Use the back of a spoon to make a well near the perimeter and crack the egg directly into it. Gently spoon a bit of the tomato mixture over the whites to help contain the egg. Repeat with the remaining 4 to 5 eggs, depending on how many you can fit. Sprinkle a little salt and pepper over the eggs.

Carefully transfer the skillet to the oven (it's heavy) and bake for 8 to 12 minutes, checking often once you reach 8 minutes. They're done when the egg whites are an opaque white and the yolks have risen a bit but are still soft. They should still jiggle in the centers when you shimmy the pan (keep in mind that they'll continue cooking after you pull the dish out of the oven).

STEAK AND EGGS

Nutrition: Cal 210;Fat 36 g;Carb 3 g;Protein 44 g
Serving 1; Cook time 15 min

Ingredients

1 tablespoon butter

3 eggs

4 ounces sirloin

1/4 avocado

Salt, Pepper

Instructions

1. Melt butter in a pan and fry 2-3 eggs until the whites are set and the yolk is cooked to your desired doneness. Season with salt and pepper.
2. In another pan, cook your sirloin (or favorite cut of steak) until it reaches your desired doneness. Then, slice it into bite-sized strips and season with salt and pepper.

Slice up some avocado and serve it together with the steak and eggs.

FARMER CHEESE PANCAKES

Nutrition: Cal 200;Fat 12 g;Carb 2,5 g;Protein 18 g
Serving 5; Cook time 20 min

Ingredients

- 1 lb Farmer Cheese
- 1 cup coconut flour
- 2 eggs
- Pinch of salt, to taste (optional)
- 1 tsp Stevia, to taste (optional)

Instructions

1. Mix farmer cheese, coconut flour, salt, and 2 eggs. Mixture should be like paste texture.
2. Form pancakes into round shape. Dust it just a bit with coconut flour.

Fry till both sides are golden brown.

FRENCH OMELET

Nutrition: Cal 186;Fat 9 g;Carb 4 g;Protein 22 g
Serving 2; Cook time 10 min

Ingredients

- 2 large eggs
- 4 large egg whites
- 1/4 cup fat-free milk
- 1/8 teaspoon salt
- 1/8 teaspoon pepper
- 1/4 cup cubed fully cooked ham

- 1 tablespoon chopped onion
- 1 tablespoon chopped green pepper
- 1/4 cup shredded reduced-fat cheddar cheese

Instructions

1. Whisk together first five ingredients.
2. Place a 10-in. skillet coated with cooking spray over medium heat. Pour in egg mixture. Mixture should set immediately at edges. As eggs set, push cooked portions toward the center, letting uncooked eggs flow underneath.

When eggs are thickened and no liquid egg remains, top one half with remaining ingredients. Fold omelet in half. Cut in half to serve.

SOUTHWESTERN OMELET

Nutrition: Cal 390;Fat 31 g;Carb 7 g;Protein 22 g
Serving 4; Cook time 10 min

Ingredients

- 1/2 cup chopped onion
- 1 jalapeno pepper, minced
- 1 tablespoon canola oil
- 6 large eggs, lightly beaten
- 6 bacon strips, cooked and crumbled
- 1 small tomato, chopped
- 1 ripe avocado, cut into 1-inch slices
- 1 cup shredded Monterey Jack cheese, divided
- Salt and pepper, to taste
- Salsa (optional)

Instructions

1. Heat oil in a large skillet and sauté onion and jalapeño until they become tender. Use a slotted spoon to remove the mixture and set it aside. In the same skillet, pour the beaten eggs, cover, and cook over low heat for 3-4 minutes.
2. Sprinkle the cooked onion mixture, bacon, tomato, avocado, and half a cup of cheese over the partially cooked eggs. Season with salt and pepper to taste.

Fold the omelet in half, covering the filling. Continue cooking, covered, for an additional 3-4 minutes or until the eggs are fully set. Sprinkle the remaining cheese on top. Serve with salsa if desired.

BROCCOLI & CHEESE OMELET

Nutrition: Cal 230;Fat 17 g;Carb 5 g;Protein 15 g
Serving 4; Cook time 15 min

Ingredients

- 2-1/2 cups fresh broccoli florets
- 6 large eggs
- 1/4 cup 2% milk
- 1/2 teaspoon salt
- 1/4 teaspoon pepper
- 1/3 cup grated Romano cheese
- 1/3 cup sliced pitted Greek olives
- 1 tablespoon olive oil
- Shaved Romano cheese and minced fresh parsley

Instructions

1. In a small bowl, whisk together eggs, green onion, milk, and seasonings until well blended. Heat butter in a large nonstick skillet over medium-high heat. Pour the egg mixture into the skillet. The mixture should immediately start setting at the edges.
2. As the eggs begin to set, gently push the cooked portions toward the center, allowing the uncooked eggs to flow underneath. Continue this process until the eggs are thickened and no liquid egg remains. Once cooked, place cheese and ham on one side of the omelet.

Fold the omelet in half and cut it into two portions. Slide the omelet onto plates and top with tomato. Just before serving, drizzle with vinaigrette.

HAM & FETA OMELET

Nutrition: Cal 290;Fat 20 g;Carb 5 g;Protein 21 g
Serving 2; Cook time 15 min

Ingredients

- 4 large eggs
- 1 green onion, chopped
- 1 tablespoon 2% milk
- 1/4 teaspoon dried basil
- 1/4 teaspoon dried oregano
- Dash of garlic powder
- Dash of salt
- Dash of pepper
- 1 tablespoon butter
- 1/4 cup crumbled feta cheese
- 3 slices deli ham, chopped
- 1 plum tomato, chopped
- 2 teaspoons balsamic vinaigrette

Instructions

1. In a small bowl, whisk together eggs, green onion, milk, and seasonings until well blended. Heat butter in a large nonstick skillet over medium-high heat. Pour the egg mixture into the skillet. The mixture should immediately start setting at the edges.
2. As the eggs begin to set, gently push the cooked portions toward the center, allowing the uncooked eggs to flow underneath. Continue this process until the eggs are thickened and no liquid egg remains. Once cooked, place cheese and ham on one side of the omelet.

Fold the omelet in half and cut it into two portions. Slide the omelet onto plates and top with tomato. Just before serving, drizzle with vinaigrette.

BACON AND MUSHROOM OMELETTE

Nutrition: Cal 313;Fat 24 g;Carb 1,5 g;Protein 23 g
Serving 2; Cook time 10 min

Ingredients

- 3 medium mushrooms, raw
- 2 slices bacon
- 3 eggs
- 2 tbsp onion, chopped
- 2 slices cheddar cheese
- Lettuce or watercress, to taste (optional)
- Pinch salt
- Pinch pepper

Instructions

1. Finely dice the onion into a brunoise cut. Slice the mushrooms and bacon into small chunks as well.
2. Heat a non-stick skillet, approximately 8 inches in diameter, coated with cooking spray over medium-high heat. Cook the onion and bacon in the pan. Once the bacon is toasted to your liking, add the mushrooms and remove from heat.
3. In a mixing bowl, beat the eggs. Season with sea salt and black pepper, then add the cooked bacon, mushrooms, and onion.
4. Gently pour the egg mixture into the skillet. As the omelette begins to firm up, use a spatula to ease around the edges. Place the slices of cheddar cheese on one half of the omelette. Fold the other half onto the cheese.

5. Leave the omelette in the pan for an additional 2 minutes, allowing it to cook through. Then, carefully slide the cooked omelette onto a plate.
6. If desired, fill the inside of the omelette with lettuce leaves for added freshness. Serve immediately while the omelette is still crispy and warm.

SCRAMBLED EGGS WITH MUSHROOMS AND COTTAGE CHEESE

Nutrition: Cal 210;Fat 19 g;Carb 3 g;Protein 9 g
Serving 3; Cook time 20 min

Ingredients

- 3 eggs
- 1 cup button mushrooms, rinsed and sliced
- 1/2 medium-sized onion, finely chopped
- 3 tbsp olive oil
- 1/4 tsp oregano
- 1/4 cup cottage cheese
- 1/2 tsp sea salt
- 1/4 tsp black pepper

Instructions

1. Heat a large skillet over medium-high heat and add olive oil. Once the oil is hot, sauté the finely chopped onions until they become translucent. Add the sliced mushrooms and let them simmer until the liquid in the pan evaporates. Stir in oregano, pepper, and salt to season. Set the mixture aside.

In a bowl, beat the eggs. Season with a dash of salt and pepper to taste. Pour the beaten eggs into the skillet and cook, using a wooden spoon to fold and scramble them for about a minute, leaving them slightly underdone.

BACON AND EGG STUFFED ZUCCHINI BOATS

Nutrition: Cal 280;Fat 21 g;Carb 4 g;Protein 19 g
Serving 2; Cook time 30 min

Ingredients

- 2 medium zucchini
- 4 slices bacon, cooked and crumbled
- 4 large eggs
- Salt and pepper to taste
- Chopped chives (optional, for garnish)

Instructions

1. Preheat the oven to 375°F (190°C). Slice the zucchini in half lengthwise and scoop out the center to create a hollow "boat."
2. Place the zucchini boats on a baking sheet lined with parchment paper. Sprinkle with salt and pepper.
3. Crack an egg into each zucchini boat. Season with additional salt and pepper.
4. Bake in the preheated oven for 12-15 minutes or until the eggs are cooked to your desired doneness.

Remove from the oven and top with crumbled bacon and chopped chives, if desired. Serve hot.

BACON AND ZUCCHINI EGG MUFFINS

Nutrition: Cal 180;Fat 12 g;Carb 5 g;Protein 14 g
Serving 2; Cook time 30 min

Ingredients

- 4 slices bacon, cooked and crumbled
- 1 medium zucchini, grated and excess moisture squeezed out
- 4 large eggs
- 1/4 cup sour cream
- Salt and pepper to taste
- Chopped fresh herbs (such as parsley or chives) for garnish

Instructions

1. Preheat the oven to 350°F (175°C). Grease a muffin tin or line with muffin liners.
2. In a bowl, whisk together the eggs and sour cream. Season with salt and pepper.
3. Stir in the grated zucchini and crumbled bacon until well combined.
4. Pour the mixture evenly into the prepared muffin tin, filling each cup about 3/4 full.
5. Bake for 15-18 minutes or until the egg muffins are set and slightly golden on top.

Remove from the oven and let cool for a few minutes. Garnish with chopped fresh herbs. Serve warm or at room temperature.

DENVER OMELET SALAD

Nutrition: Cal 230;Fat 14 g;Carb 7 g;Protein 17 g
Serving 4; Cook time 10 min

Ingredients

- 8 cups fresh baby spinach
- 1 cup chopped tomatoes
- 2 tablespoons olive oil, divided
- 1-1/2 cups chopped fully cooked ham
- 1 small onion, chopped
- 1 small green pepper, chopped
- 4 large eggs
- Salt and pepper, to taste

Instructions

1. Place spinach and tomatoes on a platter and set it aside. In a large skillet, heat 1 tablespoon of olive oil over medium-high heat. Add ham, onion, and green pepper, and sauté until the ham is heated through and the vegetables are tender, which should take about 5-7 minutes. Spoon the mixture over the spinach and tomatoes.
2. In the same skillet, heat the remaining olive oil over medium heat. Crack the eggs, one at a time, into a small cup, and gently slide them into the skillet.
3. Immediately reduce the heat to low and season the eggs with salt and pepper. To prepare sunny-side-up eggs, cover the pan and cook until the egg whites are completely set and the yolks have thickened but are not hard. Top the salad with the fried eggs.

TURKEY BREAKFAST SAUSAGE

Nutrition: Cal 85;Fat 5 g;Carb 2 g;Protein 10 g
Serving 8; Cook time 10 min

Ingredients

- 1 pound lean ground turkey
- 3/4 teaspoon salt
- 1/2 teaspoon rubbed sage
- 1/2 teaspoon pepper
- 1/4 teaspoon ground ginger

Instructions

1. Crumble turkey into a large bowl. Add the salt, sage, pepper, and ginger. Shape into eight 2-inch patties.

In a nonstick skillet coated with cooking spray, cook patties over medium heat for 4-6 minutes on each side or until a thermometer reads 165° and juices run clear.

CHICKEN AVOCADO SALAD

Nutrition: Cal 400;Fat 24 g;Carb 10 g;Protein 35 g
Serving 2; Cook time 25 min

Ingredients

- 2 boneless, skinless chicken breasts
- 2 avocados, pitted and mashed
- 1 cup cherry tomatoes, halved
- 1/2 cup red onion, thinly sliced
- 4 cups mixed salad greens
- 2 tablespoons olive oil
- 1 tablespoon lemon juice
- Salt and pepper to taste

Instructions

1. Preheat the grill or a skillet over medium-high heat. Season the chicken breasts with salt and pepper.
2. Cook the chicken for about 6-8 minutes per side, or until cooked through. Let it rest for a few minutes, then slice it into strips.
3. In a large bowl, combine the mashed avocados, cherry tomatoes, red onion, mixed salad greens, olive oil, lemon juice, salt, and pepper. Toss until well coated.
4. Divide the salad mixture between two plates and top with the sliced chicken.

Serve the Chicken Avocado Salad with Fresh Vegetables immediately.

SPINACH-MUSHROOM SCRAMBLED EGGS

Nutrition: Cal 200;Fat 11 g;Carb 2 g;Protein 14 g
Serving 2; Cook time 10 min

Ingredients

- 2 large eggs
- 2 large egg whites
- 1/8 teaspoon salt
- 1/8 teaspoon pepper
- 1 teaspoon butter
- 1/2 cup thinly sliced fresh mushrooms
- 1/2 cup fresh baby spinach, chopped
- 2 tablespoons shredded provolone cheese

Instructions

1. In a small bowl, whisk together eggs, egg whites, salt, and pepper until well blended. In a small nonstick skillet, heat butter over medium-high heat.
2. Add mushrooms to the skillet and cook, stirring, for 3-4 minutes or until they become tender. Then, add spinach and continue cooking and stirring until the spinach wilts. Reduce the heat to medium.

Pour the egg mixture into the skillet and cook, stirring, just until the eggs are thickened and no liquid egg remains. Stir in the cheese until melted and well incorporated.

EGGS FLORENTINE CASSEROLE

Nutrition: Cal 271;Fat 20 g;Carb 7 g;Protein 17 g
Serving 12; Cook time 30 min

Ingredients

- 1 pound bulk pork sausage
- 2 tablespoons butter
- 1 large onion, chopped
- 1 cup sliced fresh mushrooms
- 1 package (10 ounces) frozen chopped spinach, thawed and squeezed dry
- 12 large eggs
- 2 cups 2% milk
- 1 cup shredded Swiss cheese
- 1 cup shredded sharp cheddar cheese
- 1/4 teaspoon paprika

Instructions

1. Preheat the oven to 350°F. In a large skillet, cook the sausage over medium heat for 6-8 minutes or until no longer pink, breaking it into crumbles. Drain the sausage and transfer it to a greased 13 x 9-inch baking dish.
2. In the same skillet, heat butter over medium-high heat. Add onion and mushrooms and cook, stirring, for 3-5 minutes or until tender. Stir in spinach. Spoon the vegetable mixture over the sausage in the baking dish.

In a large bowl, whisk together eggs and milk until blended. Pour the egg mixture over the vegetables. Sprinkle with cheeses and paprika.

Bake, uncovered, for 30-35 minutes or until the center is set and a thermometer inserted into the center reads 165°F. Let it stand for 10 minutes before serving.

TACO BREAKFAST SKILLET

Nutrition: Cal 523;Fat 44 g;Carb 9 g;Protein 22 g

Serving 6; Cook time 45 min

Ingredients

- 1 pound ground beef
- 4 tablespoons taco seasoning
- 2/3 cup water
- 10 large eggs
- 1 1/2 cups shredded sharp cheddar cheese, divided
- 1/4 cup heavy cream
- 1 roma tomato, diced
- 1 medium avocado, peeled, pitted, and cubed
- 1/4 cup sliced black olives
- 2 green onions, sliced
- 1/4 cup sour cream
- 1/4 cup salsa
- 1 jalapeno, sliced (optional)
- 2 tablespoons torn fresh cilantro (optional)

Instructions

1. Brown the ground beef in a large skillet over medium-high heat. Drain the excess fat.
2. Stir in the taco seasoning and water. Reduce the heat to low and let it simmer until the sauce thickens and coats the meat, which should take about 5 minutes. Remove half of the seasoned beef from the skillet and set it aside.
3. Crack the eggs into a large mixing bowl and whisk them. Add 1 cup of cheddar cheese and the heavy cream to the eggs and whisk to combine.
4. Preheat the oven to 375°F.
5. Pour the egg mixture over the remaining meat in the skillet and stir to mix the meat into the eggs. Bake for 30 minutes or until the egg bake is cooked all the way through and fluffy.
6. Top with the remaining ground beef, the remaining ½ cup of cheddar cheese, tomato, avocado, olives, green onion, sour cream, and salsa.

Garnish with jalapeno and cilantro, if using.

CHORIZO BREAKFAST BAKE

Nutrition:Cal 212;Fat 11 g;Carb 11 g;Protein 9 g

Serving 4; Cook time 50 min

Ingredients

- 2 tablespoon olive oil
- 1 red bell pepper
- 1 yellow bell pepper
- 200 grams (7 ounces) chorizo sausage
- 6 large eggs
- 2 large red onion (cut into wedges)
- 2 cloves garlic (minced)
- ½ cup coconut milk
- Salt and pepper

Instructions

1. Preheat the oven to 425 degrees Fahrenheit (220 degrees Celsius).
2. Halve the bell peppers, remove the seeds and stem, and place them on a baking tray. Drizzle the halves with 1 tablespoon of olive oil and roast them in the oven for 20 minutes. After 10 minutes of baking, add the red onion wedges to the tray, drizzle them with a splash of olive oil, and continue cooking for another 10 minutes. The peppers are ready when they are soft and have a slightly charred skin. Once done, transfer the peppers to a cutting board, cover them with a bowl to trap the steam, and let them rest for 5 minutes. This will make it easier to peel off the skin.
3. Heat 1 tablespoon of olive oil in a cast iron skillet over medium-high heat. Stir in the minced garlic and cook for 20 seconds until fragrant. Then, add the chopped chorizo and cook for 5 minutes until the chorizo is fully cooked. Remove the skillet from the heat.
4. While the chorizo is cooking, peel the skin off the roasted bell peppers and slice them into thin strips.
5. In a bowl, whisk together the eggs, coconut milk, paprika, cayenne, salt, and pepper.

Add the sliced bell peppers and red onion to the cast iron skillet, then pour the egg mixture over the ingredients. Transfer the skillet to the oven and bake for 20-25 minutes until the eggs have set and the top of the frittata is firm to the touch.

Sprinkle with chopped parsley before serving.

SPINACH AND CHEESE EGG BAKE

Nutrition: Cal 260;Fat 20 g;Carb 4 g;Protein 20 g

Serving 2; Cook time 20 min

Ingredients

- 4 large eggs
- 1 cup fresh spinach leaves, chopped
- 1/2 cup shredded cheddar cheese
- Salt and pepper to taste
- 2 tbsp. butter or olive oil

Instructions

1. Preheat your oven to 375°F (190°C). Grease a 9-inch (23 cm) baking dish with butter or olive oil.
2. In a large bowl, whisk the eggs and add the chopped spinach, shredded cheese, salt, and pepper. Mix well.
3. Pour the egg mixture into the prepared baking dish and bake in the oven for 15-20 minutes, or until the eggs are set and the top is golden brown.

Remove from the oven and let cool for a few minutes before slicing and serving.

KETO BREAKFAST CASSEROLE

Nutrition: Cal 200;Fat 15 g;Carb 4 g;Protein 13 g

Serving 10; Cook time 70 min

Ingredients

- Drizzle of oil
- ½ cup onion
- 1 tablespoon garlic, minced
- 1 pound breakfast sausage
- 12 eggs
- ½ cup almond milk
- 2 teaspoons mustard powder
- 1 teaspoon oregano
- ¼ teaspoon salt
- Pepper, to taste
- 1½ cups broccoli florets
- 1 zucchini, diced
- 1 red bell pepper, diced (or 3–4 cups veggies of choice)

Instructions

1. Preheat oven to 375°F (190°C).
2. In a skillet over medium heat, add a drizzle of oil and sauté onion and garlic.
3. Once transparent, add sausage and cook until browned, 7–10 minutes.
4. Add to a 13×9-inch casserole or baking dish and set aside.
5. In a large bowl, whisk together eggs, milk of choice, and seasonings. Stir in chopped veggies.
6. Pour mixture over sausage.
7. Bake until firm and cooked through, 30–40 minutes.
8. Allow to cool slightly before slicing into squares, serving, and enjoying!

Store leftovers in the fridge for up to 5 days, and reheat individual portions in the microwave.

AVOCADO OMELETTE

Nutrition: Cal 310;Fat 23 g;Carb 11 g;Protein 16 g

Serving 2; Cook time 5 min

Ingredients

- 3 eggs, lightly beaten
- 3 tablespoons almond milk
- Nonstick cooking spray, as needed
- 1/2 cup tofu cheese
- 1 tablespoon sliced green onion
- 1/4 cup chopped red bell pepper
- 1 ripe, fresh avocado; seeded, peeled, and cubed

Instructions

1. Mix eggs and milk.
2. Spray a large skillet with nonstick cooking spray and heat over medium low heat. Pour egg mixture into skillet. Cook eggs until top is almost set.
3. Sprinkle with cheese and green onion. Cook, about 2 minutes.

Top with red pepper and avocado, fold over, and serve immediately.

BRUSCHETTA WITH AVOCADO AND EGG

Nutrition: Cal 330;Fat 23 g;Carb 15 g;Protein 14 g

Serving 2; Cook time 15 min

Ingredients

- 1 medium avocado
- 4 slices of keto-friendly bread (e.g., almond flour bread or cloud bread)
- 1 ripe avocado
- 2 eggs
- 1 tablespoon olive oil
- 1 clove garlic, minced
- Salt and pepper to taste

- Optional toppings: chopped tomatoes, sliced radishes, microgreens

Instructions

1. Preheat your oven to 350°F (175°C).
2. In a small bowl, mash the avocado until smooth. Add minced garlic, salt, and pepper to taste. Mix well.
3. Brush the bread slices with olive oil and place them on a baking sheet. Toast them in the oven for about 8-10 minutes or until they become crispy.
4. While the bread is toasting, heat a non-stick skillet over medium heat. Crack the eggs into the skillet and cook them to your desired doneness (e.g., sunny-side up or over-easy).
5. Once the bread is toasted, remove it from the oven and spread the avocado mixture evenly on each slice.
6. Place a cooked egg on top of each avocado-covered bread slice.
7. If desired, add additional toppings like chopped tomatoes, sliced radishes, or microgreens for added freshness and flavor.

Season with a sprinkle of salt and pepper, and serve immediately.

LEMON POPPY RICOTTA PANCAKES

Nutrition: Cal 370;Fat 26 g;Carb 6,5 g;Protein 29 g
Serving 2; Cook time 20 min

Ingredients
- 1 large lemon, juiced and zested
- 6 ounces whole milk ricotta
- 3 large eggs
- 10 to 12 drops liquid stevia
- ¼ cup almond flour
- 1 scoop egg white protein powder
- 1 tablespoon poppy seeds
- ¾ teaspoons baking powder
- ¼ cup powdered erythritol
- 1 tablespoon heavy cream

Instructions

1. In a food processor, combine the ricotta, eggs, liquid stevia, half of the lemon juice, and lemon zest. Blend well until smooth, then pour the mixture into a bowl.
2. Whisk in the almond flour, protein powder, poppy seeds, baking powder, and a pinch of salt.
3. Heat a large nonstick pan over medium heat.

4. Spoon about ¼ cup of batter per pancake onto the pan.
5. Cook the pancakes until bubbles form on the surface of the batter, then flip them.
6. Let the pancakes cook until the bottom is browned, then transfer them to a plate.
7. Repeat with the remaining batter.
8. Whisk together the heavy cream, powdered erythritol, and the reserved lemon juice and zest.

Serve the pancakes hot, drizzled with the lemon glaze.

EGG STRATA WITH BLUEBERRIES AND CINNAMON

Nutrition: Cal 188;Fat 15 g;Carb 4 g;Protein 8 g
Serving 4; Cook time 20 min

Ingredients
- 6 large eggs
- 2 tbsp softened butter
- 1 tsp vanilla
- 1/2 cup blueberries (or 1/4 cup, depending upon taste)
- 1/2 tsp cinnamon (you could probably double this if you like cinnamon)
- 1 tbsp coconut oil

Instructions

1. Preheat oven to 375°F.
2. In an 8" - 9" cast iron skillet (or any oven-proof skillet), heat coconut oil over medium heat.
3. In a medium bowl beat eggs, butter, cinnamon, and vanilla together with a hand mixer until combined and fluffy (about 1-2 minutes).
4. Pour egg mixture into heated pan and allow bottom to cook slightly (about 2 minutes). Gently drop blueberries into egg mixture and place pan in oven. Cook for 15-20 or until cooked through and browned on top (but not burned).

Remove from oven and allow to cool slightly.

SWEET BLUEBERRY COCONUT PORRIDGE

Nutrition: Cal 390;Fat 22 g;Carb 12 g;Protein 10 g
Serving 2; Cook time 15 min

Ingredients
- 1 cup unsweetened almond milk
- ¼ cup canned coconut milk
- ¼ cup coconut flour

- ¼ cup ground flaxseed
- 1 teaspoon ground cinnamon
- ¼ teaspoon ground nutmeg
- Pinch salt
- 60 grams fresh blueberries
- ¼ cup shaved coconut

Instructions
1. Warm the almond milk and coconut milk in a saucepan over low heat.
2. Whisk in the coconut flour, flaxseed, cinnamon, nutmeg, and salt.
3. Turn up the heat and cook until the mixture bubbles.
4. Stir in the sweetener and vanilla extract, then cook until thickened to the desired level.
5. Spoon into two bowls and top with blueberries and shaved coconut.

SWEET APPLE CINNAMON COCONUT PORRIDGE

Nutrition: Cal 390;Fat 22 g;Carb 12 g;Protein 10 g
Serving 2; Cook time 15 min

Ingredients
- 1 cup unsweetened coconut milk
- 1/2 cup shredded unsweetened coconut
- 2 tablespoons ground flaxseed
- 1/4 cup chopped walnuts
- 1/2 teaspoon ground cinnamon
- 1 small apple, diced
- 1 tablespoon butter or coconut oil
- Optional toppings: additional shredded coconut, sliced almonds, chia seeds, or a drizzle of sugar-free maple syrup

Instructions
1. In a saucepan, combine the coconut milk, shredded coconut, ground flaxseed, chopped walnuts, and ground cinnamon.
2. Bring the mixture to a gentle simmer over medium heat, stirring occasionally. Allow it to cook for about 5 minutes until it thickens slightly.
3. While the porridge is simmering, heat a separate pan over medium heat and melt the butter or coconut oil.
4. Add the diced apple to the pan and sauté until it becomes slightly soft, about 3-4 minutes.
5. Once the porridge has thickened, remove it from the heat and divide it between two bowls.

6. Top each bowl of porridge with the sautéed apples.
7. If desired, sprinkle additional shredded coconut, sliced almonds, or chia seeds on top for added texture and flavor.
8. Serve the sweet apple cinnamon coconut porridge warm and enjoy!

LOW-CARB BREAKFAST QUICHE

Nutrition: Cal 450;Fat 36 g;Carb 6 g;Protein 24 g
Serving 4; Cook time 55 min

Ingredients
- 1 lb ground Italian sausage
- 1.5 cups shredded cheddar cheese
- 8 large eggs
- 1 tbsp ranch seasoning
- 1 cup sour cream

Instructions
1. Preheat oven to 350°F.
2. In an oven-safe skillet, brown ground sausage and drain the grease.
3. In a large bowl, whisk together egg, sour cream, and ranch seasoning. You may want to use a hand mixer.
4. Mix in cheddar cheese.
5. Pour egg mixture into pan and stir until everything is fully blended.
6. Cover with foil and bake for 30 minutes.
7. Remove foil and bake for another 25 minutes or until golden brown.

QUICHE WITH BOILED CHICKEN BREAST AND MUSHROOM

Nutrition: Cal 340;Fat 23 g;Carb 3 g;Protein 29 g
Serving 2; Cook time 40 min

Ingredients
- 4 large eggs
- 1/4 cup heavy cream
- 1/2 cup shredded cheese (e.g., cheddar or mozzarella)
- 1 cup sliced mushrooms
- 1 cup boiled chicken breast, shredded
- 1/4 cup chopped onion
- 1 tablespoon butter or olive oil
- Salt and pepper to taste
- Optional garnish: fresh parsley or chives

Instructions
1. Preheat your oven to 350°F (175°C).

2.In a skillet, heat the butter or olive oil over medium heat. Add the chopped onion and sliced mushrooms. Sauté until the mushrooms become tender and any excess liquid has evaporated.

3.In a mixing bowl, whisk together the eggs and heavy cream. Season with salt and pepper.

4.Grease a 9-inch pie dish or any oven-safe baking dish with butter or cooking spray.

5.Spread the sautéed mushrooms and onions evenly on the bottom of the greased dish.

6.Sprinkle the shredded chicken breast on top of the mushrooms and onions.

7.Pour the egg and cream mixture over the mushrooms, onions, and chicken. Ensure the mixture covers the ingredients evenly.

8.Sprinkle the shredded cheese over the top of the quiche.

9.Bake in the preheated oven for approximately 25-30 minutes or until the quiche is set and the top is golden brown.

10. Remove from the oven and let it cool for a few minutes. Slice into portions and garnish with fresh parsley or chives, if desired.

COCONUT FLOUR PANCAKES

Nutrition: Cal 274;Fat 23g;Carb 8g;Protein 8g
Serving 2; Cook time 20 min

Ingredients
MAIN INGREDIENTS:
- 2 tbsp coconut flour
- 2 eggs
- ½ tbsp So Nourished Erythritol or a dash of stevia extract
- ¼ tsp baking powder
- 2 tbsp sour cream
- 2 tbsp melted butter
- ½ tsp vanilla extract

FOR THE TOPPING:
- 50 g strawberries
- 1 tbsp shredded coconut
- 1 tbsp almond slices
- 1 tbsp maple syrup (optional)

Instructions
1.In a bowl, combine the eggs, sour cream, 1 ½ tablespoons of melted butter (save the rest for frying the pancakes), and vanilla extract. Mix everything well.

2.Add the coconut flour, baking powder, and erythritol to the mixture. Mix again until well combined. Allow the mixture to sit for about 15 minutes. If the batter is too thick, add a small amount of water (around 20-30 ml) and mix until you achieve the desired consistency.

Heat a pan over medium heat and add butter for frying. Spoon the batter onto the pan to form pancakes. The size and number of pancakes will depend on your preference. With this recipe, you can make approximately 6 pancakes.

PEPPERONI, HAM & CHEDDAR STROMBOLI

Nutrition: Cal 525;Fat 37 g;Carb 16 g;Protein 32 g
Serving 3; Cook time 40 min

Ingredients
- 1 ¼ cups shredded mozzarella cheese
- ¼ cup almond flour
- 3 tablespoons coconut flour
- 1 teaspoon dried Italian seasoning
- Salt and pepper
- 1 large egg, whisked
- 6 ounces sliced deli ham
- 2 ounces sliced pepperoni
- 4 ounces sliced cheddar cheese
- 1 tablespoon melted butter
- 6 cups fresh salad greens

Instructions
1.Preheat your oven to 400°F (200°C) and line a baking sheet with parchment paper.

2.Place the shredded mozzarella cheese in a microwave-safe bowl and heat it in the microwave until melted and smooth.

3.In a separate bowl, combine the almond flour, coconut flour, and dried Italian seasoning.

4.Pour the melted cheese into the flour mixture and season with salt and pepper. Mix everything together until a dough forms.

5.Transfer the dough onto a piece of parchment paper. Place another piece of parchment paper on top and roll out the dough into an oval shape.

6.Use a knife to make diagonal slits along the edges of the dough, leaving the middle 4 inches untouched.

7.Arrange the sliced deli ham and cheddar cheese in the middle of the dough. Then add the sliced pepperoni on top.

8. Fold the strips of dough over the filling, creating a braided appearance.
9. Brush the top of the dough with melted butter.
10. Bake in the preheated oven for 15 to 20 minutes, or until the dough is golden brown and crispy.

Slice the Stromboli into portions and serve it with a side of fresh salad greens.

EGGS AND ASPARAGUS BREAKFAST BITES

Nutrition: Cal 426;Fat 35 g;Carb 6 g;Protein 20 g
Serving 2; Cook time 25 min

Ingredients
• 4 medium eggs
• 100 g asparagus, fresh or canned
• 1 tbsp butter, melted
• ¼ tsp baking powder
• 1 tbsp coconut flour
• 80 g cream cheese
• 40 g shredded cheddar cheese
• Salt, to taste

Instructions
1. If you are using fresh asparagus, chop them into approximately 2-cm long pieces. Heat a pan and melt butter in it. Pan-fry the asparagus pieces in the melted butter for about 5 minutes until they are tender. If you are using canned asparagus, simply chop them into pieces. Set them aside.
2. In a bowl, combine the remaining ingredients and mix them well. Allow the mixture to sit for 10 minutes, allowing the flavors to blend.
3. Brush a generous amount of oil onto the baking molds to prevent sticking. Place some pieces of asparagus in the molds, then pour the reserved mixture over them. Be careful not to fill the molds up to the brim, as the mixture will expand during baking.
4. Preheat your oven to 350°F (175°C). Place the filled molds in the preheated oven and bake for approximately 20 minutes. Check occasionally to ensure that the asparagus bites are thoroughly cooked.

Once the asparagus bites are done, carefully remove them from the molds and transfer them to a serving plate. They are now ready to be enjoyed as a delicious appetizer or side dish.

CHEDDAR BISCUITS

Nutrition: Cal 284;Fat 25 g;Carb 2 g;Protein 20 g
Serving 4; Cook time 20 min

Ingredients
• 1 cup cheddar cheese, shredded
• 1/4 cup butter melted and slightly cooled
• 4 eggs
• 1/3 cup coconut flour
• 1/4 teaspoon baking powder
• 1/4 teaspoon garlic powder
• 1 teaspoon dried parsley (optional)
• 1/4 teaspoon Old Bay Seasoning (optional)
• 1/4 teaspoon salt

Instructions
1. Preheat the oven to 400°F (200°C).
2. Crack the eggs into a bowl. Add garlic powder, melted butter, dried parsley, and seasoning powder (if desired). Season with salt to taste.
3. Combine the cheese, baking powder, and coconut flour with the egg mixture. Fold until you have a lump-free batter.
4. Grease a cookie sheet and drop ice cream-sized scoops of the batter onto it.
5. Bake the biscuits in the oven for about 15 minutes or until they are lightly browned.
6. Serve the biscuits with any meal or enjoy them on their own.

If you want to store them for later, allow the biscuits to cool completely before transferring them to a jar to maintain their crispness.

VEGETABLE TART

Nutrition: Cal 250;Fat 22 g;Carb 5.5 g;Protein 10 g
Serving 8; Cook time 70 min

Ingredients
• 6 eggs
• ½ cup heavy cream
• 8 oz cream cheese
• ½ cup shredded cheese
• ½ cup almond milk (or coconut milk)
• 12 oz zucchini
• 4 oz cauliflower
• 2 oz broccoli
• 8 oz red pepper
• 3 oz jalapeno
• 3 oz onion
• 3 cloves garlic
• Seasoning of your choice

Instructions

1. Finely mince the cauliflower, broccoli, garlic, onion, red pepper, jalapeño, and dice the zucchini.
2. Heat oil in a large skillet and sauté the diced vegetables until they become soft but not mushy. Remove from heat and set aside.
3. Crack the eggs into a separate bowl. Add almond milk, softened cream cheese, and heavy cream. Mix well to combine all ingredients.
4. Add the sautéed vegetables to the cream cheese mixture. Stir in the cheese and your choice of seasonings. Fold everything together until well combined.
5. Line the base of a springform pan with foil to prevent the mixture from seeping through. Cover the base and sides with parchment paper, then brush with oil. Pour the batter into the prepared pan. Preheat the oven to 350°F and bake for approximately one hour, or until the surface of the tart is golden brown.

Once baked, generously sprinkle cheese on top.

Slice the tart into wedges and serve.

KETO SAUSAGE BREAKFAST SANDWICH

Nutrition: Cal 350;Fat 25 g;Carb 2 g;Protein 12 g
Serving 3; Cook time 20 min

Ingredients
- 6 large eggs
- 2 tbsp. heavy cream
- Pinch red pepper flakes
- Kosher salt
- Freshly ground black pepper
- 1 tbsp. butter
- 3 slices cheddar
- 6 frozen sausage patties, heated according to package instructions
- 1 Avocado, sliced

Instructions
1. In a small bowl, whisk together eggs, heavy cream, and red pepper flakes. Season the mixture generously with salt and pepper. Heat butter in a non-stick skillet over medium heat. Pour approximately one-third of the egg mixture into the skillet.
2. Place a slice of cheese in the center and let it cook for about 1 minute. Fold the sides of the egg over the cheese, covering it completely.
3. Remove the folded omelet from the pan and repeat the process with the remaining eggs.

To serve, sandwich the folded omelets between two sausage patties and top with avocado.

CABBAGE HASH BROWNS

Nutrition: Cal 250;Fat 22 g;Carb 5.5 g;Protein 10 g
Serving 2; Cook time 35 min

Ingredients
- 2 large eggs
- 1/2 tsp. garlic powder
- 1/2 tsp. kosher salt
- Freshly ground black pepper
- 2 c. shredded cabbage
- 1/4 small yellow onion, thinly sliced
- 1 tbsp. vegetable oil

Instructions
1. In a large bowl, whisk together eggs, garlic powder, salt, and black pepper. Add cabbage and onion to the egg mixture and toss to combine.
2. Heat oil in a large skillet over medium-high heat. Divide the mixture into 4 patties in the pan and press them with a spatula to flatten. Cook until golden and tender, approximately 3 minutes per side.

OMELET-STUFFED PEPPERS

Nutrition: Cal 280;Fat 12 g;Carb 8 g;Protein 25 g
Serving 4; Cook time 60 min

Ingredients
- 2 bell peppers, halved and seeds removed
- 8 eggs, lightly beaten
- 1/4 c. milk
- 4 slices bacon, cooked and crumbled
- 1 c. shredded cheddar
- 2 tbsp. finely chopped chives, plus more for garnish
- Kosher salt
- Freshly cracked black pepper

Instructions
1. Preheat the oven to 400°F. Place the peppers cut side up in a large baking dish. Add a small amount of water to the dish and bake the peppers for 5 minutes.
2. In a separate bowl, beat together the eggs and milk. Stir in the bacon, cheese, chives, and season with salt and pepper.

Once the peppers are done baking, pour the egg mixture into the peppers. Place the dish back in the oven and bake for an additional 35 to 40 minutes, or until the eggs are set. Garnish with additional chives and serve.

BACON AVOCADO BOMBS

Nutrition: Cal 250;Fat 19 g;Carb 2,5 g;Protein 17 g
Serving 4; Cook time 30 min

Ingredients
- 2 avocados
- 1/3 c. shredded Cheddar
- 8 slices bacon

Instructions
1. Heat broiler and line a small baking sheet with foil.
2. Slice each avocado in half and remove the pits. Peel the skin off of each avocado.
3. Fill two of the halves with cheese, then replace with the other avocado halves. Wrap each avocado with 4 slices of bacon.
4. Place bacon-wrapped avocados on the prepared baking sheet and broil until the bacon is crispy on top, about 5 minutes. Very carefully, flip the avocado using tongs and continue to cook until crispy all over, about 5 minutes per side.

Cut in half crosswise and serve immediately.

HAM & CHEESE EGG CUPS

Nutrition: Cal 340;Fat 30 g;Carb 10 g;Protein 12 g
Serving 12; Cook time 30 min

Ingredients
- Cooking spray, for pan
- 12 slices ham
- 1 c. shredded cheddar
- 12 large eggs
- Kosher salt
- Freshly ground black pepper
- Chopped fresh parsley, for garnish

Instructions
1. Preheat the oven to 400°F and lightly grease a 12-cup muffin tin with cooking spray. Place a slice of ham in each cup, ensuring it covers the bottom and sides. Sprinkle shredded cheddar cheese on top of the ham. Crack one egg into each ham cup and season with salt and pepper.
2. Bake the ham and egg cups in the preheated oven for approximately 12 to 15 minutes, or until the eggs are cooked to your desired level of doneness. Keep in mind that a shorter baking time will result in runnier yolks, while a longer baking time will yield firmer yolks.

3. Once cooked, garnish the ham and egg cups with fresh parsley for added flavor and presentation. Serve them warm and enjoy!

KETO PIZZA EGG WRAP

Nutrition: Cal 350;Fat 10 g;Carb 2 g;Protein 25 g
Serving 1; Cook time 15 min

Ingredients
- 2 large eggs
- ½ tbsp butter
- ½ tbsp tomato sauce
- ½ oz. (2 tbsp) mozzarella cheese, shredded
- 1½ oz. salami, sliced

Instructions
1. Heat a large non-stick frying pan over medium heat and add the butter, allowing it to melt and coat the pan.
2. Crack the eggs into a bowl and whisk them until they are smooth and well combined.
3. Slowly pour the beaten eggs into the pan, ensuring that the mixture spreads evenly to the edges of the pan.
4. Cook the eggs until the edges start to lift off the sides of the frying pan. Using a spatula, gently lift the edges of the egg and tilt the pan to allow the uncooked mixture to flow underneath.
5. Once the bottom side is cooked and set, carefully flip the omelette using a spatula or by gently sliding it onto a plate and then flipping it back into the pan. Cook the other side for approximately 30 seconds to ensure it is cooked through.
6. Remove the omelette from the pan and place it on a clean surface. Spread tomato sauce, mozzarella cheese, and salami slices in the center of the omelette. Carefully roll the omelette into a wrap, enclosing the filling.

GREEN EGGS

Nutrition: Cal 300;Fat 20 g;Carb 8 g;Protein 18 g
Serving 2; Cook time 20 min

Ingredients
- 1½ tbsp rapeseed oil , plus a splash extra
- 2 trimmed leeks , sliced
- 2 garlic cloves , sliced
- ½ tsp coriander seeds
- ½ tsp fennel seeds
- pinch of chilli flakes , plus extra to serve
- 200g spinach

- 2 large eggs
- 2 tbsp Greek yogurt
- squeeze of lemon

Instructions

1. Heat the oil in a large frying pan over medium heat. Add the leeks and a pinch of salt, and cook them until they become soft and translucent. Stir in the garlic, coriander, fennel seeds, and chili flakes. Once the seeds start to crackle, add the spinach to the pan and reduce the heat. Mix everything together until the spinach wilts and reduces in volume. Push the spinach mixture to one side of the pan. Drizzle a little more oil into the empty side of the pan and crack the eggs into it. Fry the eggs to your desired level of doneness.

2. Stir the yogurt into the spinach mixture and season it to taste. Divide the mixture onto two plates. Top each portion with a fried egg. Squeeze a little lemon juice over the dish and season with black pepper and chili flakes to serve.

MASALA FRITTATA WITH AVOCADO SALSA

Nutrition: Cal 350;Fat 25 g;Carb 12 g;Protein 16 g
Serving 4; Cook time 40 min

Ingredients

- 2 tbsp rapeseed oil
- 3 onions, 2½ thinly sliced, ½ finely chopped
- 1 tbsp Madras curry paste
- 500g cherry tomatoes, halved
- 1 red chilli, deseeded and finely chopped
- small pack coriander, roughly chopped
- 8 large eggs, beaten
- 1 avocado, stoned, peeled and cubed
- juice 1 lemon

Instructions

1. Heat the oil in a medium-sized non-stick, ovenproof frying pan. Add the sliced onions and cook them over medium heat for approximately 10 minutes until they become soft and golden. Stir in the Madras paste and cook for an additional minute, then add half of the tomatoes and half of the chili. Cook until the mixture thickens and the tomatoes have burst.

2. Preheat the grill to high. Add half of the coriander to the beaten eggs and season with salt and pepper. Pour the egg mixture over the spicy onion mixture in the frying pan. Stir gently once or twice, then cook over low heat for 8-10 minutes until the frittata is almost set. Transfer the pan to the grill and cook for an additional 3-5 minutes until the frittata is fully set.

3. To make the salsa, mix together the avocado, remaining chili and tomatoes, chopped onion, remaining coriander, and lemon juice. Season with salt and serve the salsa alongside the frittata.

KETO BREAKFAST PARFAIT

Nutrition: Cal 335;Fat 29 g;Carb 10 g;Protein 11 g
Serving 2; Cook time 10 min

Ingredients

- ½ cup Greek Yogurt full fat
- ¼ cup Heavy Cream
- 1 teaspoon Vanilla Essence
- ½ cup Keto Chocolate Almond Clusters
- 2 Strawberries diced
- 8 Blueberries

Instructions

1. In a mixing bowl, combine the Greek yogurt, heavy cream, and vanilla extract. Whisk together until the mixture becomes thick and smooth.

2. Spoon half of the yogurt mixture into two glasses, creating a bottom layer. Sprinkle half of the Keto Chocolate Almond Clusters over the yogurt layer.

3. Add the remaining yogurt mixture on top, followed by the remaining Keto Chocolate Almond Clusters.

4. Finish off by topping the parfaits with the diced strawberries and blueberries.

5. Enjoy this delicious and satisfying dessert!

KETO SAUSAGE & EGG BOWLS

Nutrition: Cal 435;Fat 29 g;Carb 8 g;Protein 27 g
Serving 2; Cook time 10 min

Ingredients

- 1/4 cup sausage – cooked and crumbled
- 2 whole eggs
- sprinkle of cheddar cheese
- salt & pepper to taste

- 1 tbs butter

Instructions

1. Begin by cracking two eggs into a bowl and whisking them together until well mixed.
2. Heat butter in a skillet over medium-high heat.
3. Once the butter has melted, add the scrambled eggs to the pan, stirring them frequently to ensure even cooking. Be careful not to overcook the eggs.
4. When the eggs are mostly set but still slightly glossy, add the sausage and cheese to the pan.
5. Remove the skillet from the heat and mix the sausage and cheese into the eggs until well combined.

Season with salt and pepper according to your taste preferences.

CHEESE AND EGG STUFFED PEPPERS

Nutrition: Cal 285;Fat 7 g;Carb 7 g;Protein 14 g
Serving 8; Cook time 50 min

Ingredients

- 4 large bell peppers, cut in half lengthwise and remove inner seeds and stems
- 1 tablespoon olive oil
- 1 cup white onion
- 1 pound gluten free pork sausage, casing removed
- 2 cups spinach
- 4 large eggs
- 1/4 teaspoon salt & pepper, each
- 3/4 cup shredded mozzarella

Instructions

1. Preheat your oven to 350°F (180°C) and lightly grease a 9x13 baking dish.
2. Place the bell peppers, cut side up, in the greased baking dish. Set aside.
3. In a large skillet, warm the olive oil over medium heat. Add the onions and cook for about 5 minutes until softened. Add the sausage and cook until no longer pink. Stir in the spinach and cook for an additional 1-2 minutes until wilted. Remove from heat.
4. In a medium-sized mixing bowl, whisk together the eggs, salt, and pepper. Stir in 1/2 cup of the cheese.
5. Spoon the sausage mixture evenly into the prepared peppers. Pour the egg mixture over the top of the sausage. Sprinkle with the remaining 1/4 cup of cheese.

4. Place the baking dish in the oven and bake for an additional 35-40 minutes until the cheese has golden.

EGG WRAPS WITH HAM AND GREENS

Nutrition: Cal 371;Fat 26 g;Carb 5 g;Protein 28 g
Serving 6; Cook time 20 min

Ingredients

- 8 large eggs
- 4 teaspoons water
- 2 teaspoons all-purpose flour or cornstarch
- 1/2 teaspoon fine salt
- 4 teaspoons vegetable or coconut oil
- 1 1/3 cups shredded Swiss cheese
- 4 ounces very thinly sliced ham
- 1 1/3 cups loosely packed watercress

Instructions

1. In a medium bowl, combine the eggs, water, flour or cornstarch, and salt. Whisk the mixture until the eggs are broken up and the flour or cornstarch is completely dissolved.
2. Heat 1 teaspoon of oil in a 12-inch nonstick frying pan over medium heat until it shimmers. Swirl the pan to coat the bottom with oil. Pour 1/2 cup of the egg mixture into the pan, swirling it to create a thin, even layer on the bottom. Cook the wrap until the edges and bottom are completely set, and the top is mostly set but may still be slightly wet, which usually takes 3 to 6 minutes.
3. Using a flat spatula, loosen the edges of the wrap and slide it underneath, making sure it can move freely around the pan. Flip the wrap with the spatula. Immediately sprinkle 1/3 cup of cheese over the wrap and cook for about 1 minute until the second side is set. Slide the wrap onto a work surface or cutting board (the cheese may not be fully melted yet). While the wrap is still warm, place a single layer of ham over the eggs and arrange 1/3 cup of watercress across the center of the wrap. Roll it up tightly.
4. Repeat the process of cooking and filling the remaining wraps. Once all the wraps are done, use a serrated knife to cut each wrap crosswise into 6 pieces, resulting in bite-sized portions.

KETO CROQUE MADAME

Nutrition: Cal 566;Fat 47 g;Carb 3 g;Protein 33 g
Serving 4; Cook time 30 min

Ingredients
CHAFFLES:
- 2 large egg
- 1 cup cheddar cheese, grated

SANDWICH:
- 4 slice deli-sliced black forest ham
- 2/3 cup gruyere cheese, shredded
- 2 tablespoon butter
- 4 large egg

BECHEMEL SAUCE:
- 1/2 cup heavy cream
- 1/4 cup parmesan cheese
- 1/3 cup gruyere cheese, shredded

Instructions
1. Gather and prepare all the ingredients. Preheat the oven to 425°F (220°C).
2. In a bowl, whisk together the eggs and grated cheese to make the chaffle batter.
3. Grease a small waffle iron and pour the chaffle batter onto it. Cook the chaffles according to the waffle iron instructions.
4. Place the cooked chaffles on a parchment-lined baking sheet. Top each chaffle with deli-sliced ham and shredded Gruyere cheese. Bake in the oven for 10-15 minutes, or until the cheese is melted.
5. While the chaffles are baking, fry the eggs in a frying pan with butter. Once cooked, place a fried egg on top of each baked chaffle.
6. In a saucepan over medium heat, prepare the béchamel sauce by adding the heavy cream. Slowly add in the Parmesan cheese and Gruyere cheese, a small handful at a time, and wait until each batch is melted before adding more.
7. Drizzle the béchamel sauce over the chaffles, serve with a small side salad, and enjoy!

KETO SPINACH SHAKSHUKA

Nutrition: Cal 318;Fat 23 g;Carb 5 g;Protein 19 g
Serving 4; Cook time 25 min

Ingredients
- 3 tablespoon olive oil
- 1/2 medium onion, minced
- 2 teaspoon fresh garlic, minced
- 1 medium jalapeno pepper, seeded + minced
- 16 ounce frozen spinach, thawed
- 1 teaspoon cumin
- 3/4 teaspoon ground coriander
- 2 tablespoon harissa
- Salt and pepper to taste
- 1/2 cup vegetable broth
- 8 large eggs
- 1/4 cup fresh parsley, chopped, for garnish
- 1 teaspoon crushed red pepper flakes, for garnish

Instructions
1. Gather and prepare all the ingredients. Preheat the oven to 350°F (175°C).
2. Heat the olive oil in a skillet over medium heat. Add the minced onion and sauté until fragrant.
3. Add the thawed spinach to the skillet and let it cook until wilted.
4. Stir in the cumin, coriander, harissa, salt, and pepper. Mix well and cook for an additional 1-2 minutes.
5. Transfer the seasoned spinach mixture to a food processor. Pulse until coarse. Then, add the vegetable broth and pulse until smooth. Wipe out the skillet.
6. Drizzle oil in the bottom of the skillet or spray with cooking spray. Pour the smooth spinach mixture into the skillet. Using a spoon, create small wells in the mixture.
7. Gently crack the eggs into these wells. Cook in the oven until the egg whites are set and the yolk is slightly runny, about 20-25 minutes.

KETO SAUSAGE CREAM CHEESE ROLLS

Nutrition: Cal 203;Fat 16 g;Carb 3 g;Protein 12 g
Servig 10; Cook time 25 min

Ingredients
FOR THE ROLLS:
- 2 cups shredded mozzarealla cheese
- 2 ounces cream cheese
- 3/4 cup almond flour
- 2 tablespoons ground flax meal

FOR THE FILLING:
- 1/2 pound cooked breakfast sausage, drained
- 3 ounces of cream cheese

Instructions
Preheat oven to 400F.

FOR THE ROLLS:

1. In a microwave-safe mixing bowl, combine the shredded mozzarella cheese and cream cheese. Heat in 30 second increments, stirring in between until completely melted.
2. Add the almond flour and ground flax meal.
3. Mix the dough well until you have a soft ball
4. Between two silicone baking mats or parchment paper roll the dough into a rectangle roughly 12x9 inches.

FOR THE FILLING:
1. Combine the sausage and cream cheese.
2. Spread the sausage cream cheese mixture evenly on the dough.
3. Starting at one end roll the dough as tightly as you can into a log.
4. Slice into rolls about the width of two fingers, be careful not to slice them too thick because it will be difficult for the dough in the center to cook through.
5. Place the rolls on a greased baking sheet.
6. Bake 12-15 minutes until golden brown.

KETO BISCUITS AND GRAVY

Nutrition: Cal 203;Fat 16 g;Carb 3 g;Protein 12 g
Serving 6; Cook time 40 min

Ingredients
Keto Biscuits

- ¼ cup unsalted butter melted
- 4 large eggs
- ⅓ cup coconut flour
- 1 cup cheddar cheese shredded
- 1 tbsp cream cheese
- ¼ tsp salt
- ¼ tsp baking powder

KETO SAUSAGE GRAVY

- 1 lb ground sausage
- ½ cup chicken broth
- 1 cup heavy cream
- salt & pepper to taste
- 4 tbsp cream cheese
- ½ tsp chili flakes optional
- ¼ tsp xanthan gum optional

Instructions
TO MAKE THE KETO BISCUITS
1. Preheat the oven to 350°F / 180°C and line a baking sheet with parchment paper.
2. In a large bowl add the eggs, one tablespoon cream cheese, and salt. Whisk for 30 seconds.
3. Pour the melted butter over the egg mixture and continue whisking.

4. Add the shredded cheddar cheese, coconut flour, and baking powder and combine well. Let the biscuits dough sit for about 5 minutes so the coconut flour can absorb the liquid and make the dough thick.
5. Divide the dough into 9 equal biscuits. Place them 2 inches apart on the baking sheet.
6. Bake in the preheated oven for about 15 minutes or until they get a beautiful golden color.

TO MAKE THE SAUSAGE GRAVY
1. In a large skillet add the ground sausage. Brown and crumble the meat into smaller pieces over medium heat until fully cooked.
2. Add the chicken broth, cream cheese and whipping cream. Stir to combine well and let it simmer until it becomes thicker. Season with salt and pepper to taste (if necessary).
3. Serve one or two keto biscuits with 1/2 cup of gravy. Enjoy!

PROTEIN BREAKFAST SCRAMBLE

Nutrition: Cal 511;Fat 41 g;Carb 6 g;Protein 28 g
Serving 4; Cook time 20 min

Ingredients

- 6 links breakfast sausage sliced
- 6 slices bacon chopped
- 4 oz hard salami (such as Genoa) cubed
- 1 small onion sliced
- 1 medium bell pepper sliced
- 6 large eggs
- ¼ cup sour cream
- ½ cup cheddar cheese grated
- 2 stalks green onion (scallion) sliced
- salt and pepper

Instructions
1. Place a frying pan over medium-high heat and let it heat up. Once hot, add the raw sliced bacon and sausage to the pan. Fry them until they are cooked through, and just starting to brown and crisp, which should take about 5-8 minutes.
2. Use 6 slices of bacon for this step.
3. Add chopped salami to the pan and continue frying until the salami, bacon, and sausage reach the desired level of crispness. If the pan contains a lot of rendered fat, you can drain off a portion now to avoid a greasy result. This step typically takes around 2-3 minutes.
4. For this recipe, use 6 links of breakfast sausage and 4 ounces of hard salami, such as Genoa.

5. Next, add the sliced onions and peppers to the pan and fry them until they are softened, which should take about 1 minute.

6. Use 1 small onion and 1 medium bell pepper for this step.

7. Stir in the egg mixture and, using a spatula, begin to combine and scramble everything in the pan. Cook the eggs to your desired level of doneness, which usually takes around 3-5 minutes.

8. Stir in grated cheese, then top the mixture with sliced green onions. Finally, season the dish to taste with salt and pepper.

9. Use 2 stalks of green onion (scallion) for this step, and season with salt and pepper according to your preference.

RADISH AND TURNIP HASH WITH FRIED EGGS

Nutrition: Cal 391;Fat 34 g;Carb 10 g;Protein 12 g
Serving 2; Cook time 20 min

Ingredients

- 2 to 3 small turnips, trimmed, peeled, and cut into 3/4-inch cubes (about 1 1/2 cups cubed)
- 4 to 5 small radishes, scrubbed and trimmed, and cut into 3/4-inch cubes (about 1 1/2 cups cubed)
- Coarse sea salt
- Freshly ground pepper
- 2 tablespoons grapeseed oil, or other neutral, heat-tolerant oil
- 1 stalk green garlic, trimmed and chopped (white and light green parts only)
- 2 tablespoons unsalted butter
- 4 eggs
- 1 tablespoon minced parsley

Instructions

1. Fill a large saucepan with water and bring it to a boil. Add 2 teaspoons of sea salt. Boil the cubes of turnip for just 3 to 4 minutes, or until they are tender. Using a slotted spoon, transfer the turnip cubes to a bowl, drain any excess water, and set them aside.

2. Next, briefly boil the radishes for 30 to 60 seconds, then transfer them to a bowl using a slotted spoon, drain any excess water, and set them aside.

3. Place a large cast iron skillet over medium-high heat. Add grapeseed oil to the skillet and let it heat up. Once hot, add the turnips and radishes to the skillet, along with a pinch of

sea salt and pepper. Cook the vegetables for about 8 minutes, turning them only once or twice, until they become golden-brown. Reduce the heat to medium and stir in the green garlic, cooking for approximately 1 minute.

4. Push the vegetables to the sides of the pan, melt butter in the center of the pan, and crack the eggs into the melted butter. Season each egg with salt individually. For over-easy eggs, cook them uncovered for 4 to 6 minutes.

5. For over-medium eggs, cover the pan for 3 minutes, then uncover and continue cooking until the whites are set, which should take about 2 to 3 minutes more. Finish by sprinkling minced parsley, sea salt, and pepper to taste over the dish. Serve immediately.

KALE AND GOAT CHEESE FRITTATA CUPS

Nutrition: Cal 179;Fat 14,7 g;Carb 1 g;Protein 10 g
Serving 8; Cook time 40 min

Ingredients

- 2 cups chopped lacinato kale
- 1 garlic clove, thinly sliced
- 3 tablespoons olive oil
- 1/4 teaspoon red pepper flakes
- 8 large eggs
- 1/4 teaspoon salt
- Dash ground black pepper
- 1/2 teaspoon dried thyme
- 1/4 cup goat cheese, crumbled

Instructions

1. Preheat the oven to 350°F. Prepare 2 cups of kale by removing the leaves from the kale ribs. Wash and dry the leaves, then cut them into 1/2-inch-wide strips.

2. In a 10-inch nonstick skillet, heat 1 tablespoon of oil over medium-high heat. Add the garlic and cook for 30 seconds. Add the kale and red pepper flakes, and cook until the kale is wilted, which takes about 1 to 2 minutes.

3. In a medium bowl, beat the eggs and season with salt and pepper. Add the cooked kale and thyme to the egg mixture, stirring to combine.

4. Grease 8 cups of a 12-cup muffin tin using the remaining 2 tablespoons of oil. Alternatively, you can use butter or nonstick spray. Divide the egg and kale mixture among the greased cups. Sprinkle the tops with goat cheese. Bake in the preheated oven until the frittatas are set in the center, which typically takes about 25 to 30 minutes.

5. Frittatas are best enjoyed warm from the oven or within the next day. However, if you have leftovers, you can refrigerate them and reheat them for up to a week.

ROASTED RADISH AND HERBED RICOTTA OMELET

Nutrition: Cal 350;Fat 27 g;Carb 5 g;Protein 20 g
Serving 2; Cook time 15 min

Ingredients

FOR THE ROASTED RADISHES:

- 1 cup thinly-sliced French Breakfast radishes, or other radish variety
- 2 teaspoons olive oil
- 1/4 teaspoon sea salt

FOR THE RICOTTA:

- 1/4 cup plus 2 tablespoons fresh whole milk ricotta
- 2 teaspoons minced fresh chives
- 1 teaspoon minced fresh thyme
- 1 teaspoon minced fresh flat leaf parsley, plus extra for topping

FOR THE EGGS:

- 4 large or extra-large eggs
- 2 tablespoons whole milk
- 1/2 teaspoon sea salt
- 1/4 teaspoon black pepper
- 1 tablespoon butter

Instructions

1. To prepare the radishes, preheat the oven to 400°F. In a bowl, toss the radishes with olive oil and salt. Spread them in a thin layer on a roasting dish and bake for 10 to 12 minutes, until they become soft and tender. Be cautious not to overcook them, as they may turn into radish chips.

2. In a small bowl, combine the ricotta cheese with the minced herbs.

3. To make the omelet, whisk together the eggs, milk, salt, and pepper. Heat 1/2 tablespoon of butter in an 8-inch non-stick skillet over medium-low heat. Pour in half of the egg mixture and cook for 1 to 2 minutes, allowing the bottom to set slightly. Use a spatula to lift the edges and tilt the pan to allow the uncooked eggs to flow underneath the cooked part. Repeat this process until the majority of the egg is set. Carefully flip the omelet and remove it from the heat.

4. Spread half of the ricotta mixture over half of the omelet and sprinkle it with half of the roasted radishes. Fold the omelet over the filling and garnish with a few more roasted radish slices and minced parsley.

5. Repeat the steps to make the second omelet. Serve both omelets immediately.

MIXED MUSHROOM EGG BAKES

Nutrition: Cal 287;Fat 21 g;Carb 8 g;Protein 16 g
Serving 4; Cook time 35 min

Ingredients

- Butter or cooking spray
- 2 tablespoons extra-virgin olive oil
- 1/3 cup minced shallot (from about 2 small shallots)
- 8 ounces sliced mixed fresh mushrooms (cremini, oyster or shiitake, stems removed before slicing)
- 2 tablespoons chopped fresh thyme
- 6 large eggs
- 3/4 cup whole milk
- 1/2 teaspoon kosher salt
- 1/2 teaspoon ground black pepper
- 1/2 cup shredded mozzarella cheese

Instructions

1. Position a rack in the middle of the oven and preheat it to 400°F. Grease 4 (8-ounce) ramekins with a small amount of butter, or use cooking spray as an alternative. Place the ramekins on a rimmed baking sheet for easier handling. Set them aside.

2. In a medium saucepan, heat the olive oil over medium-high heat until it shimmers. Add the shallot and sauté until it becomes soft and translucent, which should take about 3 minutes. Add the mushrooms and a pinch of salt, and continue cooking until the mushrooms have softened and become fragrant, approximately 5 minutes. Stir in the thyme and remove the saucepan from the heat.

3. In a medium bowl, whisk together the eggs, milk, salt, and pepper. Divide the mushroom mixture evenly among the ramekins. Sprinkle the cheese over the mushrooms. Pour the egg mixture over the top, leaving a small space below the rim of each ramekin.

4. Place the baking sheet with the ramekins in the oven and bake for 20 to 25 minutes, or until the tops are golden and have slightly puffed up, and the eggs are completely set.

CHICKEN AND CHEESE BREAKFAST BOWLS

Nutrition: Cal 240;Fat 15 g;Carb 2 g;Protein 30 g
Serving 2; Cook time 20 min

Ingredients
- •4 ounces cooked chicken breast, diced
- •4 large eggs
- •1/2 cup shredded cheddar cheese
- •Salt and pepper to taste
- •2 tbsp. butter or olive oil

Instructions
1. Begin by preheating your oven to 375°F (190°C). Take a 9-inch (23cm) baking dish and grease it with butter or olive oil to prevent sticking.

2. In a large bowl, whisk the eggs thoroughly. Then, add the diced chicken, shredded cheese, salt, and pepper to the bowl. Mix all the ingredients together until well combined.

3. Pour the egg mixture into the prepared baking dish, ensuring it is spread evenly. Place the dish in the preheated oven and bake for approximately 15-20 minutes. Keep an eye on it and remove it from the oven when the eggs are fully set and the top has turned a golden brown color.

4. Once cooked, take the dish out of the oven and allow it to cool for a few minutes. This will make it easier to slice and serve. Enjoy your delicious baked chicken and cheese dish!

SPICY CHICKEN BREAKFAST BOWLS

Nutrition: Cal 260;Fat 18 g;Carb 5 g;Protein 37 g
Serving 2; Cook time 20 min

Ingredients
- •2 boneless, skinless chicken breasts, diced
- •1 tbsp. olive oil
- •1 tsp. chili powder
- •1 tsp. paprika
- •Salt and pepper to taste
- •2 cups fresh spinach leaves
- •2 tbsp. sour cream
- •2 tbsp. sliced jalapeños

Instructions
1. Start by heating the olive oil in a large pan over medium heat. Once the oil is hot, add the diced chicken to the pan. Season the chicken with chili powder, paprika, salt, and pepper. Cook the chicken for about 5-7 minutes, or until it is browned and fully cooked.

2. Next, divide the cooked chicken evenly between two bowls. On top of each bowl, add a cup of fresh spinach leaves for a refreshing touch. Then, spoon a tablespoon of sour cream over the spinach, followed by a tablespoon of sliced jalapeños to add some heat and flavor.

3. Enjoy your delicious and flavorful chicken bowls with a delightful combination of ingredients!

KETO BREAKFAST SANDWICH

Nutrition: Cal 603;Fat 54 g;Carb 4 g;Protein 22 g
Serving 2; Cook time 35 min

Ingredients
- •4 sausage patties
- •2 egg
- •2 tbsp cream cheese
- •4 tbsp sharp cheddar
- •1/2 medium avocado, sliced
- •1/2–1 tsp sriracha (to taste)
- •Salt, pepper to taste

Instructions
1. In a skillet over medium heat, cook the sausages according to the package instructions. Once cooked, set them aside.

2. In a small bowl, place cream cheese and sharp cheddar. Microwave for 20-30 seconds until the cheese is melted.

3. Mix the melted cheese with sriracha sauce, and set it aside.

4. In another bowl, beat the egg and season it with your preferred seasoning. Cook a small omelette using the beaten egg.
5. Fill the omelette with the cheese sriracha mixture, and assemble it into a sandwich using the cooked sausages.

POACHED EGGS MYTILENE

Nutrition: Cal 275;Fat 23 g;Carb 6 g;Protein 13 g
Serving 1; Cook time 20 min

Ingredients

- 4 sausage patties
- 2 egg
- 2 tbsp cream cheese
- 4 tbsp sharp cheddar
- 1/2 medium avocado, sliced
- 1/2−1 tsp sriracha (to taste)
- Salt, pepper to taste

Instructions

1. In a skillet over medium heat, cook the sausages according to the package instructions. Once cooked, set them aside.
2. In a small serving bowl, combine lemon juice and oil. Whisk them together until well combined.
3. In a medium sauté pan or small saucepan, add water and vinegar and bring it to a slow boil. Crack one egg into a small bowl, being careful not to break the yolk. Gently slip the egg into the simmering water, holding the bowl just above the surface of the water. Repeat this step with the remaining egg.
4. Cook the eggs until the whites are firm and the yolks are lightly cooked on the outside but still liquid inside, which usually takes about 2 to 3 minutes. Use a slotted spoon to remove the eggs from the water and place them into a serving bowl.
5. Break the yolks with a fork and drizzle them with the lemon juice mixture. Stir the yolks twice, and season them with salt and pepper.

HEALTHY BREAKFAST CHEESECAKE

Nutrition: Cal 152;Fat 12 g;Carb 3 g;Protein 6 g
Serving 1; Cook time 1 hour 5 min

Ingredients

- Crust Ingredients:
- 2 cups whole almonds
- 2 tablespoon Joy Filled Eats Sweetener (or see alternatives in recipe notes)
- 4 tablespoon salted butter

FILLING INGREDIENTS:

- 16 oz 4% fat cottage cheese
- 8 oz cream cheese
- 6 eggs
- ¾ cup Joy Filled Eats Sweetener (or see alternatives in recipe notes)
- ½ teaspoon almond extract
- ½ teaspoon vanilla extract

TOPPING WHEN SERVING:

- ¼ cup frozen mixed berries per cheesecake thawed

Instructions

1. Preheat the oven to 350 degrees Fahrenheit. In a large food processor, pulse the almonds, 2 tablespoons of sweetener, and 4 tablespoons of butter until a coarse dough forms. Grease two twelve-hole standard silicone muffin pans or line metal tins with paper or foil cupcake liners. If using silicone muffin pans, the cheesecakes will pop out easily. Divide the dough between the 24 holes and press it into the bottom to form a crust. Bake for 8 minutes.
2. While the crust is baking, combine the Friendship Dairies 4% cottage cheese and cream cheese in the food processor (no need to wash the bowl). Pulse the cheeses until smooth. Add the sweetener and extracts. Mix until well combined.
3. Add the eggs to the mixture and blend until smooth, scraping down the sides of the bowl as needed. Divide the batter between the muffin cups.
4. Bake for 30-40 minutes, or until the centers of the cheesecakes no longer jiggle when the pan is lightly shaken. Allow them to cool completely. If you did not use paper or foil liners, refrigerate for at least 2 hours before attempting to remove them from the pan. Serve with thawed frozen berries.

BLUEBERRY PANCAKES

Nutrition: Cal 202;Fat 16 g;Carb 9 g;Protein 10 g
Serving 3; Cook time 10 min

Ingredients

- 2 eggs
- 2/3 cup almond flour
- 1 tsp baking powder
- 1/2 tsp vanilla
- 1 tsp Swerve sweetener
- 3 tbsp milk or almond milk
- 1/4 cup blueberries
- Keto pancake syrup for serving, optional

Instructions

1. In a bowl, whisk together the eggs. Add vanilla, Swerve, and milk, and mix until combined. Add almond flour and baking powder, and mix until well combined. Stir in the blueberries.
2. Spray a non-stick frying pan or pancake griddle with a non-stick cooking spray and heat it over medium-high heat. Using a ladle, pour the pancake batter onto the frying pan, making 6 small pancakes.
3. Cook the pancakes for 3-4 minutes, or until the bottom is golden-brown and bubbles begin to form on top of the pancakes. Then, carefully flip the pancakes over with a spatula and cook for another 2 minutes, or until the other side is golden-brown.

LOW CARB PUMPKIN CHEESECAKE PANCAKES

Nutrition: Cal 202;Fat 16 g;Carb 9 g;Protein 10 g
Serving 16; Cook time 10 min

Ingredients

- 4 ounces Cream Cheese
- 4 large Eggs
- 2 Tablespoons Pure Pumpkin Puree
- 1 teaspoon Pure Vanilla Extract
- 1 teaspoon Pyure Sugar Substitute (or your choice)
- 1/2 teaspoon Baking Powder
- 1/4 teaspoon Pumpkin Pie Spice
- 1/8 teaspoon Ground Cinnamon
- 2 teaspoons Butter

Instructions

1. Place all the ingredients, except for the butter, in a blender and process until smooth. Let the mixture sit while you heat the skillet.
2. Heat a cast iron skillet or griddle over medium heat until hot. Add 1 teaspoon of butter to the skillet and let it melt.
3. Slowly pour the pancake batter into the skillet to make 3-inch pancakes. When bubbles start to form on the surface, flip the pancakes. Continue cooking until all the batter has been used. Use the second teaspoon of butter, halfway through, to grease the pan.
4. Serve the pancakes with butter and maple syrup.

TURKISH-STYLE BREAKFAST RECIPE

Nutrition: Cal 359;Fat 27 g;Carb 7 g;Protein 17 g
Serving 4; Cook time 25 min

Ingredients

- 4 eggs
- 250g halloumi, sliced thickly into 8 pieces
- 250g yogurt
- 400g tomatoes, roughly chopped
- 400g cucumber, sliced

For The Zhoug:

- 1 bunch parsley
- ½ bunch coriander
- 2 green chillies
- 2 cloves garlic
- 200ml olive oil
- Pinch of sugar
- ½ tsp ground cumin
- ¼ tsp cardamom

Instructions

1. To prepare the zhoug, blend all the ingredients in a food processor until finely chopped, adding water to achieve a loose pesto-like consistency. Season the zhoug to taste.
2. Place a pan of water on the stove and bring it to a rolling boil. Carefully add the eggs and cook for 6 minutes for soft-boiled eggs. Immediately transfer the eggs to a bowl of cold water and peel them.
3. Heat a griddle pan over high heat. Add the halloumi and cook on each side for 2 minutes, until golden and slightly charred.
4. Swirl the zhoug into the yogurt and spoon it onto plates. Top with the tomatoes, cucumber, and halloumi.

POACHED EGG AND BACON SALAD

Nutrition: Cal 311;Fat 22 g;Carb 12 g;Protein 15 g
Serving 2; Cook time 20 min

Ingredients

- 100g (3½oz) unsmoked bacon lardons
- 1 slice bread, cut into small cubes
- 2 medium or large eggs
- 2 good handfuls of mixed salad leaves (we used rocket and chard)
- 10 baby plum tomatoes, halved
- 1 stick celery, chopped
- **For The Dressing:**
- 1tbsp olive oil
- 1tsp white wine vinegar
- ½tsp Dijon mustard
- Salt and ground black pepper

Instructions

1. Heat a frying pan over medium heat. Add the bacon and fry until golden and crispy. Remove the bacon from the pan using a slotted spoon and set it aside. In the same pan, add the bread cubes and fry them in the bacon fat until they are browned and crispy.
2. While the bread is frying, prepare the poached eggs. Fill a small pan with boiling water, about 10cm (4in) deep, and place it over high heat. Add a dash of white wine vinegar. Once the water comes to a boil again, carefully crack an egg into the pan.
3. As the water returns to a gentle boil, use a slotted spoon to gather the egg whites around the yolk. Reduce the heat and let the egg simmer for about a minute for a soft poached egg, or longer for a firmer one.
4. Lift the poached egg out of the pan using the slotted spoon and place it in a bowl of warm water if you're cooking more than one or two eggs. Repeat the process with another egg in the pan. Here's a video on how to poach an egg if you need visual guidance.
5. Prepare the dressing by mixing together the ingredients. On two plates, arrange a generous handful of salad leaves. Divide the bacon, croutons, tomatoes, and celery between the plates. Place the drained poached eggs on top, drizzle the salad with the dressing, and sprinkle with salt and pepper.

SPINACH PANCAKES

Nutrition: Cal 186;Fat 15 g;Carb 5 g;Protein 7 g
Serving 4; Cook time 15 min

Ingredients
For The Batter:

- 30 g or ⅓ cup gram (chickpea) flour
- 85 ml/⅓ cup water
- A pinch of sea salt
- 1 garlic clove
- 2 handfuls of spinach
- 2 tbsp olive oil
- 1 tbsp no-taste coconut oil or unrefined rapeseed oil

For The Filling:

- 50 g Parmesan cheese, grated
- ½ avocado, sliced lengthways
- 1 tbsp chopped chives
- Chopped chillies (if liked)

Instructions

1. In a blender, combine all of the batter ingredients and blend until smooth. Heat coconut oil or rapeseed oil in a frying pan.
2. Pour a thin layer of the batter mixture into the pan. Top with most of the avocado slices, chives, and grated cheese, reserving some for garnishing later.
3. Cook for a few minutes until the edges start to loosen. Use a spatula to flip the pancake over.
4. Sprinkle the remaining cheese, chives, and avocado slices on top of the pancake, and add a few slices of red chili if desired, for an extra kick.

PECAN & COCONUT ' N ' OATMEAL

Nutrition: Cal 312;Fat 25 g;Carb 7 g;Protein 14 g
Serving 1; Cook time 10 min

Ingredients

- ½ cup coconut or almond milk
- 2 teaspoons chia seeds
- 2 tablespoons almond flour
- 1 tablespoon flax meal
- 2 tablespoons hemp hearts
- ¼ teaspoon ground cinnamon
- ¼ teaspoon pure vanilla extract
- 1 tablespoon pecans, toasted and chopped
- 1 tablespoon coconut flakes

Instructions

1. In a small pot, combine the milk, chia seeds, almond flour, flax meal, hemp hearts, cinnamon, and vanilla. Cook the mixture over low heat, stirring constantly, until it thickens. This usually takes about 5 minutes.

2. Once the mixture has thickened, spoon it into a bowl. Top it with pecans and coconut flakes for added flavor and texture. You can enjoy it immediately while it's still warm and creamy.
3. Sit back, relax, and savor the delicious and nutritious chia seed pudding with the delightful crunch of pecans and coconut flakes.

CHEDDAR CHIVE BAKED AVOCADO EGGS

Nutrition: Cal 257;Fat 22 g;Carb 2 g;Protein 13 g
Serving 2; Cook time 15 min

Ingredients

- 2 eggs
- 2 ounces cheddar cheese, shredded
- 2 teaspoons heavy cream
- 1 teaspoon fresh chopped chives
- Sea salt and freshly ground black pepper to taste
- 1 avocado, cut in half and pitted

Instructions

1. Preheat your oven to 425°F (220°C).
2. In a medium bowl, combine the eggs, cheddar cheese, cream, half of the chives, salt, and pepper. Use a fork to beat the mixture until well mixed.
3. Arrange the avocados in a small rimmed baking dish, cut side up, ensuring they fit snugly to prevent rolling. Pour the egg filling into the center of each avocado half.
4. Bake for 12 minutes or until the filling is lightly golden on top. Remove from the oven and serve hot, garnished with the remaining chives.

KETO EGG ROLL IN A BOWL

Nutrition: Cal 346 Fat 7 g;Carb 8 g;Protein 22 g
Serving 6; Cook time 25 min

Ingredients

- 1 pound ground pork
- Salt and pepper, to taste
- 2 cloves garlic, finely minced
- 1 tablespoon ginger paste (or 1 teaspoon ground ginger)
- 6 ounces coleslaw mix
- 6 ounces broccoli slaw (or more coleslaw mix)
- ⅓ cup soy sauce
- 1 tablespoon garlic chili sauce, optional

- 1 tablespoon toasted sesame seeds, for garnish, optional
- 2 tablespoons toasted sesame oil
- 2 scallions, sliced on the bias or chopped, optional

Instructions

1. Heat a large skillet over medium heat and add the ground pork. Cook the pork until fully cooked and no pink remains, usually about 7-10 minutes. Use a spatula to break the meat into small pieces. If there is excess grease, drain it. Next, add the garlic, ginger, and a light sprinkle of salt and pepper to the skillet.
2. Add the coleslaw mix to the cooked pork. If needed, switch to a larger pan at this point. The cabbage will cook down, so in a few minutes, it will fit better in the pan. Cook the cabbage until it begins to soften and becomes translucent.
3. Incorporate the broccoli slaw into the pan. If you're using shredded cabbage instead, add it now. Continue cooking the vegetables for about 5-7 minutes until they are softened but still retain some texture.
4. Pour the soy sauce into the mixture and gently stir. This is also the time to adjust the seasoning with additional salt and pepper to your preferred taste.
5. Optional: Add the chili sauce to the skillet and stir to combine. The dish should come together and the meat and vegetables should be well mixed. If you prefer a bit of crunch, you can slightly undercook the vegetables.
6. Garnish the dish with toasted sesame seeds, a drizzle of sesame oil, and green onions. Serve the stir-fry warm and store any leftovers in the refrigerator for up to 3 days for the best taste.

KETO PIGS IN A BLANKET

Nutrition: Cal 333;Fat 26 g;Carb 7 g;Protein 17 g
Serving 4; Cook time 30 min

Ingredients

- 1 cup shredded mozzarella cheese
- ½ cup blanched, finely ground almond flour
- 1 ounce cream cheese
- ½ teaspoon baking soda
- 1 egg yolk
- 4 beef hot dogs
- ½ teaspoon sesame seeds or everything bagel seasoning (optional)
- Ketchup or Mustard for dipping (optional)

Instructions

1. Preheat the oven to 400°F (200°C) and line a medium-sized baking sheet with parchment paper.
2. In a large microwave-safe bowl, combine the mozzarella and almond flour. Break the cream cheese into small pieces and add them to the bowl. Microwave for 30 to 45 seconds, or until the cheese is melted.
3. Stir the mixture with a fork until a soft ball of dough forms. Sprinkle the dough with baking soda and add the egg yolk. Break the yolk with a fork and stir it into the dough until a smooth ball forms.
4. Lay a piece of parchment paper on a flat work surface. Wet your hands with a bit of water and flatten the dough to about 3 x 4 inches and about 1/2 inch thick.
5. Use a knife to cut the dough into four even pieces. Pat the hot dogs with a paper towel to remove surface moisture, and gently wrap a piece of dough around each, leaving the ends exposed and pinching at the seam to close. The dough will expand a bit during baking, so try to wrap each as closely as possible without breaking the dough.
6. Place all the wrapped hot dogs on the baking sheet and sprinkle with sesame seeds. Bake for 18-20 minutes until the dough turns golden and firm. Remove from the oven and allow to cool for at least 10 minutes; otherwise, the dough may fall apart.
7. Serve with your favorite dipping sauces, such as mustard or ketchup.

KETO MEAL PREP BREAKFAST BOMBS

Nutrition: Cal 333;Fat 26 g;Carb 7 g;Protein 17 g
Serving 4; Cook time 30 min

Ingredients
- 2 Cups Blanched Finely Ground Almond Flour
- 2 Teaspoons Baking Powder
- ¼ Teaspoon Baking Soda
- 4 Tablespoons Cold Butter, Cubed
- ⅓ Cup Sour Cream
- 1 Large Egg
- ½ Teaspoon Apple Cider Vinegar
- Pinch of Salt
- 6 Ounces of Cooked Breakfast Sausage, crumbled
- 6 Large Eggs, Scrambled
- 4 Slices Cooked Bacon, Crumbled
- ½ Cup Shredded Cheddar Cheese

- Sugar-Free Syrup (Optional)

Instructions
1. Preheat the oven to 350 degrees Fahrenheit (175 degrees Celsius).
2. In a food processor, combine almond flour, baking powder, and baking soda. Pulse a few times to combine.
3. Add the butter to the food processor and process on low for 20 seconds or until large crumbs form.
4. While still processing on low, add sour cream, egg, and apple cider vinegar. Sprinkle in a bit of salt to taste.
5. Turn off the food processor and let the mixture sit for 5 minutes.
6. In a large bowl, toss the sausage, eggs, bacon, and cheese. Scoop the biscuit mixture into the large bowl and gently toss to combine with the other ingredients. You can use your hands for better mixing.
7. Spray a muffin tin with non-stick spray, then scoop about 1/4 cup of the mixture into each section.
8. Bake for 12-15 minutes or until golden brown around the edges. Let cool for at least 15 minutes before serving.
9. Store the biscuit muffins in an airtight container in the fridge for up to 4 days for the best taste. To reheat, microwave for 20-30 seconds.

KETO CAULIFLOWER BUNS

Nutrition: Cal 150 Fat 10 g;Carb 6 g;Protein 10 g
Serving 8; Cook time 30 min

Ingredients
- 12 Ounces Cauliflower
- ½ Cup Mozzarella Cheese, shredded
- ¼ cup Cheddar Cheese, shredded
- ¼ cup Almond Flour
- 1 Egg

Instructions
1. Preheat the oven to 400°F (200°C).
2. Cook the cauliflower using your preferred method. Allow it to cool, and then wring out any excess moisture using a cheesecloth or kitchen towel.
3. In a food processor, combine the cooked cauliflower with all the other ingredients. Pulse until well combined, about 30-45 seconds. Make sure to scrape down the sides to ensure the entire mixture is combined.

4. Scoop the mixture onto a parchment-lined baking sheet in 1/4 cup measurements. Shape and flatten the mixture to form buns.
5. Bake for 12-15 minutes or until the tops of the buns begin to lightly brown.
6. Remove from the oven and allow the buns to cool before using them.

KETO THREE CHEESE CAULIFLOWER MAC AND CHEESE CUPS

Nutrition: Cal 391 Fat 29 g;Carb 7 g;Protein 24 g
Serving 4; Cook time 35 min

Ingredients
- 1 medium head fresh cauliflower
- 2 tablespoons salted butter
- 2 tablespoons diced onion
- 2 cloves garlic, minced
- 2 ounces cream cheese, softened
- ¼ cup heavy whipping cream
- ½ teaspoon Italian seasoning of choice
- Salt and Pepper, to taste
- ¼ teaspoon xanthan gum
- 1 cup spinach, sliced into strips
- ¾ cup white cheddar, shredded
- ¼ cup mozzarella, shredded
- 12 slices prosciutto
- 6 tablespoons Parmesan cheese, shredded

Instructions
1. Preheat oven to 400 degrees.
2. Add a couple cups of water to a large pot, place steamer basket into pot above water, and bring to boil. While the water is heating, prepare cauliflower.
3. Remove core and leaves from cauliflower. Chop into bite-size pieces. When water is boiling, carefully add cauliflower to steamer basket. Cover and let steam for 5-7 minutes or until fork tender.
4. Prepare sauce while cauliflower is steaming. When finished, turn off heat and set aside until ready to add to sauce.

SAUCE
1. In skillet over medium-low heat melt butter. Add onion and cook for 2-4 minutes until onion is tender and becoming translucent.
2. Add garlic and softened cream cheese. Softened cream cheese will be easier to smooth into sauce. Using wooden spoon or rubber spatula, press cream cheese flat into pan to help smooth as it warms and gently stir.
3. Pour in heavy whipping cream, seasoning, and xanthan gum. Stir ingredients until smooth, raising temperature slightly if needed to get sauce fully mixed.
4. Add spinach, white cheddar, mozzarella to sauce and turn off heat. Continue stirring for a few minutes, until spinach begins to wilt and cheeses are fully melted and smooth.
5. Add steamed cauliflower to pan and fold into cheese sauce. I did not remove any moisture from mine. (See notes section)
6. Using large muffin tin (1 cup capacity) place two slices of prosciutto in X to cover the bottom of the tin and stretch up around the sides as much as possible. It may rip a little, that's ok. Just be sure the bottom is covered.
7. Place ½ cup of cheesy cauliflower mixture into prosciutto cups and top with 1 tablespoon of Parmesan.
8. Bake for 15-20 minutes or until bubbly and brown. Serve warm.

KETO YOGURT PARFAIT

Nutrition: Cal 335;Fat 29 g;Carb 10 g;Protein 11 g
Serving 2; Cook time 10 min

Ingredients
- ½ cup Greek Yogurt full fat
- ¼ cup Heavy Cream
- 1 teaspoon Vanilla Essence
- ½ cup Keto Chocolate Almond Clusters
- 2 Strawberries diced
- 8 Blueberries

Instructions
1. In a mixing bowl, combine the yogurt, cream, and vanilla. Whisk together until thick and smooth.
2. Spoon half of the yogurt mixture into two glasses, then sprinkle half of the granola on top.
3. Add the remaining yogurt mixture to the glasses, followed by the remaining granola.
4. Top with berries of your choice.
5. Enjoy your delicious yogurt parfait.

KETO HOT POCKET

Nutrition: Cal 283;Fat 12 g;Carb 1 g;Protein 14 g
Serving 6; Cook time 10 min

Ingredients

- 3 eggs, separated
- 2 TBS unflavored egg white
- 3 ounces cream cheese, warmed (or reserved yolks if dairy free)
- 1/2 tsp onion powder (optional)

FILLING:

- 6 egg, scrambled
- 6 slices bacon, cooked (or ham)
- 6 (1 ounce) slices cheddar cheese

Instructions

1. To start, separate the eggs, placing the egg whites in a mixing bowl. Whip the egg whites until they form stiff peaks. Gradually fold in the whey protein and, if desired, onion powder.
2. Carefully fold in the cream cheese into the whipped egg whites, making sure not to deflate them. Thoroughly grease a cookie sheet and spoon the mixture onto the sheet, forming six large mounds.
3. Top each mound with scrambled eggs, cheese, and chopped ham or bacon. Cover them with additional egg white batter and smooth it out with a spatula. Bake at 375 degrees Fahrenheit for approximately 25 minutes, or until the mixture is lightly browned.
4. Once done, indulge in the delicious flavors of your fluffy and protein-packed breakfast creation.

KETO BREAKFAST CHILI

Nutrition: Cal 634;Fat 38 g;Carb 15 g;Protein 16 g
Serving 8; Cook time 2 hours 20 min

Ingredients

- 2 pounds ground grass fed beef
- 1 pound ground chorizo or Italian sausage
- 4 cups tomato sauce (preferably homemade organic or from a glass jar)
- 1/2 yellow onion, chopped
- 3 stalks celery, chopped
- 1 green bell pepper, seeded and chopped
- 1 red bell pepper, seeded and chopped
- 2 green chile peppers, seeded and chopped
- 2 slices bacon
- 1 cup organic beef broth (homemade broth is best: I always store extra in my freezer)
- 1/4 cup chili powder
- 1 TBS minced garlic
- 3 TBS fresh oregano
- 2 tsp ground cumin
- 3 TBS fresh basil
- 1 tsp Celtic sea salt
- 1 tsp ground black pepper
- 1 tsp cayenne pepper
- 1 tsp paprika

TOPPINGS:

- Fried Eggs
- Avocado, cubed into 1 cm chunks
- Bacon, fried and crumbled
- If desired, serve in a bread bowl:

BREAD BOWL:

- 3 eggs, separated
- 1/2 tsp cream of tartar
- 1/4 cup unflavored egg white or whey protein
- 3 oz organic sour cream or cream cheese (or yolks if dairy sensitive)

Instructions

1. To prepare this hearty and flavorful chili, start by heating a large stock pot over medium-high heat. Crumble the ground chuck, bacon, and sausage into the hot pan and cook until evenly browned. Remove any excess grease and pour in the tomato sauce. Add onion, celery, green and red bell peppers, chili peppers, and broth. Season with chili powder, garlic, oregano, cumin, basil, salt, pepper, cayenne, and paprika.
2. Stir the mixture to blend all the ingredients and simmer over low heat for at least 2 hours, stirring occasionally. For even richer flavors, you can simmer it for a longer time. Adjust the salt, pepper, and chili powder if necessary. Remove from heat and serve immediately or refrigerate for later. To enhance the taste and nutrition, top the chili with a fried egg, avocado, and bacon pieces.
3. For the bread bowl, preheat the oven to 350 degrees Fahrenheit. Separate the eggs, keeping the yolks reserved. In a clean, dry bowl, whip the egg whites and cream of tartar until stiff peaks form. Mix in the protein powder until the mixture is smooth. Carefully fold in the cream cheese and sour cream, or yolks if sensitive to dairy, using a spatula to prevent the whites from breaking down.
4. Grease muffin tins and spoon the mixture into the pan, creating 12 medium bowls or 24 mini bowls with a dip in the center. Bake at 350

degrees for 12-15 minutes. Once they come out of the oven, you may need to push down the center to create space for the chili filling.

BIG MAC BREAKFAST PIE

Nutrition: Cal 387;Fat 33 g;Carb 3 g;Protein 20 g
Serving 8; Cook time 41 min

Ingredients
- 1 pound ground beef
- ½ cup chopped onions
- 1 clove garlic, minced
- 2 teaspoons Redmond Real salt, divided (use code Maria15 for 15% off
- ¼ cup Primal Kitchen Ketchup (or tomato sauce)
- 8 large eggs, beaten
- ¾ cup shredded cheddar cheese (about 3 ounces)
- 2 tablespoons Primal Kitchen mayo
- 2 teaspoons yellow mustard
- ¼ teaspoon black pepper
- Garnish:
- 2 tablespoons Toasted sesame seeds, for garnish
- 12 slices dill pickles, for garnish
- 6 Cherry tomatoes, halved

SPECIAL SAUCE:
- ½ cup Primal Kitchen mayonnaise
- ¼ cup chopped dill pickles
- 3 tablespoons Primal Kitchen Ketchup
- 2 tablespoons Swerve (or ½ teaspoon stevia glycerite or a few drops liquid stevia)
- ⅛ teaspoon fine sea salt
- ⅛ teaspoon fish sauce (optional, for umami flavor)

Instructions
1. To make this dish, preheat the oven to 350°F. In a large oven-safe skillet over medium heat, cook ground beef, onions, and garlic. Season with 1½ teaspoons of salt. Cook, crumpling the beef with a wooden spoon, until the beef is fully cooked and the onions are translucent, approximately 7 minutes. Stir in the tomato sauce and mix well.
2. In a large bowl, combine the eggs, cheese, mayo, mustard, ½ teaspoon of salt, and pepper. Add the beef mixture to the egg mixture and stir to combine. Pour the mixture into a greased casserole dish. Spray the top with Primal Kitchen Avocado Oil Spray.

3. Place the dish in the oven and bake for 25 minutes, or until the eggs are cooked through in the center. Remove from the oven and let it rest for 10 minutes. Then, slice and serve. If desired, garnish with fresh sesame seeds and pickles, and serve with secret sauce.
4. Store any leftovers in an airtight container in the fridge for up to 3 days. To reheat, either place in a preheated 350°F oven for 3 minutes or microwave for 30 seconds, or until heated through.

CREAM OF WHEAT CEREAL

Nutrition: Cal 172;Fat 5 g;Carb 17 g;Protein 15 g
Serving 2; Cook time 10 min

Ingredients
- ¾ cup of warm unsweetened vanilla or chocolate almond milk (or coconut milk)
- 1-2 tsp psyllium husk
- 1 scoop vanilla or chocolate (egg white or whey) protein powder
- 1 TBS vanilla extract
- 1 drop of stevia glycerite
- ½ tsp of nutmeg
- ½ tsp cinnamon
- Optional: you can add some coconut flakes, nuts or peanut butter to this recipe.

Instructions
1. In a bowl, combine warm milk, whey protein, stevia, cinnamon, nutmeg, and any other desired toppings.
2. Stir the mixture well to ensure all the ingredients are thoroughly combined. Allow the mixture to sit for a few minutes until it thickens to a consistency similar to oatmeal.

GREEN EGGS AND HAM: AVOCADO HOLLANDAISE

Nutrition: Cal 351;Fat 28 g;Carb 4 g;Protein 21 g
Serving 4; Cook time 10 min

Ingredients
- 1 ripe medium avocado, peeled and chopped
- 2 egg yolks
- 1 TBS fresh lime or lemon juice
- 2 TBS MCT oil, heated (or bacon fat, heated)
- ½ tsp Celtic sea salt
- ¼ tsp cayenne pepper (if desired)
- 8 poached eggs
- 8 thin slices of ham or Canadian bacon

•4 Protein Buns
Instructions

1. To make Avocado Hollandaise, begin by placing the avocado, yolks, and lime juice in a blender and puree until smooth and fluffy. This process should take about 2 minutes.
2. While the blender is running, slowly drizzle in the very hot oil and continue to puree until everything is well combined.
3. Once everything is blended, season with salt. If you like a little heat, you can also add cayenne pepper.
4. To serve, spoon the Hollandaise over poached eggs, ham, and a toasted Protein bun. Enjoy your delicious and healthy Green Eggs and Ham!

DUTCH BABY

Nutrition: Cal 251;Fat 20 g;Carb 2 g;Protein 16 g
Serving 2; Cook time 25 min

Ingredients

•3 large eggs
•¾ cup unsweetened cashew/almond milk (hemp milk if nut free)
•¼ cup unflavored egg white protein powder
•1 tsp baking powder
•1 tsp Redmond Real salt
•2 TBS coconut oil (or butter if not dairy sensitive)
•2 tablespoons chopped dill (or other herbs)
•8 sprigs asparagus
•Parmesan cheese (Nutritional Yeast if dairy free)

Instructions

1. To make a delicious and healthy pancake, you will need an 8-inch cast iron skillet and an oven preheated to 425 degrees F (400 degrees F in convection ovens). The first step is to ensure the skillet preheats and gets very hot.
2. In a blender, combine the eggs, almond milk, protein powder, baking powder, and salt. Blend for about 1 minute or until foamy.
3. Using an oven mitt, remove the skillet from the oven and place the coconut oil into the skillet. Swirl the skillet to coat the inside of the skillet. Next, pour the batter into the skillet. Arrange asparagus on top of the batter (they may fall into the batter which is fine). Sprinkle with Parmesan or Nutritional Yeast.
4. Bake for about 18-20 minutes or until the pancake is puffed and golden brown. When it's done, remove the pancake from the oven, spread additional butter or coconut oil on the pancake, cut it into wedges, and enjoy!

CARNIVORE QUICHE

Nutrition: Cal 421;Fat 30 g;Carb 2 g;Protein 34 g
Serving 8; Cook time 65 min

Ingredients
CRUST:

•1 ¼ cups powdered pork rinds
•1 ¼ cups freshly grated Parmesan (or hard Gouda) cheese
•1 egg, beaten

FILLING:

•½ cup chicken or beef bone broth
•1 cup grated Swiss cheese (or Muenster cheese)
•4 oz cream cheese
•1 tablespoon butter, melted
•½ cup diced ham
•4 eggs, beaten
•½ tsp Redmond Real salt

Instructions

1. To prepare a pork rind crust quiche, preheat the oven to 325 degrees F. Begin by making the tart shell. Combine the pork rinds and cheese in a bowl and mix well. Add an egg and mix until the dough is stiff and well combined. If necessary, add more powdered pork rinds. Press the pie crust into a 9-inch pie dish and bake it for 12 minutes or until it begins to lightly brown.
2. To make the filling, take a medium-sized bowl and combine broth, Swiss cheese, butter, and cream cheese. Stir well to combine. Add in the ham, eggs, and salt. Pour the mixture into the pre-baked crust.
3. Bake the quiche in the oven or air fryer for 15 minutes. Then, reduce the heat to 300 degrees F (150 degrees C) and bake for an additional 30 minutes, or until a knife inserted 1 inch from the edge comes out clean. You may have to cover the edges with foil to prevent over-browning.
4. Once the quiche is done, allow it to sit for 10 minutes before cutting into wedges. This will allow the quiche to set properly and make it easier to cut. Serve and enjoy your delicious pork rind crust quiche!

HUEVOS RANCHEROS WITH A PROTEIN-SPARING TWIST

Nutrition: Cal 436;Fat 24 g;Carb 8 g;Protein 45 g
Serving 2; Соок time 20 min

Ingredients
TORTILLAS:
- 1 tablespoon Coconut oil/ghee/butter (for frying)
- 3 egg, separated
- 2 TBS unflavored egg white protein
- 1 tsp onion powder
- Optional: 1 tsp Mexican spices

TOPPING:
- ½ cup 85% lean ground beef (OR my Chili Recipe), browned
- 4 Fried Eggs
- ½ sliced Avocado
- ½ cup Salsa
- 1 whole Green Onions, sliced

Instructions
1. In a bowl, use an electric hand mixer or stand mixer to whisk the egg whites until they form stiff peaks. Make sure no egg yolks are included in the mixture as it may affect the outcome of the recipe.
2. Gradually add the unflavored protein powder and seasonings to the whipped egg whites, mixing slowly until everything is well combined.
3. Heat a small skillet over medium-high heat with oil.
4. Take the tortilla dough and fry them one at a time in the skillet, cooking until they are firm but not crispy. Once cooked, remove the tortillas onto paper towels to eliminate excess oil.
5. While the tortillas fry, prepare the beef and any other desired toppings.
6. Once the tortillas are done, proceed to cook eggs over easy in the same skillet.
7. To assemble the dish, place the tortillas on plates and top them with a layer of meat.
8. Add your preferred toppings such as chili, crumbled bacon, avocado, fried egg, and salsa to complete the dish.

PROTEIN SPARING PANCAKES

Nutrition: Cal 62;Fat 2 g;Carb 1 g;Protein 12 g
Serving 2; Соок time 7 min

Ingredients
- 3 egg whites
- 1 tablespoon Further Food gelatin
- ¼ teaspoon Redmond Real Salt
- 2 tablespoons Further Food vanilla collagen
- 1 teaspoon vanilla extract (or other extract: almond, coconut, maple)
- Avocado Oil Spray

GARNISH:
- Cinnamon and Swerve confectioners, if desired

Instructions
1. To make the Protein Sparing pancakes, separate the eggs (save the yolks for a different recipe). Place the whites in a clean, dry, cool bowl. Add the gelatin and salt and whip on high for a few minutes until very stiff.
2. Gently fold in the Further Food collagen, and extract.
3. Heat a non-stick pan to medium high heat. Spray with avocado oil spray and place a circle of dough on the pan. Fry until golden brown, about 1 minute. Flip and соок another minute or until golden. Remove from heat and place on a plate.
5. Sprinkle the protein sparing pancakes with cinnamon and Swerve confectioners or кeto pancake syrup if desired. Enjoy!

POULTRY

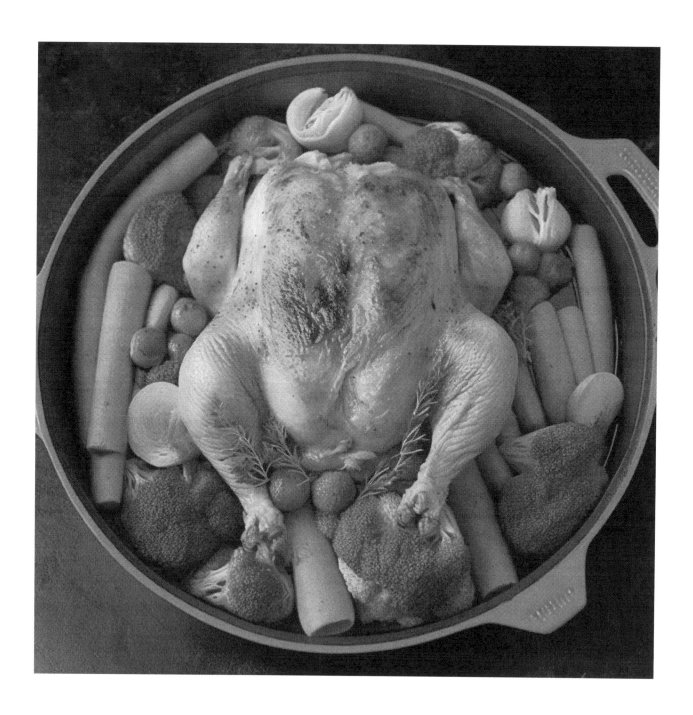

PAPRIKA CHICKEN

Nutrition: Cal 390;Fat 30 g; Carb 4 g;Protein 25 g
Serving 4; Cook time 35 min

Ingredients

- 4 (4-ounce) chicken breasts, skin-on
- Sea salt
- Freshly ground black pepper
- 1 tablespoon olive oil
- ½ cup chopped sweet onion
- ½ cup heavy (whipping) cream
- 2 teaspoons smoked paprika
- ½ cup sour cream
- 2 tablespoons chopped fresh Parsley

Instructions

1. Season the chicken lightly with salt and pepper.
2. Place a large skillet over medium-high heat and add the olive oil.
3. Sear the chicken on both sides until almost cooked through, approximately 15 minutes in total. Remove the chicken to a plate.
4. Add the onion to the skillet and sauté until tender, about 4 minutes.
5. Stir in the cream and paprika, bringing the liquid to a simmer.
6. Return the chicken and any accumulated juices to the skillet and simmer for 5 minutes until completely cooked.
7. Stir in the sour cream and remove the skillet from the heat.
8. Serve the dish topped with parsley.

STUFFED CHICKEN BREASTS

Nutrition: Cal 390;Fat 30 g; Carb 3 g;Protein 25 g
Serving 4; Cook time 30 min

Ingredients

- 1 tablespoon butter
- ¼ cup chopped sweet onion
- ½ cup goat cheese, at room temperature
- ¼ cup Kalamata olives, chopped
- ¼ cup chopped roasted red pepper
- 2 tablespoons chopped fresh basil
- 4 (5-ounce) chicken breasts, skin-on
- 2 tablespoons extra-virgin olive oil

Instructions

1. Preheat the oven to 400°F.
2. In a small skillet over medium heat, melt the butter and add the onion. Sauté until tender, approximately 3 minutes.

3. Transfer the onion to a medium bowl and add the cheese, olives, red pepper, and basil. Stir until well blended, then refrigerate for about 30 minutes.
4. Cut horizontal pockets into each chicken breast and stuff them evenly with the filling. Secure the two sides of each breast with toothpicks.
5. Place a large ovenproof skillet over medium-high heat and add the olive oil.
6. Brown the chicken on both sides, about 10 minutes in total.

Place the skillet in the oven and roast until the chicken is just cooked through, about 15 minutes. Remove the toothpicks and serve.

BACON-WRAPPED CHICKEN WITH SHRIMP

Nutrition: Cal 625;Fat 47 g; Carb 11 g;Protein 42 g
Serving 2; Cook time 25 min

Ingredients

- 2 chicken fillets (about 8 oz each)
- 4 slices of bacon
- 8 medium-sized shrimp, peeled and deveined
- 1 avocado, diced
- 1/4 cup cherry tomatoes, halved
- 1/4 cup red onion, diced
- 2 tbsp olive oil
- 1 tbsp lemon juice
- 1/2 tsp garlic powder
- 1/2 tsp salt
- 1/4 tsp black pepper

Instructions

1. Preheat the oven to 375°F.
2. Carefully make a pocket in the side of each chicken fillet, ensuring not to cut through the other side.
3. Season the chicken fillets with garlic powder, salt, and black pepper.
4. Stuff four shrimp into the pocket of each chicken fillet, pressing them down firmly.
5. Wrap each chicken fillet with two slices of bacon, tucking the ends of the bacon under the chicken to secure it.
6. Heat the olive oil in a large skillet over medium-high heat. Once hot, add the chicken fillets and cook for 2-3 minutes on each side or until the bacon is lightly browned.

7. Transfer the chicken fillets to a baking sheet and bake in the preheated oven for 15-20 minutes or until the chicken is cooked through and the bacon is crispy.

8. In a small bowl, whisk together the lemon juice, garlic powder, salt, and black pepper.

9. In a separate bowl, combine the diced avocado, cherry tomatoes, and red onion. Drizzle with the lemon dressing and toss gently to combine.

10. Serve the chicken fillets hot with the avocado salad on the side.

BACON-WRAPPED BLUE CHEESE CHICKEN

Nutrition: Cal 525;Fat 35 g; Carb 2 g;Protein 51 g
Serving 2; Cook time 25 min

Ingredients
- 2 chicken fillets (about 8 oz each)
- 4 slices of bacon
- 1/4 cup crumbled blue cheese
- 1/4 tsp garlic powder
- 1/4 tsp salt
- 1/8 tsp black pepper
- 1 tbsp olive oil

Instructions
1. Preheat the oven to 375°F.
2. Carefully create a pocket in the side of each chicken fillet, being cautious not to cut through the other side.
3. In a small bowl, combine the blue cheese, garlic powder, salt, and black pepper.
4. Stuff the blue cheese mixture into the pockets of each chicken fillet.
5. Wrap each chicken fillet with two slices of bacon, securing the ends of the bacon under the chicken.
6. Heat the olive oil in a large skillet over medium-high heat. Once hot, add the chicken fillets and cook for 2-3 minutes on each side or until the bacon is lightly browned.
7. Transfer the chicken fillets to a baking sheet and bake in the preheated oven for 15-20 minutes or until the chicken is cooked through and the bacon is crispy.
Allow the chicken to rest for a few minutes before serving.

GARLIC CHICKEN WITH ROASTED VEGETABLES

Nutrition: Cal 610;Fat 44 g; Carb 12 g;Protein 42 g
Serving 2; Cook time 45 min

Ingredients
- 2 chicken thighs, bone-in and skin-on (about 8 oz each)
- 2 small zucchinis, sliced
- 2 garlic cloves, minced
- 4 cherry tomatoes, halved
- 1/2 bell pepper, sliced
- 1 small carrot, peeled and sliced
- 2 tbsp olive oil
- 1 tsp dried oregano
- 1 tsp salt
- 1/2 tsp black pepper

Instructions
1. Preheat the oven to 375°F.
2. In a large bowl, combine the zucchini, garlic, cherry tomatoes, bell pepper, carrot, olive oil, dried oregano, salt, and black pepper. Toss to coat the vegetables evenly with the seasoning.
3. Spread the vegetables in a single layer on a baking sheet.
4. Place the chicken thighs on top of the vegetables, skin side up.
5. Bake in the preheated oven for 35-40 minutes or until the chicken is cooked through and the vegetables are roasted and tender.
6. Serve the garlic chicken hot with the roasted vegetables on the side.

CREAM CHEESE STUFFED CHICKEN

Nutrition: Cal 565;Fat 38 g; Carb 8 g;Protein 46 g
Serving 2; Cook time 30 min

Ingredients
- 2 chicken fillets (about 8 oz each)
- 2 oz cream cheese, softened
- 1/2 tsp garlic powder
- 1/2 tsp salt
- 1/4 tsp black pepper
- 8 asparagus spears, trimmed
- 1 small cucumber, sliced
- 2 tbsp olive oil
- 1 tbsp lemon juice
- 1/2 tsp Dijon mustard
- 1/4 tsp salt

•1/8 tsp black pepper

Instructions

1. Preheat the oven to 375°F.
2. Carefully make a pocket in the side of each chicken fillet without cutting through the other side.
3. In a small bowl, combine the cream cheese, garlic powder, salt, and black pepper.
4. Stuff the cream cheese mixture into the pockets of each chicken fillet.
5. Place the stuffed chicken fillets in a baking dish and bake in the preheated oven for 25-30 minutes or until the chicken is cooked through.
6. In another small bowl, whisk together the olive oil, lemon juice, Dijon mustard, salt, and black pepper to make the dressing for the salad.
7. Blanch the asparagus in boiling water for 2-3 minutes or until tender. Drain and set aside.
8. Arrange the sliced cucumbers and blanched asparagus on a plate and drizzle with the dressing. Serve the cream cheese stuffed chicken hot with the asparagus and cucumber salad on the side.

ONE PAN KETO CHEESY JALAPEÑO CHICKEN

Nutrition: Cal 425;Fat 26 g;Carb 5 g;Protein 40 g
Serving 4; Cook time 25 min

Ingredients

4 small chicken breast (this was about 1.5 pounds for me)
1 teaspoon cumin
1/2 teaspoon chili powder
1/2 teaspoon garlic powder
1/2 teaspoon salt
1/2 teaspoon pepper
1 tablespoon butter
1/2 cup chopped onion (half of one small onion)
2 jalapenos, seeded and diced
1 teaspoon minced garlic
1/4 cup heavy cream
1/3 cup chicken broth
2 ounces cream cheese
1 cup shredded cheddar cheese (divided)

Instructions

Combine the cumin, chili powder, garlic powder, salt, and pepper in a small bowl. Set the spice mixture aside.

Heat a 12-inch skillet over medium heat and either spray it with nonstick spray or add up to 1 tablespoon of olive oil.

Sprinkle each side of the chicken breast with the spice mixture, ensuring even coverage.

Sear the chicken in the skillet for 2-3 minutes on each side until nicely browned. Once browned, remove the chicken from the skillet and set it aside.

Add 1 tablespoon of butter to the skillet and then add the onion, jalapenos, and garlic. Sauté the mixture for 3-4 minutes, stirring occasionally.

Reduce the heat to low and add the cream, broth, and cream cheese to the skillet. Stir the mixture until the cream cheese melts completely.

Add 1/2 cup of the shredded cheese to the sauce and stir well until it is melted and the sauce is smooth.

Return the chicken to the skillet and cover it with the remaining shredded cheese.

Place a lid on the skillet and let it simmer over low heat for 6-8 minutes, allowing the cheese to melt and the flavors to meld together.

KETO CRACK CHICKEN

Nutrition: Cal 242;Fat 20 g;Carb 2 g;Protein 40 g
Serving 4; Cook time 25 min

Ingredients

For the chicken

4 small chicken breasts
1/4 teaspoon salt
1/4 teaspoon pepper
1/2 teaspoon garlic powder
1 teaspoon oil
4 slices bacon chopped
1 tablespoon butter
6 ounces shredded cheese

For the cream cheese filling

4 ounces cream cheese softened
1/2 teaspoon onion powder
1/4 teaspoon garlic powder
1/8 teaspoon celery salt
1/4 teaspoon dried dill

Instructions

Preheat the oven to 200°C/400°F and generously grease a 13 x 9-inch baking dish. Set the dish aside.

Using a meat mallet, gently pound the four chicken breasts until they reach a thickness of approximately ¼ inch. Season the chicken breasts with salt, pepper, and garlic powder.

Heat olive oil in a non-stick pan over medium heat. Add the diced bacon and cook until it turns crispy. Remove the bacon from the pan, but leave the bacon grease behind. Add butter to the pan and let it heat up. Place the chicken breasts in the pan and cook them for about 2-3 minutes per side, until they develop a golden brown color.

Transfer the cooked chicken breasts into the prepared baking dish and pour the pan juices over them.

In a small bowl, whisk together the cream cheese and spices until well combined.

Evenly spread the cream cheese mixture over the top of each chicken breast. Sprinkle half of the cooked bacon on top, followed by the shredded cheese.

Bake the dish for approximately 15 minutes, or until the chicken is cooked through and the cheese has melted and turned golden. Remove from the oven and serve immediately.

CHICKEN FLORENTINE

Nutrition: Cal 295;Fat 22 g;Carb 6 g;Protein31 g
Serving 4; Cook time 25 min

Ingredients
For the chicken
2 large chicken breasts
1/2 teaspoon salt
1/2 teaspoon pepper
1/2 cup almond flour
2 tablespoons parmesan cheese
1 tablespoon olive oil
1 tablespoon butter
For the florentine sauce
1 tablespoon butter
2 cloves garlic minced
3/4 cup chicken broth
1 tablespoon Italian seasonings
1 cup heavy cream
1/4 cup parmesan cheese
2 cups baby spinach loosely packed
Instructions
Begin by slicing the two chicken breasts lengthwise to create four thin pieces of chicken. Season these four chicken pieces with salt and pepper, and set them aside.

In a small bowl, whisk together the almond flour and Parmesan cheese. Dip each chicken fillet into the flour mixture, ensuring that every piece is thoroughly coated.

Heat the oil and one tablespoon of butter in a skillet over medium heat. Once the skillet is hot, add the chicken and cook for 8-10 minutes, flipping halfway through, until the chicken is golden on the outside. Remove the chicken from the heat.

Add the extra butter to the pan, along with the garlic, and cook for 30 seconds before adding the chicken broth and Italian seasoning. Allow it to simmer for 5-6 minutes or until the liquid has noticeably reduced. Next, add the cream and bring it to a boil. Finally, incorporate the Parmesan cheese and spinach.

Return the chicken back into the pan and let it simmer for 5 minutes, allowing the sauce to thicken.

Serve the chicken along with the Florentine sauce immediately.

HUNAN CHICKEN

Nutrition: Cal 358;Fat 22 g;Carb 8 g;Protein 26 g
Serving 4; Cook time 15 min

Ingredients
For the chicken
1 lb chicken thigh skinless, chopped into bite sized pieces
1 tablespoon almond flour or cornstarch
1 tablespoon oil
For the stir fry
1 tablespoon sesame oil
2 cloves garlic minced
1 tablespoon ginger minced
3 cups broccoli chopped
1 large bell pepper chopped
1 medium zucchini chopped
For the Hunan sauce
1/2 cup chicken broth
3 tablespoon soy sauce
1 tablespoon fish sauce
1 tablespoon white vinegar
2 tablespoon brown sugar substitute
2 tablespoon chili paste I used sambal oelek
1/2 teaspoon xanthan gum or cornstarch
Instructions
Prepare the Hunan sauce by whisking together all the ingredients until well combined. Set the sauce aside.

In a bowl, combine the chopped chicken and almond flour, and gently mix them together.

Heat the oil in a non-stick pan or wok over medium heat. Stir-fry the chicken until it is mostly cooked. Once done, remove the chicken from the pan and set it aside.

Add the sesame oil to the pan and heat it up. Then, add the minced garlic and ginger, and stir-fry for several minutes until fragrant. Next, add the remaining vegetables and continue cooking until they are mostly tender. Return the chicken to the pan, and pour in the Hunan sauce. Allow the sauce to bubble and thicken for several minutes, while stirring occasionally. Once the desired consistency is reached, remove the pan from the heat.

Serve the dish over cauliflower rice or your preferred low-carb side dish of choice.

KETO ORANGE CHICKEN

Nutrition: Cal 280;Fat 14 g;Carb 13 g;Protein 23 g
Serving 4; Cook time 20 min

Ingredients
For the chicken
1 1/2 lbs skinless chicken breasts chopped into bite sized pieces
3 large eggs
1/4 cup heavy cream
1 cup coconut flour
1/4 teaspoon salt
1/4 teaspoon pepper
3 tablespoons oil to fry
For the keto orange sauce
1 cup orange juice no added sugar
1/2 cup brown sugar substitute or granulated sweetener of choice
2 tablespoons white vinegar
2 tablespoons soy sauce
2 cloves garlic minced
1 teaspoon xanthan gum optional

Instructions
Begin by preparing the sauce. In a small saucepan, combine the orange juice, brown sugar substitute, vinegar, soy sauce, and garlic. Heat the mixture for 3-4 minutes. Add the xanthan gum and whisk vigorously to ensure there are no clumps. Let the sauce simmer for 5-6 minutes until it thickens and becomes sticky.

In a bowl, whisk together the eggs and heavy cream, then add the chopped chicken. In a large plate, combine the coconut flour, salt, and pepper, and mix until well combined.

Take each piece of chicken and individually coat it in the flour mixture, making sure each piece is fully coated.

Heat oil in a large pan over medium heat. Once the oil reaches around 350F, add enough chicken to fill the pan without overcrowding. Fry the chicken for 2-3 minutes, then flip and cook for an additional minute. Remove the chicken from the pan and place it on a plate lined with paper towel. Repeat the process until all the chicken has been fried.

Once all the chicken is cooked, toss it in the orange sauce until fully coated. Serve immediately.

CHICKEN WITH CREAMY PEPPER SAUCE

Nutrition: Cal 490;Fat 38 g; Carb 3 g;Protein 30 g
Serving 2; Cook time 35 min

Ingredients
- 2 chicken thighs, boneless and skinless (about 8 oz total)
- 1/2 cup shredded mozzarella cheese
- 1/4 cup heavy cream
- 2 tbsp unsalted butter
- 1/4 cup diced onion
- 1 garlic clove, minced
- 1/4 tsp black pepper
- Salt, to taste
- Fresh parsley, chopped (optional)

Instructions
1. Preheat the oven to 375°F.
2. Season the chicken thighs with salt and black pepper. Place them in a baking dish and bake for 25-30 minutes, or until fully cooked.
3. While the chicken is cooking, melt the butter in a saucepan over medium heat. Add the diced onion and minced garlic, and sauté until softened and fragrant.
4. Stir in the heavy cream and black pepper, and let the mixture come to a simmer. Let it cook for 3-4 minutes, or until the sauce has thickened slightly.
5. Remove the chicken from the oven and top each thigh with shredded mozzarella cheese. Return the chicken to the oven and bake for an additional 5-7 minutes, or until the cheese is melted and bubbly.
6. Spoon the creamy pepper sauce over the chicken thighs, and garnish with fresh parsley if desired.

CHICKEN AND EGGPLANT CURRY WITH ALMONDS

Nutrition: Cal 555;Fat 42 g; Carb 12 g;Protein 28 g
Serving 2; Соок time 25 min

Ingredients
- 2 chicken thighs, boneless and skinless (about 8 oz total)
- 1 small eggplant, diced
- 1/2 cup coconut cream
- 1/4 cup sliced almonds
- 1 tbsp olive oil
- 2 garlic cloves, minced
- 1 tsp ground cumin
- 1 tsp ground coriander
- 1/2 tsp ground turmeric
- 1/4 tsp cayenne pepper
- 1/2 tsp salt
- 1/4 tsp black pepper
- Fresh cilantro, chopped (optional)

Instructions

1. In a large skillet, heat the olive oil over medium heat. Add the chicken thighs and cook for 5-6 minutes on each side, until they are browned and fully cooked. Remove the chicken from the skillet and set it aside.
2. In the same skillet, add the diced eggplant and sauté for 2-3 minutes, until it is slightly softened.
3. Add the minced garlic, ground cumin, ground coriander, ground turmeric, cayenne pepper, salt, and black pepper to the skillet. Cook for 1-2 minutes, until the spices become fragrant.
4. Pour in the coconut cream and stir to combine. Bring the mixture to a simmer and let it cook for 5-7 minutes, until the eggplant is tender and the sauce has thickened.
5. Return the cooked chicken thighs to the skillet and coat them in the curry sauce. Let everything simmer for a few more minutes until the chicken is heated through.
6. Toast the sliced almonds in a dry skillet over medium heat for 2-3 minutes, until they are lightly browned.
7. Serve the chicken and eggplant curry hot, sprinkled with the toasted almonds and chopped cilantro if desired.

COCONUT BREADED CHICKEN

Nutrition: Cal 564;Fat 41 g; Carb 12 g;Protein 45 g
Serving 2; Соок time 30 min

Ingredients
- 2 chicken fillets (about 8 oz each)
- 1/2 cup coconut flour
- 1/2 cup unsweetened shredded coconut
- 1 tsp garlic powder
- 1/2 tsp salt
- 1/4 tsp black pepper
- 2 eggs
- 2 tbsp coconut oil

Instructions

1. Preheat the oven to 375°F.
2. Cut the chicken fillets into small strips or nuggets.
3. In a small bowl, whisk the eggs together.
4. In a separate bowl, combine the coconut flour, shredded coconut, garlic powder, salt, and black pepper.
5. Dip each chicken strip into the egg mixture and then coat with the coconut flour mixture, pressing it onto the chicken to adhere well.
6. Heat the coconut oil in a large skillet over medium-high heat. Once hot, add the chicken strips and cook for 2-3 minutes on each side or until golden brown.
7. Transfer the chicken strips to a baking sheet and bake in the preheated oven for 10-15 minutes or until cooked through and crispy.

Serve hot with your favorite keto-friendly dipping sauce, such as mayonnaise or hot sauce.

INDIAN-STYLE KETO CHICKEN

Nutrition: Cal 450;Fat 27 g;Carb 7 g;Protein 43 g
Serving 2; Соок time 50 min

Ingredients
- 2 boneless, skinless chicken breasts
- 1/2 cup full-fat Greek yogurt
- 1 tablespoon ghee or coconut oil
- 1 small onion, diced
- 2 garlic cloves, minced
- 1 tablespoon grated fresh ginger
- 1 teaspoon ground cumin
- 1 teaspoon ground coriander
- 1/2 teaspoon ground turmeric
- 1/4 teaspoon cayenne pepper (or to taste)
- 1/4 cup tomato sauce
- 1/4 cup heavy cream

- Salt and pepper, to taste
- Chopped fresh cilantro, for garnish

Instructions

1. Start by cutting the chicken into bite-sized pieces and season them with salt and pepper. In a bowl, mix together the yogurt, cumin, coriander, turmeric, and cayenne pepper. Add the chicken pieces to the bowl and coat them thoroughly with the spiced yogurt. Allow the chicken to marinate for at least 30 minutes (or up to 24 hours) in the refrigerator.
2. Heat ghee or coconut oil in a large skillet over medium-high heat. Add the onion and cook until softened and lightly browned, approximately 5 minutes. Stir in the garlic and ginger, and cook for an additional minute, stirring constantly.
3. Add the marinated chicken to the skillet and cook, stirring occasionally, until the chicken is browned on all sides, about 10 minutes.
4. Pour in the tomato sauce and heavy cream, and stir to combine. Reduce the heat to low and simmer for approximately 10 minutes, until the chicken is fully cooked and the sauce has thickened.
5. Serve the dish hot, garnished with chopped cilantro.

CHICKEN FRICASSEE WITH VEGETABLES

Nutrition: Cal 431;Fat 32 g;Carb 7 g;Protein 27 g
Serving 2; Cook time 35 min

Ingredients

- 2 chicken fillets, cut into bite-size pieces
- 2 tablespoons butter
- 1 small onion, chopped
- 1 celery stalk, sliced
- 1 small carrot, diced
- 1/2 cup sliced mushrooms
- 1/2 cup chicken broth
- 1/2 cup heavy cream
- 1 tablespoon chopped fresh parsley
- Salt and pepper, to taste

Instructions

1. Begin by melting the butter in a large skillet over medium heat.
2. Add the chicken to the skillet and cook until it is browned on all sides, which should take approximately 5-7 minutes.
3. Remove the chicken from the skillet and set it aside for now.

4. In the same skillet, add the onion, celery, and carrot, and sauté them until they are softened, which should take around 5 minutes.
5. Next, add the mushrooms to the skillet and cook for an additional 2-3 minutes.
6. Pour in the chicken broth and heavy cream, and stir to combine all the ingredients together.
7. Return the chicken back to the skillet and bring the mixture to a simmer.
8. Allow it to cook until the chicken is fully cooked through and the sauce has thickened, which should take approximately 10-15 minutes.
9. Finally, stir in the chopped parsley, salt, and pepper, and serve the dish.

CHICKEN STIR-FRY WITH MUSHROOMS

Nutrition: Cal 370;Fat 22 g;Carb 8 g;Protein 34 g
Serving 2; Cook time 25 min

Ingredients

- 2 chicken fillets, sliced
- 1 cup mushrooms, sliced
- 1 onion, sliced
- 1 cup soy sprouts
- 2 cloves garlic, minced
- 1 tablespoon ginger, minced
- 2 tablespoons coconut oil
- 2 tablespoons soy sauce
- 1 tablespoon sesame oil
- Salt and pepper, to taste
- Chopped scallions for garnish

Instructions

1. Begin by heating the coconut oil in a wok or large skillet over high heat.
2. Add the sliced chicken to the wok and stir-fry it until it is browned and fully cooked.
3. Incorporate the mushrooms, onion, garlic, and ginger into the wok, and continue to stir-fry for an additional 2-3 minutes until the vegetables are slightly softened.
4. Introduce the soy sauce, sesame oil, soy sprouts, salt, and pepper to the wok, and stir-fry for another 1-2 minutes until all the ingredients are well combined.

Remove the wok from the heat and garnish the dish with chopped scallions.

GRILLED CHICKEN FILLET WITH CREAMY WINE SAUCE

Nutrition: Cal 324;Fat 20 g;Carb 32 g;Protein 32 g
Serving 2; Cook time 1 hour 15 min

Ingredients
• 2 boneless chicken fillets (about 6 oz each)
• 1 tbsp fresh thyme, chopped
• 1 tbsp fresh rosemary, chopped
• 1 tbsp fresh basil, chopped
• 3 cloves garlic, minced
• 2 tbsp balsamic vinegar
• Salt and pepper, to taste
• 1/4 cup dry white wine
• 1/4 cup heavy cream
• 1 tbsp butter

Instructions
1. Combine the chopped thyme, rosemary, basil, minced garlic, balsamic vinegar, salt, and pepper in a small bowl.
2. Place the chicken fillets in a resealable plastic bag and pour the marinade over the chicken.
3. Seal the bag and let the chicken marinate in the refrigerator for at least 1 hour, or overnight for maximum flavor.
4. Preheat a grill to medium-high heat.
5. Remove the chicken from the marinade and discard the remaining marinade.
6. Grill the chicken fillets for 6-8 minutes per side, or until they are fully cooked and no longer pink.
7. In a small saucepan, heat the white wine over medium heat and let it simmer until it reduces by half.
8. Stir in the rosemary, heavy cream, and butter to the saucepan, continuously stirring until the sauce thickens. Season with salt and pepper to taste.
9. Serve the grilled chicken fillets with the creamy wine sauce drizzled over the top.

CHICKEN FILLET STUFFED WITH SHRIMP

Nutrition: Cal 380;Fat 21 g;Carb 2 g;Protein 47 g
Serving 3; Cook time 45 min

Ingredients
• 2 boneless chicken fillets (about 6 oz each)
• 1/2 lb shrimp, peeled and deveined
• 3 tbsp unsalted butter, melted
• 3 cloves garlic, minced
• 2 tbsp fresh parsley, chopped
• Salt and pepper, to taste

Instructions
1. Preheat your oven to 375°F (190°C).
2. Butterfly the chicken fillets by making a horizontal cut through the middle, ensuring not to cut all the way through, and open them like a book.
3. Season both sides of the chicken fillets with salt and pepper.
4. In a small bowl, combine the melted butter, minced garlic, and chopped parsley.
5. Brush the butter mixture onto the inside of the chicken fillets.
6. Place the shrimp on top of one half of each chicken fillet, then fold the other half over to create a pocket.
7. Secure the chicken fillets with toothpicks.
8. Arrange the stuffed chicken fillets in a baking dish and bake in the oven for 25-30 minutes, or until the chicken is cooked through and no longer pink.
9. Before serving, remember to remove the toothpicks.

CHICKEN SALAD PUFFS

Nutrition: Cal 109;Fat 13 g;Carb 2 g;Protein 15 g
Serving 12; Cook time 20 min

Ingredients
PUFFS
• 3 eggs separated
• 1/2 tsp cream of tartar
• 3 oz cream cheese softened (or you could use 2 tablespoons allulose to keep it dairy free and lower fat for PSMF macros)
• 1/2 cup unflavored egg white or whey protein
CHICKEN SALAD FILLING:
• 1 chicken thigh cooked and shredded
• 2 pieces sugar free bacon
• 2 oz blue cheese crumbled (if not dairy sensitive)
• 4 ounces homemade mayo

Instructions
1. To prepare these delicious protein sparing bread puffs, begin by preheating your oven to 375 degrees Fahrenheit. Set aside the egg yolks for another recipe.
2. In a large bowl, whip the egg whites and cream of tartar until they form stiff peaks. Add the protein powder and gently fold in the cream cheese or allulose using a spatula, being careful not to deflate the whites.

3. Grease a baking sheet or use a mini muffin tin and place rounded balls of dough onto it. Bake the puffs at 375 degrees Fahrenheit for 10 minutes. Once done, keep the oven closed and allow the puffs to cool inside.
4. For the chicken salad filling, combine all the ingredients in a large bowl, seasoning with salt and pepper to taste. Stuff the filling into the protein sparing bread puffs and savor the deliciousness!

SESAME CHICKEN AVOCADO SALAD

Nutrition: Cal 540;Fat 47 g;Carb 10 g;Protein 23 g
Serving 2; Cook time 10 min

Ingredients:
- 1 tablespoon sesame oil
- 8 ounces boneless chicken thighs, chopped
- Salt and pepper
- 4 cups fresh spring greens
- 1 cup sliced avocado
- 2 tablespoons olive oil
- 2 tablespoons rice wine vinegar
- 1 tablespoon sesame seeds

Instructions:
1. Heat the sesame oil in a skillet over medium-high heat until it's hot and shimmering.
2. Season the chicken with salt and pepper, then add it to the skillet.
3. Cook the chicken, stirring often, until it is browned and fully cooked.
4. Remove the chicken from the heat and let it cool slightly.
5. Divide the spring greens onto two salad plates and place avocado slices on top.
6. Drizzle the salads with olive oil and rice wine vinegar for added flavor.
7. Top the salads with the cooked chicken and sprinkle sesame seeds over them before serving.

EASY CASHEW CHICKEN

Nutrition: Cal 330;Fat 24 g; Carb 8 g;Protein 22 g
Serving 3; Cook time 15 min

Ingredients
- 3 raw chicken thighs, boneless and skinless
- 2 tablespoons coconut oil (for cooking)
- 1/4 cup raw cashews
- 1/2 medium green bell pepper
- 1/2 teaspoon ground ginger
- 1 tablespoon rice wine vinegar
- 1 1/2 tablespoons liquid aminos
- 1/2 tablespoon chili garlic sauce
- 1 tablespoon minced garlic
- 1 tablespoon sesame oil
- 1 tablespoon sesame seeds
- 1 tablespoon green onions
- 1/4 medium white onion
- Salt and pepper, to taste

Instructions
1. Begin by heating a pan over low heat. Toast the cashews in the pan for about 8 minutes, or until they turn lightly brown and become fragrant. Once toasted, remove them from the pan and set them aside.
2. Dice the chicken thighs into 1-inch chunks. Cut the onion and pepper into equally sized chunks as well.
3. Increase the heat to high and add coconut oil to the pan.
4. Once the oil reaches the desired temperature, add the chicken thighs to the pan and allow them to cook through, which should take about 5 minutes.
5. Once the chicken is fully cooked, add the pepper, onions, garlic, chili garlic sauce, and seasonings such as ginger, salt, and pepper. Cook on high heat for 2-3 minutes.
6. Add liquid aminos, rice wine vinegar, and the toasted cashews to the pan. Cook on high heat and allow the liquid to reduce down until it reaches a sticky consistency. There should not be any excess liquid remaining in the pan upon completing the cooking process.

KETO PESTO STUFFED CHICKEN BREASTS

Nutrition: Cal 415;Fat 30 g; Carb 5 g;Protein 33 g
Serving 4; Cook time 525 min

Ingredients
- 4 boneless, skinless chicken breasts
- 1/2 cup homemade or store-bought pesto
- 1/2 cup almond flour
- 1/2 tsp garlic powder
- 1/2 tsp paprika
- Salt and pepper, to taste
- 2 tbsp olive oil

Instructions
1. Preheat the oven to 375°F.

2. Butterfly the chicken breasts by slicing them horizontally, but not all the way through, so they open like a book.
3. Spread about 2 tablespoons of pesto onto the inside of each chicken breast, then fold them back up and secure with toothpicks.
4. In a shallow bowl, mix together the almond flour, garlic powder, paprika, salt, and pepper.
5. Coat each chicken breast in the almond flour mixture, shaking off any excess.
6. Heat the olive oil in an oven-safe skillet over medium-high heat. Add the chicken breasts and cook for 2-3 minutes per side, until golden brown.
7. Transfer the skillet to the oven and bake for 15-20 minutes, until the chicken is cooked through and the internal temperature reaches 165°F.
8. Let the chicken rest for a few minutes, then remove the toothpicks and slice.

SMOKED CHICKEN SALAD SANDWICH

Nutrition: Cal 299;Fat 13 g; Carb 3 g;Protein 24 g
Serving 4; Cook time 3 hours 50 min

Ingredients
- 4 cups cubed, smoked chicken meat
- 1 cup homemade baconnaise OR organic mayonnaise
- 1 tsp paprika
- 1 green onion, chopped
- 1 tsp Celtic sea salt
- ground black pepper to taste
- OPTIONAL: Sliced hard boiled eggs, 1 cup chopped celery, 1/2 cup minced green pepper
- 8 Protein Buns

Instructions
1. To prepare smoked chicken sandwiches, begin by properly cleaning and portioning a whole chicken into thighs, breasts, and wings. Soak wood chips and place them in the bottom of your smoker.
2. Next, position the chicken on the racks and smoke it outdoors according to the manufacturer's instructions, typically for a duration of 3-4 hours.
3. Once the chicken has finished smoking, preheat your oven to 250 degrees F and transfer the chicken to the oven to complete the cooking process for approximately 30 minutes or until it reaches a deep golden color.

4. While the chicken is cooking, you can prepare the flavorful filling for your sandwiches. In a medium bowl, combine mayonnaise with paprika and salt. Incorporate finely chopped onion and any other preferred additions such as celery or green pepper.
7. Add the diced poultry to the mixture and thoroughly combine all ingredients. Adjust the seasoning with black pepper to your taste and consider incorporating sliced hard-boiled eggs if desired.

THAI CHICKEN LETTUCE WRAPS

Nutrition: Cal 270;Fat 14 g; Carb 12 g;Protein 21 g
Serving 4; Cook time 10 min

Ingredients
- 1 lb ground chicken
- 1 tablespoon olive oil
- 2 tablespoons red curry paste
- 1 tablespoon ginger, minced
- 4 cloves garlic, minced
- 1 red bell pepper, sliced thinly
- 4 green onions, chopped
- 1 cup cabbage, shredded or coleslaw mix
- 1/4 cup hoisin sauce
- 1/4 teaspoon salt, or to taste
- 1/4 teaspoon pepper, or to taste
- 5 leaves basil, chopped
- 1/2 head iceberg lettuce, cut into half

Instructions
1. Add olive oil to a large skillet and heat until oil is very hot. Add ground chicken and cook until no longer pink and starts to brown, break it up with a wooden spoon as necessary. Should take about 3 minutes.
2. Add red curry paste, ginger, garlic, peppers, coleslaw mix, and stir-fry for another 3 minutes. Add hoisin sauce and green onions, and toss. Remove from heat then add basil and toss. Transfer cooked chicken to a bowl.
3. Serve by placing spoonfuls of chicken into pieces of lettuce, fold lettuce over like small tacos, and eat.

GARLIC, LEMON & THYME ROASTED CHICKEN BREASTS

Nutrition: Cal 230;Fat 27 g; Carb 4 g;Protein 26 g
Serving 4; Cook time 2 hours 45 min

Ingredients

- 4 boneless skinless chicken breasts
- zest of 1 lemon
- juice of 1 lemon
- 1/2 cup extra virgin olive oil
- 4 cloves garlic minced
- 1 tablespoon fresh thyme
- 1 teaspoon salt
- 1/2 teaspoon ground black pepper
- 1 tablespoon olive oil for sauteing

Instructions

1. Begin by preparing the marinade. In a mixing bowl, combine the lemon juice, lemon zest, 1/2 cup of olive oil, minced garlic, thyme, salt, and pepper. Stir well to ensure the ingredients are fully incorporated. Place the chicken breasts in a non-reactive glass dish or a plastic zip-top bag, and pour the marinade over the chicken. Make sure the chicken is evenly coated with the marinade. Cover the dish or seal the bag, then refrigerate for a minimum of 2 hours to allow the flavors to infuse.
2. Preheat your oven to 400 degrees Fahrenheit (200 degrees Celsius). Remove the chicken breasts from the marinade and use a paper towel to gently wipe off any excess marinade. Heat 1 tablespoon of olive oil in a skillet over medium-high heat. Once the oil is hot, add the chicken breasts to the skillet and sear them for approximately 2 minutes on each side, or until they turn a golden brown color. The purpose of searing is to enhance the flavor and texture of the chicken.
3. Transfer the seared chicken breasts to a baking sheet lined with a baking rack. Place the sheet in the preheated oven and roast the chicken at 400 degrees Fahrenheit for 20-30 minutes, depending on the thickness of the chicken breasts. Cook until the internal temperature of the chicken reaches 165 degrees Fahrenheit (75 degrees Celsius) when measured with a meat thermometer. This ensures that the chicken is fully cooked and safe to eat.

GRILLED CHICKEN KABOBS

Nutrition: Cal 278;Fat 12 g; Carb 26 g;Protein 27 g
Serving 2; Cook time 30 min

Ingredients

- 0.5 pound boneless skinless chicken breasts cut into 1 inch pieces
- 0.13 cup olive oil
- 0.17 cup soy sauce
- 0.13 cup honey
- 0.5 teaspoon minced garlic
- salt and pepper to taste
- 0.5 red bell pepper cut into 1 inch pieces
- 0.5 yellow bell pepper cut into 1 inch pieces
- 1 small zucchini cut into 1 inch slices
- 0.5 red onion cut into 1 inch pieces
- 0.5 tablespoon chopped parsley

Instructions

1. Place the olive oil, soy sauce, honey, garlic and salt and pepper in a large bowl.
2. Whisk to combine.
3. Add the chicken, bell peppers, zucchini and red onion to the bowl. Toss to coat in the marinade.
4. Cover and refrigerate for at least 1 hour, or up to 8 hours.
5. Soak wooden skewers in cold water for at least 30 minutes. Preheat grill or grill pan to medium high heat.
6. Thread the chicken and vegetables onto the skewers.
7. Cook for 5-7 minutes on each side or until chicken is cooked through.
8. Sprinkle with parsley and serve.

CHICKEN ENCHILADA BOWL

Nutrition: Cal 356;Fat 35 g; Carb 6 g;Protein 28 g
Serving 4; Cook time 30 min

Ingredients

- 2 tablespoons coconut oil (for searing chicken)
- 1 pound of boneless skinless chicken thighs
- 3/4 cup red enchilada sauce
- 1/4 cup water
- 1/4 cup chopped onion
- 1 4 ounce can diced green chiles

Toppings (feel free to customize)

- 1 whole avocado, diced
- 1 cup shredded cheese (I used mild cheddar)
- 1/4 cup chopped pickled jalapenos
- 1/2 cup sour cream

• 1 roma tomato, chopped

Instructions

1. In a pot or Dutch oven over medium heat, melt the coconut oil. Once hot, sear the chicken thighs until lightly browned.
2. Pour in the enchilada sauce and water, then add the onion and green chiles. Reduce the heat to a simmer, cover the pot, and cook the chicken for 17-25 minutes or until it is tender and fully cooked through, reaching an internal temperature of at least 165°F.
3. Carefully remove the chicken from the pot and place it on a work surface. Chop or shred the chicken according to your preference, then add it back into the pot. Let the chicken simmer uncovered for an additional 10 minutes to allow it to absorb the flavors and for the sauce to reduce slightly.
4. To serve, top the dish with avocado, cheese, jalapeno, sour cream, tomato, and any other desired toppings. Feel free to customize these toppings to your preference. You can serve the dish alone or over cauliflower rice if desired, just make sure to adjust your personal nutrition information as needed.

CHICKEN PHILLY CHEESESTEAK

Nutrition: Cal 263;Fat 12 g; Carb 5 g;Protein 27 g
Serving 3; Соок time 15 min

Ingredients

• 10 ounces boneless chicken breasts (about 2)
• 2 tablespoons worcestershire sauce
• 1/2 teaspoon onion powder
• 1/2 teaspoon garlic powder
• 1 dash of ground pepper
• 2 teaspoons olive oil, divided
• 1/2 cup diced onion, fresh or frozen
• 1/2 cup diced bell pepper, fresh or frozen
• 1/2 teaspoon minced garlic
• 3 slices provolone cheese or queso melting cheese

Instructions

1. Begin by slicing the chicken breasts into very thin pieces. You can freeze them slightly beforehand to make the slicing easier. Place the sliced chicken in a medium bowl and add the next four ingredients: Worcestershire sauce, garlic powder, onion powder, and ground pepper. Stir well to coat the chicken with the marinade.

2. Heat one teaspoon of olive oil in a large ovenproof skillet, preferably 9 inches in diameter. Add the chicken pieces to the skillet and cook them until they are nicely browned, which should take about 5 minutes. Flip the pieces over and cook for an additional 2-3 minutes, or until they are browned on the other side. Once cooked, remove the chicken from the skillet.
3. Add the remaining teaspoon of olive oil to the warm skillet. Then, add the onions, bell peppers, and garlic. Cook and stir the vegetables until they are heated through and tender, which typically takes about 2-3 minutes.
4. Turn off the heat and return the cooked chicken back to the skillet. Stir it together with the vegetables to combine them well. Place sliced cheese over the mixture, ensuring it covers everything, and cover the skillet for 2-3 minutes to allow the cheese to melt.

DUCK ACCORDING TO UKRAINIAN RECIPE

Nutrition: Cal 450;Fat 32 g;Carb 5 g;Protein 29 g
Serving 2; Соок time 55 min

Ingredients

• 2 duск legs
• 1 tablespoon olive oil
• 1/2 teaspoon salt
• 1/4 teaspoon black pepper
• 1/2 onion, sliced
• 2 cloves garlic, minced
• 1/4 cup chicken or beef broth
• 1/4 cup dry red wine
• 1 tablespoon tomato paste
• 1 teaspoon paprika
• 1/2 teaspoon dried thyme
• 1/2 teaspoon dried rosemary
• 1 bay leaf

Instructions

1. Preheat the oven to 375°F (190°C) to ensure it reaches the desired temperature for cooking.
2. Season the duck legs with salt and pepper on both sides, ensuring an even distribution of the seasoning for enhanced flavor.
3. Heat a large oven-proof skillet over medium-high heat to provide an ideal cooking surface.
4. Add olive oil to the skillet and carefully sear the duck legs for approximately 2-3 minutes on each side, allowing them to develop a golden brown color for added visual appeal.

5. Once seared, remove the duck legs from the skillet and set them aside momentarily, ensuring they remain warm.

6. In the same skillet, add the sliced onion and garlic, and sauté them for 2-3 minutes until they become softened, releasing their aromatic flavors.

7. Introduce chicken or beef broth, dry red wine, tomato paste, paprika, dried thyme, dried rosemary, and a bay leaf to the skillet, stirring them together to create a cohesive sauce.

8. Return the seared duck legs to the skillet and spoon the sauce over the top, ensuring they are well coated for optimal flavor infusion.

9. Transfer the skillet to the preheated oven and bake for approximately 45-50 minutes, allowing the duck legs to cook through and become tender, resulting in succulent meat.

10. For a complete and satisfying meal, serve the cooked duck legs with a side of sautéed cabbage or roasted vegetables, providing contrasting textures and flavors to complement the main dish.

DUCK STEWED WITH PRUNES

Nutrition: Cal 460;Fat 26 g;Carb 21 g;Protein 27 g
Serving 2; Cook time 2 hours 15 min

Ingredients
- 2 duck legs
- 1/2 teaspoon salt
- 1/4 teaspoon black pepper
- 2 tablespoons olive oil
- 1 large onion, chopped
- 2 cloves garlic, minced
- 1 cup chicken broth
- 1 cup dry red wine
- 1 cup pitted prunes
- 2 tablespoons honey
- 1 bay leaf
- 1/2 teaspoon dried thyme
- 1/2 teaspoon dried rosemary

Instructions
1. Begin by preheating the oven to 325°F (163°C) to ensure the desired temperature is reached for cooking.

2. Season the duck legs with a sprinkle of salt and pepper on both sides, evenly distributing the seasoning for enhanced flavor.

3. Heat a large Dutch oven over medium-high heat, providing a suitable cooking vessel for the next steps.

4. Add a drizzle of olive oil to the Dutch oven, allowing it to heat up. Carefully sear the duck legs for approximately 2-3 minutes on each side until they acquire a delightful golden brown color.

5. Once seared to perfection, remove the duck legs from the Dutch oven and set them aside, ensuring they stay warm.

6. Utilizing the same Dutch oven, add the chopped onion and minced garlic. Sauté the mixture for about 2-3 minutes until the ingredients become soft and fragrant.

7. Incorporate chicken broth, dry red wine, pitted prunes, honey, bay leaf, dried thyme, and dried rosemary into the Dutch oven, stirring all the ingredients together to create a flavorful blend.

8. Return the seared duck legs to the Dutch oven, gently spooning the sauce over the top, ensuring they are well-coated with the aromatic mixture.

9. Cover the Dutch oven with its lid and transfer it to the preheated oven, allowing the duck legs to bake for approximately 2 hours. This will result in tender and succulent meat, while the sauce thickens and develops a rich consistency.

10. Before serving, remember to remove the bay leaf from the sauce, as its purpose has been fulfilled.

11. To complement the dish, serve the duck with a side of roasted root vegetables or cauliflower rice, providing a satisfying and nutritious accompaniment.

DUCK WITH STEWED CABBAGE

Nutrition: Cal 420;Fat 27 g;Carb 14 g;Protein 33 g
Serving 2; Cook time 35 min

Ingredients
- 2 duck breasts
- 1/2 head of green cabbage, chopped
- 1/2 onion, chopped
- 2 cloves garlic, minced
- 2 tablespoons olive oil
- 1/2 teaspoon salt
- 1/4 teaspoon black pepper
- 1/2 teaspoon dried thyme
- 1/2 teaspoon dried rosemary
- 1/2 cup chicken or beef broth
- 1 tablespoon apple cider vinegar

Instructions

1. Preheat the oven to 375°F (190°C) to ensure the desired temperature for cooking.
2. Heat a large oven-proof skillet over medium-high heat, ensuring it is suitable for transferring to the oven later.
3. Season the duck breasts with a sprinkling of salt and pepper on both sides, evenly distributing the seasoning for enhanced taste.
4. Add a drizzle of olive oil to the skillet and carefully sear the duck breasts for approximately 2-3 minutes on each side, allowing them to develop a beautiful golden brown color.
5. Once seared, remove the duck from the skillet and set it aside, ensuring it stays warm.
6. In the same skillet, add the chopped onion and garlic, sautéing them for about 2-3 minutes until they become softened and aromatic.
7. Introduce the chopped cabbage, dried thyme, dried rosemary, chicken or beef broth, and apple cider vinegar to the skillet, stirring all the ingredients together to achieve a harmonious blend.
8. Return the seared duck to the skillet, gently spooning the cabbage mixture over the top, ensuring the flavors are well combined.
9. Transfer the skillet to the preheated oven and bake for approximately 20-25 minutes, allowing the duck to cook through until it reaches the desired level of doneness.
10. To serve, present the duck with a generous portion of the stewed cabbage, allowing the flavors to complement each other in this delightful dish.

DUCK AND CAULIFLOWER STIR-FRY

Nutrition: Cal 531;Fat 37 g;Carb 7 g;Protein 38 g
Serving 2; Cook time 25 min

Ingredients
- 2 duck breasts, skin on
- Salt and black pepper, to taste
- 2 cups cauliflower florets
- 2 tablespoons olive oil
- 2 cloves garlic, minced
- 1/4 cup natural peanut butter (no sugar added)
- 2 tablespoons soy sauce or coconut aminos
- 1 tablespoon apple cider vinegar
- 1/4 teaspoon red pepper flakes (optional)
- 1/4 cup chopped fresh cilantro (optional)

Instructions

1. Begin by seasoning the duck breasts with a balanced amount of salt and black pepper on both sides, ensuring even distribution of the seasoning for optimal flavor.
2. Heat a large skillet over medium-high heat and place the duck breasts, skin side down, into the hot skillet. Cook them for approximately 5 minutes or until the skin turns crispy and golden brown. Flip the duck breasts over and continue cooking for another 3-5 minutes, ensuring they are cooked through. Once done, remove the duck breasts from the skillet and allow them to rest for 5 minutes. After they have cooled slightly, slice the duck meat into thin strips.
3. In the same skillet, add the cauliflower florets and cook them for about 5-7 minutes, stirring occasionally, until they are lightly browned and tender. Once cooked, remove the cauliflower from the skillet and set it aside.
4. In a small bowl, whisk together the natural peanut butter, soy sauce or coconut aminos, apple cider vinegar, and red pepper flakes (if desired), until the ingredients are well combined and form a smooth sauce.
5. Using the same skillet, heat the olive oil over medium heat. Add the minced garlic and cook it for approximately 1-2 minutes, until it becomes fragrant.
6. Return the sliced duck meat and cooked cauliflower back to the skillet. Pour the peanut butter sauce over the top and stir everything together until the meat and cauliflower are well coated with the sauce.
7. Cook for an additional 2-3 minutes, stirring occasionally, until everything is heated through and the sauce has thickened slightly.
8. Serve the duck and cauliflower stir-fry while hot, optionally garnishing it with freshly chopped cilantro for added freshness and flavor.

CREAMY DUCK WITH SPINACH RECIPE

Nutrition: Cal 593;Fat 47 g;Carb 5 g;Protein 38 g
Serving 2; Cook time 35 min

Ingredients
- 2 duck legs, skin on
- Salt and black pepper, to taste
- 1 tablespoon coconut oil
- 1/2 cup chopped onion

- 2 garlic cloves, minced
- 1/2 cup coconut cream
- 2 cups fresh spinach
- 1 tablespoon chopped fresh basil
- 1 tablespoon chopped fresh cilantro
- 1 tablespoon chopped fresh mint

Instructions

1. Preheat the oven to 375°F (190°C).
2. Season the duck legs with salt and black pepper on both sides.
3. Heat a skillet over medium-high heat and add the coconut oil. Once the oil is hot, carefully place the duck legs in the skillet, skin side down. Cook for approximately 5 minutes or until the skin becomes crispy and golden brown. Flip the duck legs over and cook for an additional 3-5 minutes until they are cooked through. Remove the duck legs from the skillet and transfer them to a baking dish.
4. In the same skillet, sauté the chopped onion and minced garlic until they become soft and fragrant.
5. Add the coconut cream to the skillet and stir to combine with the onions and garlic. Allow the sauce to simmer for a few minutes until it thickens slightly.
6. Pour the coconut cream sauce over the duck legs in the baking dish. Place the dish in the preheated oven and bake for 20-25 minutes until the sauce is bubbly and the duck is heated through.
7. While the duck is baking, thoroughly wash the spinach leaves and remove any tough stems. Roughly chop the spinach and set it aside.
8. Once the duck is done, remove it from the oven and let it cool for a few minutes to allow the flavors to settle.
9. In a separate skillet, heat a tablespoon of coconut oil over medium heat. Add the chopped spinach and cook until it wilts, which should take about 2-3 minutes.
10. To serve, place the duck legs on individual plates and drizzle them with the creamy coconut sauce. Serve alongside the sautéed spinach and garnish with freshly chopped herbs for an added burst of flavor.

DUCK AND SPINACH SALAD

Nutrition: Cal 575;Fat 42 g;Carb 6 g;Protein 41 g
Serving 3; Cook time 45 min

Ingredients

- 2 duck breasts, skin on
- Salt and black pepper, to taste
- 4 cups fresh spinach leaves
- 4 slices bacon, cooked and chopped
- 1/4 cup chopped red onion
- 1/4 cup crumbled feta cheese
- 2 tablespoons olive oil
- 1 tablespoon red wine vinegar
- 1 teaspoon Dijon mustard
- 1/2 teaspoon garlic powder

Instructions

1. Preheat your oven to 400°F (200°C).
2. Season the duck breasts with salt and black pepper on both sides.
3. Heat a skillet over medium-high heat and add the duck breasts, skin side down. Cook for approximately 5 minutes or until the skin becomes crispy and golden brown. Flip the duck breasts over and cook for an additional 3-5 minutes until they are cooked through. Remove the duck breasts from the skillet and let them rest for 5 minutes.
4. While the duck is resting, prepare the salad. Wash the spinach leaves and pat them dry. Place them in a large salad bowl.
5. Add the chopped bacon, red onion, and crumbled feta cheese to the bowl with the spinach.
6. In a separate small bowl, whisk together the olive oil, red wine vinegar, Dijon mustard, and garlic powder.
7. Slice the duck breasts into thin pieces and add them to the salad bowl.
8. Drizzle the dressing over the salad and toss gently to combine.

CREAMY DUCK SOUP

Nutrition: Cal 503;Fat 35 g;Carb 9 g;Protein 39 g
Serving 2; Cook time 45 min

Ingredients

- 2 duck breasts, skin on
- Salt and black pepper, to taste
- 1 tablespoon olive oil
- 1 small onion, chopped
- 2 garlic cloves, minced
- 8 oz mushrooms, sliced

- 1 tablespoon grated ginger
- 2 cups chicken broth
- 1/2 cup heavy cream
- 2 medium tomatoes, chopped
- 1 tablespoon chopped fresh cilantro
- Salt and black pepper, to taste

Instructions

1. Season the duck breasts with salt and black pepper on both sides.
2. Heat a skillet over medium-high heat and add the duck breasts, skin side down. Cook for approximately 5 minutes or until the skin becomes crispy and golden brown. Flip the duck breasts over and cook for another 3-5 minutes until they are cooked through. Remove the duck breasts from the skillet and let them rest for 5 minutes. Once cooled, shred the duck meat.
3. Heat a large soup pot over medium-high heat and add the olive oil. Once the oil is hot, add the chopped onion and minced garlic. Cook until soft and fragrant.
4. Add the sliced mushrooms and grated ginger to the pot and cook for about 5 minutes, stirring occasionally.
5. Pour in the chicken broth and bring it to a boil. Reduce the heat to low and simmer for about 10 minutes.
6. Add the heavy cream and chopped tomatoes to the pot and cook for another 5 minutes.
7. Use an immersion blender or transfer the soup to a blender and blend until smooth.
8. Add the shredded duck meat to the pot and let it simmer for another 5-10 minutes to allow the flavors to meld together.
9. Season the soup with salt and black pepper, to taste.
10. Serve the soup hot, garnished with chopped fresh cilantro.

KETO DUCK ROLLS

Nutrition: Cal 474;Fat 30 g;Carb 6 g;Protein 38 g
Serving 2; Cook time 25 min

Ingredients

- 2 duck breasts, skin on
- Salt and black pepper, to taste
- 1 tablespoon olive oil
- 1/2 cup sliced scallions
- 1/2 cup sliced cucumber
- 1/4 cup chopped fresh cilantro
- 1/4 cup chopped fresh mint

- 1/4 cup chopped roasted peanuts
- 4 large lettuce leaves
- 2 tablespoons fish sauce
- 2 tablespoons lime juice
- 1 tablespoon low-carb sweetener (such as monk fruit sweetener)
- 1 small red chili pepper, sliced (optional)

Instructions

1. Season the duck breasts with salt and black pepper on both sides.
2. Heat a skillet over medium-high heat and add the duck breasts, skin side down. Cook for approximately 5 minutes or until the skin becomes crispy and golden brown. Flip the duck breasts over and cook for another 3-5 minutes until they are cooked through. Remove the duck breasts from the skillet and let them rest for 5 minutes. Once cooled, slice the duck meat into thin strips.
3. In a small bowl, whisk together the fish sauce, lime juice, and low-carb sweetener until well combined.
4. Arrange the lettuce leaves on a flat surface.
5. Divide the sliced duck meat among the lettuce leaves, placing them in the center.
6. Top the duck meat with sliced scallions, sliced cucumber, chopped fresh cilantro, chopped fresh mint, and chopped roasted peanuts.
7. Drizzle the fish sauce mixture over the top of the filling.
8. Roll up the lettuce leaves tightly to form the duck rolls.
9. Serve the duck rolls immediately, garnished with sliced red chili pepper (if using).

DUCK, BACON, GREEN BEAN, AND MUSHROOM SKILLET

Nutrition: Cal 532;Fat 41 g;Carb 9 g;Protein 33 g
Serving 2; Cook time 25 min

Ingredients

- 2 duck breasts, skin on
- Salt and black pepper, to taste
- 4 slices bacon, diced
- 8 oz green beans, trimmed and cut into bite-size pieces
- 8 oz mushrooms, sliced
- 2 cloves garlic, minced
- 2 tablespoons olive oil
- 1/4 teaspoon red pepper flakes (optional)

Instructions

1. Season the duck breasts with salt and black pepper on both sides.
2. Heat a large skillet over medium-high heat and add the duck breasts, skin side down. Cook for about 5 minutes or until the skin is crispy and golden brown. Flip the duck breasts over and cook for another 3-5 minutes until cooked through. Remove the duck breasts from the skillet and let them rest for 5 minutes. Once cooled, slice the duck meat into thin strips.
3. In the same skillet, cook the diced bacon over medium heat until crispy. Remove the bacon with a slotted spoon and set it aside.
4. Add the green beans, mushrooms, minced garlic, and olive oil to the skillet. Cook for about 5-7 minutes, stirring occasionally, until the vegetables are tender and lightly browned.
5. Add the sliced duck meat and cooked bacon back to the skillet, along with the red pepper flakes (if using). Cook for another 2-3 minutes, stirring occasionally, until everything is heated through.
6. Season with additional salt and black pepper, to taste.
7. Serve the duck, bacon, green bean, and mushroom skillet hot, garnished with chopped fresh parsley if desired.

KETO DUCK DUMPLINGS

Nutrition: Cal 396;Fat 30 g;Carb 8 g;Protein 23 g
Serving 2; Cook time 25 min

Ingredients
- 1/2 lb ground duck meat
- 1/2 cup almond flour
- 1 large egg
- 2 green onions, finely chopped
- 2 cloves garlic, minced
- 1 teaspoon grated ginger
- 1/2 teaspoon salt
- 1/4 teaspoon black pepper
- 1 tablespoon coconut aminos
- 1 tablespoon sesame oil
- 2 cups chicken or beef broth
- 1 tablespoon chopped cilantro (optional)

Instructions
1. In a large mixing bowl, combine the ground duck meat, almond flour, egg, green onions, garlic, ginger, salt, black pepper, coconut aminos, and sesame oil. Thoroughly mix all the ingredients until well combined.

2. Take a tablespoon of the duck mixture and shape it into a ball. Repeat this process with the remaining mixture to create 16-18 dumplings.
3. In a large saucepan, heat the chicken or beef broth over medium-high heat until it reaches a boiling point.
4. Carefully add the duck dumplings to the broth and reduce the heat to low. Allow them to simmer for approximately 8-10 minutes or until the dumplings are fully cooked.
5. Divide the duck dumplings and broth into two bowls. Optionally, garnish with chopped cilantro, if desired. Serve the dish hot.

DUCK AND BROCCOLI "ALFREDO"

Nutrition: Cal 475;Fat 34 g;Carb 7 g;Protein 33 g
Serving 2; Cook time 25 min

Ingredients
- 2 duck breasts, skin on
- Salt and black pepper, to taste
- 2 cups broccoli florets
- 2 tablespoons butter
- 2 cloves garlic, minced
- 1/4 cup heavy cream
- 1/4 cup grated parmesan cheese
- 1/4 teaspoon dried oregano
- 1/4 teaspoon dried basil
- 1/4 teaspoon dried thyme
- Salt and black pepper, to taste
- Fresh parsley, chopped (optional)

Instructions
1. Season the duck breasts generously with salt and black pepper on both sides.
2. Heat a large skillet over medium-high heat and add the duck breasts, skin side down. Cook for approximately 5 minutes or until the skin becomes crispy and golden brown.
3. Flip the duck breasts over and continue cooking for another 3-5 minutes until they are cooked through. Remove the duck breasts from the skillet and allow them to rest for 5 minutes. Once cooled, slice the duck meat into thin strips.
4. In the same skillet, add the broccoli florets and cook for about 5-7 minutes, stirring occasionally, until they are tender.
5. In a small saucepan, melt the butter over medium heat. Add the minced garlic and cook for about 1-2 minutes until it becomes fragrant.

6. Add the heavy cream, grated Parmesan cheese, dried oregano, dried basil, dried thyme, salt, and black pepper to the saucepan. Stir everything together until well combined and the cheese has melted.
7. Add the sliced duck meat and cooked broccoli to the skillet. Pour the sauce over the top and stir everything together until well coated.
8. Cook for another 2-3 minutes, stirring occasionally, until everything is heated through and the sauce has thickened.
9. Serve the duck and broccoli "Alfredo" hot, optionally garnished with chopped fresh parsley.

DUCK A L'ORANGE RECIPE

Nutrition: Cal 405;Fat 31 g;Carb 3 g;Protein 27 g
Serving 2; Cook time 25 min

Ingredients
- 2 duck breasts
- Salt and pepper
- 1 tablespoon olive oil
- 1/4 cup chicken broth
- 1/4 cup fresh orange juice
- 1 tablespoon orange zest
- 1 tablespoon butter
- 1 tablespoon chopped fresh parsley (optional)

Instructions
1. Set the oven temperature to 400°F.
2. Make a crisscross pattern on the skin of the duck breasts with a sharp knife. Season with salt and pepper on both sides.
3. Preheat a large ovenproof skillet over medium heat and add the olive oil to it. Toss in the chicken breasts, skin side down, and cook for 6 to 8 minutes, or until the skin is golden brown and crisp.
4. Flip the chicken breasts and place the skillet in a preheated oven. Roast for 8–10 minutes, or until the duck is done to your liking.
5. Take the duck breasts out of the oven and place them on a cutting board. Create a foil tent over them and let them rest for 5 minutes.While the duck is resting, bring the skillet to the stove and place it over medium heat.
6. Pour off any excess fat. Stir in the orange juice, orange zest, and chicken broth. simmer for three to five minutes, or until the sauce has thickened.
7. Melt the butter, then stir it in until it's all incorporated

8. Cut the duck breasts in half horizontally and serve with orange sauce. Sprinkle chopped parsley on top (optional).

DUCK BREAST WITH CHERRY PORT SAUCE

Nutrition: Cal 498;Fat 35 g;Carb 6 g;Protein 37 g
Serving 2; Cook time 25 min

Ingredients
- 2 duck breasts, skin on
- Salt and pepper
- 1 tablespoon avocado oil
- 1/4 cup chicken broth
- 1/4 cup port wine
- 1/4 cup fresh cherries, pitted and halved
- 1 tablespoon unsalted butter
- Fresh thyme sprigs (optional)

Instructions
1. 1. Set the oven temperature to 400°F.
2. Cut a crosshatch pattern into the skin of the duck breasts, being careful not to cut all the way through the meat. Season with salt and pepper on both sides.
3. Place an oven-safe skillet over medium-high heat and warm the avocado oil. Place chicken breasts skin-side down in a skillet and cook over medium heat for about 5 minutes, or until the skin is crisp and golden brown.
4. After the oven has been preheated, step four is to flip the duck breasts. Cook the duck breasts for 8 to 10 minutes, or until they reach an internal temperature of 135 degrees Fahrenheit for medium-rare or 145 degrees Fahrenheit for medium
5. Take the cast-iron skillet out of the oven and place the duck breasts on a cutting board.
6. Set the skillet to medium heat on the stovetop. For around two to three minutes, or when the liquid has been reduced by half, add the chicken broth and port.
7. When the fresh cherries are soft and the sauce is thick and glossy, step seven is to add them to the skillet.
8. Take the skillet off the heat and add the unsalted butter, stirring it in until it melts and is thoroughly incorporated.
9. Slice the duck breasts and set them out on plates. To serve, spoon cherry port sauce on top and sprinkle with fresh thyme leaves.

DUCK BREAST WITH BLUEBERRY SAUCE

Nutrition: Cal 437;Fat 31 g;Carb 4 g;Protein 31 g
Serving 2; Cook time 25 min

Ingredients
- 2 duck breasts
- Salt and black pepper to taste
- 1/2 cup fresh blueberries
- 1/4 cup chicken or beef broth
- 1/4 cup dry red wine
- 1 tablespoon butter
- 1/2 teaspoon chopped fresh rosemary

Instructions
1. Preheat your oven to 400°F. Score the skin of the duck breasts with a sharp knife, being careful not to cut into the flesh. Season both sides of the duck breasts generously with salt and black pepper.
2. Place the duck breasts skin-side down in a cold oven-safe skillet or pan. Turn the heat to medium and cook for 8-10 minutes, or until the skin becomes crispy and golden brown. Flip the duck breasts over and cook for another 2-3 minutes.
3. Remove the duck breasts from the skillet and transfer them to a baking sheet. Roast in the preheated oven for 6-8 minutes or until the internal temperature reaches 135°F for medium-rare or 145°F for medium doneness.
4. While the duck breasts are roasting, prepare the blueberry sauce. In the same skillet you used to cook the duck breasts, add the blueberries, chicken or beef broth, and red wine. Bring to a boil over high heat, then reduce the heat to low and simmer for 5-7 minutes or until the sauce has slightly thickened.
5. Remove the skillet from the heat and whisk in the butter until melted and the sauce is glossy. Stir in the chopped rosemary.
6. To serve, slice the duck breasts and drizzle the blueberry sauce over the top. Enjoy your delicious and indulgent French-inspired keto meal!

CHICKEN EGG SALAD WRAPS

Nutrition: Cal 545;Fat 38 g;Carb 16 g;Protein 33 g
Serving 3; Cook time 10 min

Ingredients
- 2 romaine lettuce heads, chopped
- 2 cups chopped Baked Boneless Chicken Thighs
- 1 cup grape tomatoes
- 2 cucumbers, diced
- ½ cup chopped red onion
- 4 slices Perfectly Cooked Bacon , chopped
- ½ cup crumbled blue cheese
- 4 Hard-boiled Eggs , sliced
- ½ cup Dairy-Free Ranch Dressing

Instructions
1. Divide the lettuce equally among four storage containers, ensuring an even distribution.
2. Arrange and distribute the chicken, tomatoes, cucumbers, onion, bacon, blue cheese, and eggs evenly over the lettuce in each container.
3. Separate the dressing into 2-tablespoon servings and store them separately on the side.

CHICKEN HEARTS AND LIVER IN A CREAMY TOMATO SAUCE

Nutrition: Cal 369;Fat 27 g;Carb 8 g;Protein 26 g
Serving 4; Cook time 35 min

Ingredients
- 1 lb chicken hearts, cleaned and halved
- 1/2 lb chicken liver, cleaned and diced
- 2 tbsp olive oil
- 1/2 cup diced onion
- 1 cup canned crushed tomatoes
- 1/2 cup chicken broth
- 1/2 cup heavy cream
- 1/4 cup grated parmesan cheese
- 2 cloves garlic, minced
- 1 tsp dried oregano
- Salt and pepper to taste
- Fresh basil leaves, chopped (optional)

Instructions
1. Heat the olive oil in a large skillet over medium-high heat.
2. Add the chicken hearts and chicken liver to the skillet and cook for 8-10 minutes, stirring occasionally, until they are cooked through and slightly browned on the outside.

3. Remove the chicken hearts and liver from the skillet and set them aside.
4. In the same skillet, add the onion and garlic and sauté until the onion is translucent, about 5 minutes.
5. Add the crushed tomatoes, chicken broth, heavy cream, Parmesan cheese, oregano, salt, and pepper to the skillet. Stir to combine.
6. Bring the sauce to a simmer and cook for 5-7 minutes or until it has thickened slightly.
7. Return the chicken hearts and liver to the skillet and stir to coat them with the sauce.
8. Cook for an additional 2-3 minutes or until the chicken hearts and liver are heated through and the sauce is thick and creamy.
9. Serve garnished with fresh basil leaves, if desired.

CHICKEN HEARTS IN A CREAMY SAUCE

Nutrition: Cal 289;Fat 21 g;Carb 2 g;Protein 22 g
Serving 4; Cook time 25 min

Ingredients
- 1 lb chicken hearts, cleaned
- 1 tbsp olive oil
- 1/2 cup chicken broth
- 1/2 cup heavy cream
- 2 tbsp grated parmesan cheese
- 1 tbsp chopped fresh parsley
- 1/2 tsp garlic powder
- Salt and pepper to taste

Instructions
1. Heat the olive oil in a large skillet over medium-high heat.
2. Add the chicken hearts to the skillet and cook for 8-10 minutes, stirring occasionally, until they are cooked through and slightly browned on the outside.
3. Remove the chicken hearts from the skillet and set them aside.
4. In the same skillet, add the chicken broth, heavy cream, Parmesan cheese, garlic powder, salt, and pepper. Stir to combine.
5. Bring the sauce to a simmer and cook for 5-7 minutes or until it has thickened slightly.
6. Return the chicken hearts to the skillet and stir to coat them with the sauce.
7. Cook for an additional 2-3 minutes or until the chicken hearts are heated through and the sauce is thick and creamy.
8. Garnish with chopped parsley and serve.

KETO CHICKEN HEARTS

Nutrition: Cal 227;Fat 13 g;Carb 2 g;Protein 25 g
Serving 2; Cook time 25 min

Ingredients
- 1 lb chicken hearts, cleaned
- 1 tbsp olive oil
- 1/2 tsp salt
- 1/4 tsp black pepper
- 1/2 tsp smoked paprika
- 1/2 tsp garlic powder
- 1/4 tsp cumin

Instructions
1. Preheat your oven to 400°F (200°C).
2. In a bowl, combine the olive oil, salt, black pepper, smoked paprika, garlic powder, and cumin.
3. Toss the chicken hearts in the spice mixture until they are evenly coated.
4. Place the chicken hearts on a baking sheet lined with parchment paper.
5. Bake for 10-12 minutes, or until the chicken hearts are fully cooked and have a slight crispness on the outside.
6. Take them out of the oven and allow them to cool for a few minutes before serving.

KETO THIGH PULPS WITH MUSTARD

Nutrition: Cal 486;Fat 36 g;Carb 2 g;Protein 34 g
Serving 2; Cook time 45 min

Ingredients
- 4 chicken thigh pulps, bone-in and skin-on
- 2 tbsp Dijon mustard
- 2 tbsp mayonnaise
- 1/2 cup shredded cheddar cheese
- 2 garlic cloves, minced
- Salt and pepper to taste

Instructions
1. Preheat your oven to 375°F (190°C).
2. In a small bowl, combine Dijon mustard, mayonnaise, minced garlic, salt, and pepper.
3. Season both sides of the chicken thigh fillets with salt and pepper.
4. Place the chicken thigh fillets in a large baking dish.
5. Spread the mustard and mayonnaise mixture over the chicken thigh fillets, ensuring they are fully covered.

6. Sprinkle shredded cheddar cheese over the chicken thigh fillets.
7. Bake in the preheated oven for 35-40 minutes, or until the chicken is fully cooked and the cheese is golden brown and bubbling.

KETO CHICKEN LIVER PATE

Nutrition: Cal 285;Fat 23 g;Carb 3 g;Protein 14 g
Serving 2; Cook time 25 min

Ingredients
- 1/2 lb chicken livers
- 1/4 cup chopped onion
- 2 cloves garlic, minced
- 2 tbsp butter
- 2 tbsp heavy cream
- Salt and pepper to taste
- Fresh herbs (optional for garnish)

Instructions
1. Begin by rinsing the chicken livers and patting them dry using paper towels.
2. In a frying pan, melt the butter over medium heat. Add the chopped onion and garlic, and sauté for 2-3 minutes until they become softened.
3. Add the chicken livers to the pan and cook for 5-7 minutes until they are fully cooked through.
4. Remove the pan from the heat and allow it to cool for a few minutes.
5. Transfer the chicken liver mixture to a blender or food processor, and blend until it becomes smooth.
6. Pour in the heavy cream and blend again until the mixture is well combined.
7. Season with salt and pepper according to your taste preferences.
8. Place the pâté into a serving dish and garnish with fresh herbs if desired.
9. Refrigerate for at least 1 hour before serving to allow the flavors to meld together.

KETO WHITE CHICKEN CHILI

Nutrition: Cal 480;Fat 30 g; Carb 5 g;Protein 38 g
Serving 4; Cook time 45 min

Ingredients
- 1 lb chicken breast
- cups chicken broth
- 2 garlic cloves, finely minced
- 1 4.5 oz can chopped green chiles
- 1 diced jalapeno
- 1 diced green pepper
- 1/4 cup diced onion
- 4 tbsp butter
- 1/4 cup heavy whipping cream
- 4 oz cream cheese
- 2 tsp cumin
- 1 tsp oregano
- 1/4 tsp cayenne (optional)
- Salt and pepper to taste

Instructions
1. In a large pot, season the chicken with cumin, oregano, cayenne (if using), salt, and pepper.
2. Sear both sides of the chicken over medium heat until golden.
3. Add the broth to the pot, cover, and cook the chicken for 15-20 minutes or until fully cooked.
4. While the chicken is cooking, melt the butter in a medium skillet.
5. Add the chopped green chiles, diced jalapeno, green pepper, and onion to the skillet. Sauté until the veggies soften.
6. Add the minced garlic and sauté for an additional 30 seconds. Turn off the heat and set aside.
7. Once the chicken is fully cooked, shred it with a fork and add it back into the broth.
8. Add the sautéed veggies to the pot with the chicken and broth and simmer for 10 minutes.
9. In a medium bowl, soften the cream cheese in the microwave until you can stir it (approximately 20 seconds).
10. Mix the softened cream cheese with the heavy whipping cream.
11. Stirring quickly, add the cream cheese mixture into the pot with the chicken and veggies.
12. Simmer for an additional 15 minutes.
13. Serve the soup with your favorite toppings such as pepper jack cheese, avocado slices, cilantro, and sour cream.

GARLIC PARMESAN CHICKEN WITH BROCCOLI

Nutrition: Cal 412;Fat 24 g; Carb 8 g;Protein 43 g
Serving 4; Cook time 30 min

Ingredients
- 4 boneless, skinless chicken breasts
- 2 tablespoons olive oil

- 4 cloves garlic, minced
- 1/2 cup grated Parmesan cheese
- 1/2 teaspoon paprika
- 1/2 teaspoon dried oregano
- 1/4 teaspoon salt
- 1/4 teaspoon black pepper
- 4 cups broccoli florets

Instructions
1. Preheat the oven to 400°F (200°C).
2. Heat the olive oil in a skillet over medium heat. Add the garlic and cook for 1-2 minutes, stirring occasionally, until fragrant.
3. In a small bowl, mix together the Parmesan cheese, paprika, oregano, salt, and black pepper.
4. Dip each chicken breast in the Parmesan mixture, coating both sides.
5. Place the chicken breasts in the skillet with the garlic and cook for 4-5 minutes on each side, until golden brown.
6. Meanwhile, steam the broccoli florets in a separate pot until tender.
7. Transfer the chicken and garlic to a baking dish and bake for 10-15 minutes, or until the chicken is cooked through.
8. Serve the chicken with the broccoli on the side.

CHICKEN FILLET STUFFED WITH CHICKEN LIVER PATE

Nutrition: Cal 442;Fat 26 g;Carb 1,5 g;Protein 40 g
Serving 2; Cook time 40 min

Ingredients
- 2 chicken fillets
- 2 oz chicken liver pate(see recipe above)
- 2 oz Philadelphia cheese
- 1 tsp dried thyme
- 1 tsp garlic powder
- 1 tsp onion powder
- Salt and black pepper, to taste
- 1 tbsp olive oil

Instructions
1. Preheat your oven to 375°F (190°C).
2. Butterfly the chicken fillets by making a horizontal slice almost all the way through and opening them like a book.
3. In a small bowl, combine the chicken liver pâté, Philadelphia cheese, thyme, garlic powder, onion powder, salt, and pepper. Mix them well until fully combined.

4. Spoon the pâté mixture onto the inside of each chicken fillet, spreading it evenly.
5. Close the chicken fillets and secure them with toothpicks.
6. Season the outside of the chicken fillets with salt and pepper.
7. Heat the olive oil in a large skillet over medium-high heat.
8. Sear the chicken fillets on both sides until they are browned, approximately 3-4 minutes per side.
9. Transfer the seared chicken fillets to a baking dish and bake in the preheated oven for 15-20 minutes, or until the chicken is fully cooked and is no longer pink in the middle.

BUFFALO CHICKEN CANNOLI

Nutrition: Cal 274;Fat 10 g; Carb 2 g;Protein 22 g
Serving 6; Cook time 45 min

Ingredients
FOR THE CHICKEN:
- 3 tablespoons bacon fat lard, or ghee
- 4 chicken leg quarters about 3 pounds
- 1 1/2 teaspoons Redmond Real salt
- 1/2 teaspoon fresh ground black pepper
- ¼ cup diced yellow onions
- 1 teaspoon minced garlic
- 1/4 cup Buffalo wing–style hot sauce
- 1 cup chicken stock

CONE:
- 1 cup freshly grated hard cheese

GARNISH:
- 4 tablespoons hot sauce
- 4 tablespoons blue cheese crumbles omit if dairy sensitive
- Celery Slices

Instructions
1. To prepare the chicken: Heat the fat in a deep sauté pan over medium-high heat. Season the chicken with salt and pepper. Place the chicken in the hot fat and sauté for approximately 8 minutes or until golden brown on all sides.
2. Add the diced onion to the pan, followed by the garlic. Cook on medium heat for about 8 minutes, stirring occasionally, until the onion is golden brown. Add the hot sauce and broth, reduce the heat, and simmer for about 1½ hours or until the chicken is tender and almost falling off the bone.

3. Remove the chicken legs from the pan and allow them to cool until you can handle them. Shred the meat off the bone and set it aside.
4. To make the cannoli: Preheat the oven to 375°F. Place parchment paper on a cookie sheet and grease it with coconut oil spray. Place 3 tablespoons of cheese in a circle about 4 inches in diameter, leaving at least 2 inches of space between each cheese circle.
5. Bake for 4 to 5 minutes until the cheese circles turn golden brown. Tip: Baking one at a time helps since they harden as they cool.
6. To mold them into a cone shape, have a melted cheese round close to you. Place a round-shaped object (such as a 1-inch spice jar) nearby. Once you remove the cookie sheet from the oven, work quickly and shape the cheese around the round object. Allow it to sit for 10 minutes to cool. Once cool, fill the cone-shaped cheese with the desired filling.
7. Place each cannoli on a serving plate, drizzle with 1 tablespoon of hot sauce, and sprinkle with blue cheese crumbles. Serve with celery.

CHICKEN CHORIZO CHILI

Nutrition: Cal 288;Fat 22 g; Carb 8 g;Protein 16 g
Serving 10; Соок time 80 min

Ingredients
- 1 tablespoon coconut oil
- 2 lbs smoked chorizo sausage sliced
- 2 chicken boneless skinless chicken thighs cut into ½ inch pieces
- 1 cup chopped onion
- 1 28 oz can whole peeled tomatoes, undrained
- 3 chipotle chiles in adobo sauce
- 3 tablespoons minced garlic
- 2 tablespoons smoked paprika
- 1 tablespoon ground cumin
- 1 tablespoon dried oregano leaves
- 2 teaspoons Redmond Real salt
- 1 teaspoon cayenne pepper
- 2 cups chicken stock boxed will work, homemade preferred
- 1 can 12 oz can Lacroix lime carbonated beverage
- 1 oz unsweetened baking chocolate chopped
- ¼ cup fresh lime juice
- ¼ cup chopped fresh cilantro

Instructions

1. Heat a large soup pot over medium-high heat. Add the oil, chorizo, diced chicken, and onions. Cook until the onions are softened and the chicken is thoroughly cooked, approximately 5 minutes.
2. In the meantime, place the tomatoes with their juice and chilis in a food processor. Process until smooth. Set aside.
3. Add garlic, paprika, cumin, oregano, salt, and cayenne to the soup pot. Sauté for another minute while stirring.
4. Incorporate the tomato puree, broth, LaCroix, and chopped chocolate into the pot. Heat until it reaches a gentle boil, then reduce the heat to low and simmer for 1 hour to allow the flavors to develop. Just before serving, stir in lime juice and cilantro.

CHICKEN WINGETTES WITH CILANTRO DIP

Nutrition: Cal 296;Fat 22 g; Carb 11 g;Protein 10 g
Serving 6; Соок time 60 min

Ingredients
- 10 fresh cayenne peppers, trimmed and chopped
- 3 garlic cloves, minced
- 1 ½ cups white wine vinegar
- ½ teaspoon black pepper
- 1 teaspoon sea salt
- 1 teaspoon onion powder
- 12 chicken wingettes
- 2 tablespoons olive oil
- **DIPPING SAUCE:**
- ½ cup mayonnaise
- ½ cup sour cream
- ½ cup cilantro, chopped
- 2 cloves garlic, minced
- 1 teaspoon smoked paprika

Instructions

1. Place cayenne peppers, 3 garlic cloves, white vinegar, black pepper, salt, and onion powder in the container. Add chicken wingettes and allow them to marinate, covered, for one hour in the refrigerator.
2. Add the marinated chicken wingettes, along with the marinade and extra virgin olive oil, to the Instant Pot.
3. Secure the lid. Select the "Manual" setting and cook for 6 minutes. Once the cooking is complete, perform a quick pressure release and carefully remove the lid.

4. In a mixing bowl, thoroughly combine mayonnaise, sour cream, cilantro, garlic, and smoked paprika.
5. Serve the warm chicken with the dipping sauce on the side.

TURKEY AND CAULIFLOWER RICE BOWL

Nutrition: Cal 437 ;Fat 30 g; Carb 8 g;Protein 29 g
Serving 4; Соок time 30 min

Ingredients
- 1 lb ground turkey
- 4 cups cauliflower rice
- 1/2 cup onion, chopped
- 1/2 cup full-fat Greek yogurt
- 1/2 cup coconut cream
- 2 tbsp olive oil
- 1 tbsp grated fresh ginger
- 1 tsp ground cumin
- 1 tsp ground coriander
- 1/2 tsp turmeric
- Salt and pepper, to taste

Instructions
1. Heat the olive oil in a large skillet over medium-high heat.
2. Add the ground turkey and cook until browned and no longer pink, approximately 5-7 minutes.
3. Add the chopped onion and grated ginger to the skillet and cook for 2-3 minutes, until the onion is translucent.
4. Stir in the cauliflower rice and combine well.
5. Add the cumin, coriander, turmeric, salt, and pepper to the skillet and stir to combine.
6. Pour in the coconut cream and stir to combine.
7. Cook for an additional 5-7 minutes, until the cauliflower rice is tender and the flavors are well incorporated.
8. In a separate bowl, whisk together the Greek yogurt with a pinch of salt.
9. To serve, divide the turkey and cauliflower rice mixture into four bowls and top each with a dollop of the yogurt mixture.

FAT HEAD CHICKEN BRAID

Nutrition: Cal 290 ;Fat 22 g; Carb 4 g;Protein 19 g
Serving 8; Соок time 35 min

Ingredients
DOUGH:
- 1 3/4 cup shredded mozzarella cheese
- 2 tablespoons cream cheese
- 3/4 cup almond flour
- 1 egg
- 1/8 teaspoon Redmond Real salt
FILLING:
- 1 1/2 cups leftover chicken diced (I used Whole Foods Rotisserie chicken)
- 4 tablespoons mayo I used Primal Kitchen Mayo
- 1/2 cup shredded cheddar
- 2 slices sugar free bacon diced
- 3 tablespoons "healthified" Ranch Dressing

Instructions
1. To prepare a delicious chicken and bacon braid, preheat the oven to 400 degrees F. In a heat-safe bowl, microwave the mozzarella and cream cheese for 1-2 minutes until fully melted, then stir well. Add the almond flour, egg, and salt, and use a hand mixer to combine everything.
2. Place a greased piece of parchment paper on a pizza stone (or a cookie sheet if you don't have one), and place the dough on top. Pat it out with your hands to create an oval shape measuring about 12 inches by 8 inches, with the longer part facing you.
3. Make the filling by mixing diced chicken and mayonnaise in a bowl, then place it down the middle of the oval, lengthwise, leaving 1 ½ inches at the top and bottom, and leaving 3 inches on each side. Top with shredded cheese.

CHICKEN MILANESE

Nutrition: Cal 240 ;Fat 14 g; Carb 3 g;Protein 24 g
Serving 4; Соок time 20 min

Ingredients
- 4 boneless skinless chicken thighs, pounded thin
- Fine grain sea salt and freshly ground black pepper
- 2 eggs beaten
- 1/2 cup pork rind crumbs or grind pork rinds into fine powder

- 1/2 cup powdered Parmesan (place shredded Parmesan into a food processor until powdered)
- 3 tablespoons Primal Kitchen avocado oil or coconut oil for frying
- 2 cups leafy greens chopped
- 2 radishes sliced thin
- 4 tablespoons Primal Kitchen Ranch Dressing
- 1 lemon quartered

Instructions

1. For a delicious and easy meal, begin by placing chicken thighs between two pieces of parchment paper and gently pound them with a rolling pin until they reach about ¼ inch thickness. Season both sides generously with salt and pepper.
2. In a shallow bowl, beat the eggs and mix in a tablespoon of water. Season with salt and pepper. In another shallow bowl, combine the pork dust and powdered Parmesan.
3. Dip each chicken thigh into the beaten eggs, allowing any excess to drip off, and then coat both sides in the pork dust mixture. Heat oil in a large cast iron skillet over medium-high heat. Once hot, sear each chicken thigh until golden brown, approximately 2 minutes per side.
4. While the chicken is cooking, prepare the salad by chopping the lettuce and slicing the radish. Once the chicken is done, place it onto serving plates and divide the salad among each plate. Squeeze lemon juice over each piece of chicken and salad, then drizzle with Primal Kitchen Ranch Dressing for additional flavor. This dish is perfect for a quick and easy weeknight meal.

TURKEY AND SOY SPROUTS STIR FRY

Nutrition: Cal 496 ;Fat 131 g; Carb 9 g;Protein 41 g
Serving 2; Cook time 25 min

Ingredients

- 1 lb ground turkey
- 2 cups soy sprouts
- 4 eggs
- 1 head cauliflower, grated into rice-like texture
- 2 tbsp olive oil
- 2 cloves garlic, minced
- 1/2 tsp ginger powder
- Salt and pepper, to taste

Instructions

1. Heat the olive oil in a large skillet over medium-high heat.
2. Add the ground turkey and cook until browned and no longer pink, which should take about 5-7 minutes.
3. Incorporate the minced garlic, ginger powder, salt, and pepper into the skillet, and continue cooking for an additional 1-2 minutes until fragrant.
4. Introduce the soy sprouts to the skillet, and cook for 2-3 minutes until they begin to wilt.
5. In a separate non-stick pan, fry the eggs to your preferred level of doneness.
6. While the eggs are frying, steam the cauliflower rice in a microwave or steamer for 3-5 minutes until tender.
7. To serve, distribute the cauliflower rice evenly between two bowls, and top it with the turkey and soy sprout stir fry. Place a fried egg on top of each bowl.

TURKEY STEW RECIPE

Nutrition: Cal 386 ;Fat 20 g; Carb 12 g;Protein 36 g
Serving 5; Cook time 30 min

Ingredients

- 2 lbs turkey breast, chopped into smaller pieces
- 2 cups cherry tomatoes, chopped
- 1 onion, finely chopped
- 4 cups chicken broth
- ¾ cup heavy cream
- 2 celery stalks, chopped
- 4 tbsps. butter
- 1 tsp. dried thyme
- 1 tsp. peppercorn
- 2 tsps. Salt

Instructions

1. Combine the ingredients in the instant pot and securely seal the lid.
2. Adjust the steam release handle to the "Sealing" position and press the "Stew" button. Set the timer for twenty minutes on high heat.
3. Once the cooking is complete, allow the pressure to release naturally. Open the lid and let the mixture cool for a while. Stir in a generous amount of sour cream. To enjoy, serve it immediately.

MUSHROOM & SAGE ROLLED TURKEY BREAST

Nutrition: Cal 311;Fat 12 g;Carb 2 g;Protein 45 g
Serving 8; Cook time 1 hour 25 min

Ingredients

- ¼ cup coconut oil or butter, divided, room temperature
- 10 ounces mushrooms finely chopped
- 1 clove garlic minced
- Salt and pepper to taste
- 3 tablespoon chopped fresh sage divided
- 1 boneless butterfiled turkey breast (3 to 4 lbs)
- 1 180 F Pop Up® disposable cooking thermometer (optional, but very useful!)

Instructions

1. Preheat oven to 375F.
2. In a large saute pan over medium heat, heat 2 tablespoon butter or oil until melted and beginning to froth. Add mushrooms and cook, stirring frequently, for 2 or 3 minutes. Add garlic, sprinkle with salt and pepper, and continue to cook until most of the liquid has evaporated, 4 or 5 minutes more.
3. Add 2 tablespoon chopped sage and cook 1 minute more. Remove from heat.
4. Remove skin from turkey breast and set aside (do not discard). Lay turkey breast on a work surface and cover with plastic wrap. Pound with a kitchen mallet to an even ½ to 1-inch thickness.
5. Spread mushroom mixture evenly over turkey breast, leaving a 1 inch border and roll up from the short end tightly into a log. Wrap reserved skin over log and tie at several intervals with kitchen twine.
6. Place on a broiling pan and rub all over with remaining butter or oil. Sprinkle with remaining sage and season with salt and pepper.
7. Place pop-up timer, if using, into thickest part of the turkey roll (pierce the skin with a sharp knife if need be).
8. Roast until timer pops up or until internal temperature reaches 180F, approximately 50 to 60 minutes.

WHOLE ROASTED BRINED TURKEY

Nutrition: Cal 180;Fat 6 g;Carb 1 g;Protein 38 g
Serving 8; Cook time 4 hour 10 min

Ingredients

- Turkey Brine
- 2 cups kosher salt
- 2 gallons water
- 12lb Turkey
- Any additional Seasonings you want to add (optional)
- For the Turkey (if NOT stuffing)
- Brined Turkey
- 1 teaspoon each :
- Salt, pepper, onion powder, garlic powder, ground sage (or Bell's seasoning), paprika
- 3 tablespoon butter, melted
- 1 apple, quartered (for cooking only)
- 1 onion, quartered
- 1 stalk celery, cut into pieces

Instructions

1. The day before cooking:
2. Remove turkey from packaging. Remove gravy packet (if included) and giblets. Rinse well on the inside and outside.
3. In a large stock pot, dissolve kosher salt in water. Once the salt is completely dissolved, add the turkey to the pot. Cover and refrigerate overnight.
4. When ready to cook:
5. Preheat oven to 350 degrees.
6. Remove turkey from the brine, rinse well on the inside and outside. Pat dry. Place in a roasting pan and bend wings under the bird or cover with foil.
7. To the cavities of the turkey, add apple and vegetables. Apple will not add carbs UNLESS you are using the juice to make gravy later. If so, omit it.
8. Baste the turkey with olive oil and generously salt, pepper and seasonings on all sides. Cover with foil (remove for the last 30 minutes)
9. Place turkey in the oven and cook according to the chart below or until reaching an internal temperature of 165 degrees.
10. When done, allow the turkey to rest for 20 to 30 minutes prior to carving.

COBB SALAD

Nutrition: Cal 545;Fat 38 g;Carb 23 g;Protein 33 g
Serving 4; Cook time 20 min

Ingredients
- 1½ cups chopped Baked Boneless Chicken Thighs
- 6 Hard-boiled Eggs , chopped
- 3 celery stalks, minced
- 2 tablespoons minced red onion
- 1 tablespoon Dijon mustard
- 2 cups Mayonnaise
- Salt
- Freshly ground black pepper
- 8 leaves butter or romaine lettuce

Instructions
1. In a large bowl, combine the chicken, eggs, celery, onion, and mustard. Add the Mayonnaise and stir until mixed. Season with salt and pepper.
2. Divide the egg salad and lettuce between 3 storage containers. To serve, make egg salad wraps by filling the lettuce leaves with the salad and wrapping the lettuce around it.

JALAPENO POPPER CHICKEN

Nutrition: Cal 524;Fat 29 g;Carb 2 g;Protein 59 g
Serving 4; Cook time 20 min

Ingredients
- 4 boneless skinless chicken breasts 6-ounce
- 8 ounces cream cheese softened
- 2 jalepenos diced
- 8 strips sugar free thin-cut bacon
- Primal Kitchen Ranch Dressing for serving

Instructions
1. Begin by preheating the oven to 400°F.
2. Next, place a chicken breast on a cutting board and take a sharp knife, holding it parallel to the chicken, to make a 1-inch-wide incision at the top of the breast. Carefully cut into the chicken to form a large pocket, leaving a ½-inch border along the sides and bottom. Repeat this step with the other 3 breasts.
3. Then, place the cheese and jalapenos in a bowl and stir well to combine. Transfer the mixture to a large ziplock bag and cut a ¾-inch hole in one corner of the plastic bag. Squeeze the softened cheese into the pockets in the chicken, dividing the cheese evenly among them.
4. Wrap 2 strips of bacon around each breast and secure the ends with toothpicks. Place the bacon-wrapped chicken onto a rimmed baking sheet and place it in the oven. Cook until the bacon is crisp and the chicken is cooked through, which should take about 18-20 minutes. Timing may vary depending on how thick the chicken breast is.
5. Finally, to store any leftovers, place them in an airtight container in the refrigerator for up to 3 days. To reheat, simply place the chicken on a rimmed baking sheet and put it in a 400°F oven for 5 minutes or until it's warmed through.

CHICKEN WONTONS

Nutrition: Cal 290;Fat 22 g; Carb 1 g;Protein 11 g
Serving 12; Cook time 35 min

Ingredients
- 8 oz Cream Cheese
- 2 TBS chives chopped
- 24 pieces chicken skin about 3.5 inches in diameter OR Prosciutto
- Avocado Oil or Coconut Oil For Frying
- Redmond Real Salt if using chicken skin
- Dipping Sauce:
- 1/2 cup coconut aminos or 2 tablespoons organic Tamari sauce (aged soy sauce)
- 1/4 cup chicken bone broth homemade is naturally thick which works great for this recipe
- 2 TBS coconut vinegar or rice wine vinegar
- 1/4 cup Swerve confectioners
- 1 1/2 tsp minced garlic
- 1 1/2 tsp minced ginger
- 1/8 tsp guar gum/xathan gum natural thickener

Instructions
1. To make keto cream cheese wontons, start by combining the cream cheese and chives in a medium bowl.
2. Next, assemble the wontons by placing about 1 tablespoon of the cream cheese mixture in the center of a chicken skin or prosciutto slice. Wrap the skin around the cream cheese, making sure to use a large enough chicken skin to prevent the cream cheese from squirting out during cooking.
3. Heat 2-3 inches of oil in a large saucepan or medium skillet to just under 350 degrees Fahrenheit. Test the oil temperature with spare pieces of chicken skin to ensure it's ready. Fry the wontons in batches of 3 for 3-5 minutes, flipping them halfway through to ensure even browning. Sprinkle with salt and remove from heat.

4. While the wontons cool, make the dipping sauce by combining coconut aminos, organic broth, coconut vinegar, natural sweetener, garlic, and ginger in a small saucepan over medium-high heat. Heat until the natural sweetener is dissolved, then sift in the guar gum to prevent clumping. Adjust the amounts of each ingredient to taste.
5. Serve the dipping sauce alongside the keto cream cheese wontons for a delicious snack or appetizer.

REUBEN CHICKEN

Nutrition: Cal 584;Fat 38 g;Carb 9 g;Protein 51 g
Serving 4; Cook time 4 hours 20 min

Ingredients
THOUSAND ISLAND DRESSING:
- 1/2 cup Primal Kitchen mayo
- 1/4 cup chopped dill pickles
- 1/4 cup Primal Kitchen Ketchup
- 1/2 teaspoon stevia glycerite
- 1/8 teaspoon fish sauceor fine grain sea salt

REUBEN CHICKEN:
- 24 oz. sauerkraut drained
- 4 6 oz boneless skinless chicken breasts
- 1 1/4 teaspoons Redmond Real salt
- 1/2 teaspoon fresh ground pepper
- 4 tablespoons Primal Kitchen Dijon mustard divided

Instructions
1. To prepare this slow cooker sauerkraut and mustard chicken, start by making the dressing. Place all the ingredients in a small bowl and stir well to combine. Taste and adjust seasoning as desired, then cover and store in the fridge for up to 5 days.
2. Next, layer half the sauerkraut in the bottom of a greased 5-6 quart slow cooker. Drizzle with ⅓ of the dressing.
3. Season the chicken on all sides with salt and pepper. Place the chicken breasts on top of the sauerkraut and spread half the mustard over the chicken. Top with the remaining sauerkraut and drizzle another ⅓ of the dressing over everything, reserving the remaining dressing and mustard for serving.
4. Cover the slow cooker and cook on low for 4 hours, or until the chicken is cooked through and tender.

5. To serve, place each chicken breast on a plate. Divide the sauerkraut over the top of the chicken. Finish each plate with a drizzle of the remaining dressing and mustard.
6. Any extras can be stored in an airtight container in the fridge for up to 5 days. To reheat, simply place in a casserole dish in a 350 degree F oven for 5 minutes or until heated through.

CRACK SLAW

Nutrition: Cal 219;Fat 10 g;Carb 10 g;Protein 27 g
Serving 4; Cook time 20 min

Ingredients
- 2 tablespoons coconut oil divided
- 1/2 cup diced onion
- 1 head roasted garlic or 3 cloves minced
- 1 lb boneless skinless Chicken breast
- 1 1/2 teaspoons Redmond Real salt divided
- 5 cups shredded cabbage
- 2 tablespoons tamari sauce or 1/4 cup Coconut aminos
- 1 tablespoon grated fresh Ginger or 1/2 teaspoon dried ginger
- 1 teaspoon Redboat fish sauce or salt
- 1/2 teaspoon stevia glycerite
- Black pepper
- Garnish with sliced green onion

Instructions
1. To prepare this chicken and cabbage stir fry, begin by cutting the chicken into 3/4 inch pieces. Pat the chicken dry and season on all sides with 1 teaspoon salt.
2. Heat a tablespoon of oil in a large skillet or wok over medium heat. Add the onion and garlic, and cook for 5-7 minutes, until the onion is soft.
3. Next, increase the heat to medium-high and add the remaining oil to the skillet. Once hot, add the chicken and stir fry for 3-5 minutes, until the chicken is just golden.
4. Add the cabbage, ginger, tamari, fish sauce, stevia, 1/2 teaspoon salt, and pepper to the skillet. Stir fry for an additional 3-5 minutes, until the cabbage is tender.
5. To serve, garnish with sliced green onion. Any leftovers can be stored in an airtight container in the fridge for up to 4 days. To reheat, simply place in a greased skillet over medium heat for 3 minutes or until heated through.

KETO TANDOORI CHICKEN WINGS

Nutrition: Cal 420 ;Fat 16 g; Carb 8 g;Protein 25 g
Serving 2 Cook time 2 hours 10 min

Ingredients
- 2-1/2 lbs. chicken wings, trimmed and separated
- 1 cup Homemade Yogurt
- 2 tbsp. ginger
- 6 cloves garlic, minced
- 1-1/2 tsp. curry powder
- ¼ tsp. turmeric
- ½ tsp. cumin
- ½ tsp. dry mustard
- 2 tsp. red pepper flakes
- 1 lemon, juiced
- 3 tbsp. vegetable oil
- Salt, pepper

Instructions
1. Add all ingredients in a a bowl and mix well
2. Marinade for at least two hours at room temperature. (saving marinade)
3. Place wings on broiling rack and broil until browned, about 20 minutes
4. Baste wings with marinade about every 10 minutes.
5. Transfer to platter and serve.

YAKISOBA CHICKEN

Nutrition: Cal 317;Fat 14 g;Carb 2 g;Protein 43 g
Serving 6; Cook time 20 min

Ingredients
- 1/2 tsp sesame oil
- 1 TBS coconut oil
- 2 cloves garlic, chopped
- 4 (8 oz) chicken thighs – cut into 1-inch cubes
- 1/2 cup coconut aminos OR wheat free Tamari sauce (fermented soy sauce)
- 2 TBS hot sauce
- 1/2 teaspoon stevia glycerite (optional)
- 1 small onion, sliced lengthwise into eighths
- 1 medium head cabbage, sliced into "noodles"
- OPTIONAL: peanuts for garnish, sauteed broccoli

Instructions
1. To make this tasty stir-fry, start by combining sesame oil and coconut oil in a large skillet. Add garlic and stir-fry for a minute or two. Then, add the chicken and continue to stir-fry until it's no longer pink. Once cooked, set the mixture aside.

2. In the same skillet, add onion and cabbage noodles and stir-fry until the cabbage begins to soften. Stir in the remaining Tamari sauce, and then add the chicken mixture back into the pan. Mix everything together until well combined.

KETO RICED CAULIFLOWER & CURRY CHICKEN

Nutrition: Cal 420 ;Fat 16 g; Carb 8 g;Protein 25 g
Serving 4 Cook time 30 min

Ingredients
- 2 Lbs. of Chicken (4 breasts)
- 1 packet of Curry Paste
- 1 Cup Water
- 3 Tablespoons Ghee (can substitute butter)
- ½ Cup Heavy Cream
- 1 Head Cauliflower (around 1 kg)

Instructions
1. In a large pot, melt the ghee.
2. Add the curry paste and stir to combine.
3. Once combined, pour in the water and simmer for an additional 5 minutes.
4. Add the chicken, cover the pot, and simmer for 20 minutes.
5. Meanwhile, chop up a head of cauliflower into florets and pulse them in a food processor to make riced cauliflower (cauliflower doesn't need to be cooked).
6. Once the chicken is cooked, uncover the pot, add the cream, and cook for an additional 5 minutes.

TURKEY AND ZUCCHINI FRITTERS

Nutrition: Cal 495 ;Fat 38 g; Carb 5 g;Protein 29 g
Serving 2; Cook time 25 min

Ingredients
- 1 small zucchini, grated and drained of excess moisture
- 1/2 lb ground turkey
- 1/4 cup almond flour
- 1/4 cup grated Parmesan cheese
- 1 egg
- 1/4 tsp garlic powder
- Salt and pepper, to taste
- 2 tbsp olive oil
- 1/4 cup full-fat yogurt
- 1 tbsp chopped fresh parsley

Instructions

1. In a medium bowl, combine the grated zucchini, ground turkey, almond flour, Parmesan cheese, egg, garlic powder, salt, and pepper until thoroughly mixed.
2. Heat the olive oil in a non-stick skillet over medium heat.
3. Using a spoon, drop the turkey and zucchini mixture into the skillet, shaping them into fritters about 3 inches in diameter.
4. Cook the fritters for 3-4 minutes on each side, until they are browned and cooked through.
5. In a small bowl, mix together the yogurt and chopped parsley to create a sauce.
6. Serve the fritters hot, with a dollop of the yogurt sauce on top.

SWEET AND SOUR CHICKEN

Nutrition: Cal 252;Fat 11 g;Carb 2 g;Protein 35 g
Serving 4; Cook time 20 min

Ingredients
- 2 teaspoons avocado oil or coconut oil
- 1 pound boneless skinless chicken breasts
- Redmond Real salt
- 1/4 cup chicken bone broth
- 1/4 cup Keto Primo Ketchup
- 2 tablespoons Swerve Brown
- 1 tablespoon tamari sauce
- 1/2 tablespoon lime juice
- ¼ teaspoon fresh ginger peeled and grated
- 1 clove garlic minced

FOR GARNISH:
- Sesame seeds
- scallions sliced
- Lime wedges

Instructions
1. First, heat up some oil in a large wok or cast-iron skillet over medium-high heat. Then, pat the chicken pieces dry with a paper towel and season them well on all sides with salt.
2. Fry the chicken in the hot oil until it turns light golden brown on all sides, which should take about 4 minutes. Once done, remove the chicken from the wok and set it aside.
3. Next, add the remaining ingredients to the wok and boil over medium heat until the sauce is reduced and thickened, which should take about 10 minutes.

4. Once the sauce is ready, return the chicken to the wok and bring it to a hard boil. Reduce the heat to medium and let it simmer for 10 more minutes until the chicken is cooked through and no longer pink inside.
5. To serve, garnish the chicken with sesame seeds, sliced scallions, and lime wedges. If you have leftovers, you can store them in an airtight container in the refrigerator for up to 3 days.
6. When you're ready to reheat, simply place the chicken in a greased skillet over medium heat for 5 minutes or until it's warmed to your liking.

BAKED CHICKEN NUGGETS

Nutrition: Cal 400;Fat 26 g;Carb 2 g;Protein 43 g
Serving 4; Cook time 30 min

Ingredients:
- ¼ cup almond flour
- 1 teaspoon chili powder
- ½ teaspoon paprika
- 2 pounds boneless chicken thighs, cut into 2-inch chunks
- Salt and pepper
- 2 large eggs, whisked well

Instructions:
1. Preheat the oven to 400°F and line a baking sheet with parchment.
2. Stir together the almond flour, chili powder, and paprika in a shallow dish.
3. Season the chicken with salt and pepper, then dip in the beaten eggs.
4. Dredge the chicken pieces in the almond flour mixture, then arrange on the baking sheet.
5. Bake for 20 minutes until browned and crisp. Serve hot.

CURRIED CHICKEN SOUP

Nutrition: Cal 390;Fat 22 g;Carb 14 g;Protein 34 g
Serving 4; Cook time 30 min

Ingredients:
- 2 tablespoons olive oil, divided
- 4 boneless chicken thighs (about 12 ounces)
- 1 small yellow onion, chopped
- 2 teaspoons curry powder
- 2 teaspoons ground cumin
- Pinch cayenne
- 4 cups chopped cauliflower
- 4 cups chicken broth

- 1 cup water
- 2 cloves minced garlic
- ½ cup canned coconut milk
- 2 cups chopped kale
- Fresh chopped cilantro

Instructions:

1. Chop the chicken into bite-sized pieces then set aside.
2. Heat 1 tablespoon oil in a saucepan over medium heat.
3. Add the onions and cook for 4 minutes then stir in half of the spices.
4. Stir in the cauliflower and sauté for another 4 minutes.
5. Pour in the broth then add the water and garlic and bring to a boil.
6. Reduce heat and simmer for 10 minutes until the cauliflower is softened.
7. Remove from heat and stir in the coconut milk and kale.
8. Heat the remaining oil in a skillet and add the chicken – cook until browned.
9. Stir in the rest of the spices then cook until the chicken is done.
10. Stir the chicken into the soup and serve hot, garnished with fresh cilantro.

COCONUT CHICKEN TENDERS

Nutrition: Cal 325;Fat 9 g;Carb 2 g;Protein 45 g
Serving 4; Cook time 40 min

Ingredients:

- ¼ cup almond flour
- 2 tablespoons shredded unsweetened coconut
- ½ teaspoon garlic powder
- 2 pounds boneless chicken tenders
- Salt and pepper
- 2 large eggs, whisked well

Instructions:

1. Preheat the oven to 400°F and line a baking sheet with parchment.
2. Stir together the almond flour, coconut, and garlic powder in a shallow dish.
3. Season the chicken with salt and pepper, then dip into the beaten eggs.
4. Dredge the chicken tenders in the almond flour mixture, then arrange on the baking sheet.
5. Bake for 25 to 30 minutes until browned and cooked through. Serve hot.

TURKEY LASAGNA WITH RICOTTA

Nutrition: Cal 740 ;Fat 56 g; Carb 7.8 g;Protein 47 g
Serving 8; Cook time 60 min

Ingredients

- 2 lbs ground turkey
- 5 cups baby spinach leaves
- 1 cup ricotta
- 1 cup mozzarella cheese, grated
- 1 can crushed tomatoes
- 3 tsp dried oregano
- 2 tsp thyme
- 3 tbsp fresh parsley, finely chopped
- 1 tsp salt
- 1 tsp freshly ground black pepper
- 1 tsp onion powder
- 1 tsp garlic powder
- 8 lasagna sheets
- 3 cups water

Instructions

1. In a bowl, combine the ricotta and mozzarella cheese, and set it aside.
2. In another bowl, mix the crushed tomatoes with oregano, thyme, parsley, salt, pepper, onion powder, and garlic powder.
3. Begin layering the lasagna in a heatproof dish that fits inside the Instant Pot.
4. Start by spreading one tablespoon of the tomato sauce at the bottom of the dish and layer it with lasagna sheets. Spread more tomato sauce around the sheets and add layers of cheese, minced meat, and spinach. Top with more sauce and repeat the layering process until you have used up all the lasagna sheets. Sprinkle the remaining cheese on top and tightly cover the dish with aluminum foil.
5. Place the Instant Pot on medium heat, pour in water, and carefully place the trivet inside the pot. Position the lasagna dish on the trivet.
6. Cover the pot and manually set the timer for 30 minutes. Once the time is up, carefully release the pressure.
7. Uncover the pot and remove the foil to allow the lasagna to brown. Carefully take out the lasagna dish from the pot and serve it hot.

CREAMY TURKEY AND CAULIFLOWER SOUP

Nutrition: Cal 388 ;Fat 21 g; Carb 10 g;Protein 43 g
Serving 2; Cook time 25 min

Ingredients

- 1 lb cooked turkey, shredded
- 1 head cauliflower, chopped into florets
- 2 cups chicken broth
- 1/2 cup heavy cream
- 2 cloves garlic, minced
- 1/4 tsp dried thyme
- Salt and pepper, to taste
- Optional toppings: chopped fresh parsley, grated Parmesan cheese

Instructions

1. In a large pot, heat the chicken broth until it reaches a boiling point.
2. Add the chopped cauliflower to the pot and cook it until tender, which should take around 8-10 minutes.
3. You can use an immersion blender directly in the pot or transfer the mixture to a blender to achieve a smooth consistency.
4. Once blended, return the mixture to the pot and add the cooked turkey, minced garlic, dried thyme, salt, and pepper.
5. Cook the soup over medium heat for 5-10 minutes, stirring occasionally, until the turkey is heated through.
6. Incorporate the heavy cream into the pot and continue stirring until it is well combined.
7. To serve, divide the soup into two bowls and, if desired, add optional toppings according to personal preference.

PINE NUT BREADED BLUE CHEESE STUFFED TURKEY POCKETS

Nutrition: Cal 433 ;Fat 33 g; Carb 3 g;Protein 31 g
Serving 2; Cook time 30 min

Ingredients

- 2 thin turkey cutlets (about 4 oz each)
- 1/4 cup crumbled blue cheese
- 2 tbsp chopped pine nuts
- 2 tbsp almond flour
- 1/4 tsp garlic powder
- Salt and pepper, to taste
- 2 tbsp olive oil

Instructions

1. Preheat your oven to 375°F (190°C).
2. Place the turkey cutlets on a cutting board and season both sides with salt and pepper.
3. In a small bowl, combine the crumbled blue cheese and chopped pine nuts.
4. Spoon the blue cheese and pine nut mixture evenly onto the center of each turkey cutlet.
5. Roll up the turkey cutlets around the filling and secure them with toothpicks.
6. In another small bowl, mix together the almond flour, garlic powder, and a pinch of salt and pepper.
7. Coat the outside of the turkey pockets with the almond flour mixture.
8. Heat the olive oil in a large skillet over medium-high heat. Add the turkey pockets to the skillet and cook for 2-3 minutes on each side until browned.
9. Transfer the turkey pockets to a baking dish and bake in the oven for 10-12 minutes until cooked through and the cheese is melted.
10. Serve the dish hot and enjoy!

SALSA CHICKEN

Nutrition: Cal 244;Fat 10 g; Carb 4.2 g;Protein 30 g
Serving 6; Cook time 35 min

Ingredients

- Chicken thighs without bones (2 lbs)
- Chicken broth (1/4 cup)
- Cream cheese (4 oz.)
- Salsa (1 cup)
- Taco seasoning (3 tbsp)
- Salt, Pepper

Instructions

1. Place the chicken thighs in the pressure cooker and season them with taco seasoning, salt, and pepper.
2. Add salsa, chicken broth, and cream cheese to the cooker. Close and seal the lid. Select the "Manual" mode and set it to cook for 20 minutes on high pressure.
3. Once the cooking time is complete, allow the pressure to release naturally for 15 minutes.
4. Transfer the chicken thighs to a plate and blend the sauce until smooth.
5. Use a fork to shred the meat, then return it to the creamy sauce. Stir well to ensure the meat is coated evenly.
6. Serve the shredded chicken with lettuce, avocados, and any other desired accompaniments.

TURKEY AND SPINACH CASEROLE

Nutrition: Cal 319;Fat 20 g; Carb 5 g;Protein 29 g
Serving 2; Cook time 35 min

Ingredients
- 1 lb ground turkey
- 6 cups fresh spinach, chopped
- 1/2 cup onion, chopped
- 2 cloves garlic, minced
- 1/2 cup full-fat Greek yogurt
- 1/4 cup heavy cream
- 1/4 cup grated Parmesan cheese
- 1 tsp dried basil
- 1 tsp dried oregano
- Salt and pepper, to taste

Instructions
1. Preheat the oven to 350°F.
2. In a large skillet, cook the ground turkey over medium-high heat until it is browned and no longer pink.
3. Add the chopped onion and minced garlic to the skillet and cook for 2-3 minutes, until the onion is translucent.
4. Add the chopped spinach to the skillet and cook for another 2-3 minutes, until the spinach is wilted.
5. In a separate bowl, whisk together the Greek yogurt, heavy cream, grated Parmesan cheese, dried basil, and dried oregano.
6. Add the yogurt mixture to the skillet and stir to combine.
7. Season with salt and pepper to your taste.
8. Transfer the mixture to a 9x13-inch casserole dish and bake for 20-25 minutes, until the top is golden brown and the casserole is heated through.
9. Allow the casserole to cool for a few minutes before serving.

TURKEY AND WALNUT SALAD

Nutrition: Cal 536 ;Fat 38 g; Carb 7 g;Protein 40 g
Serving 2 Cook time 25 min

Ingredients
- 1 lb cooked turkey breast, sliced
- 2 cups mixed salad greens
- 1/2 cup walnuts, roughly chopped
- 1 avocado, sliced
- 8 oz mushrooms, sliced
- 2 tbsp olive oil
- 1 tbsp balsamic vinegar
- Salt and pepper, to taste

Instructions
1. Heat the olive oil in a large skillet over medium-high heat.
2. Add the sliced mushrooms to the skillet and cook for 5-7 minutes until they start to brown and release their moisture. Remove from heat and set aside.
3. In a large mixing bowl, combine the mixed salad greens, sliced turkey breast, chopped walnuts, and sliced avocado.
4. In a small bowl, whisk together the balsamic vinegar, salt, and pepper to make a dressing.
5. Add the cooked mushrooms to the mixing bowl with the salad ingredients and toss everything together.
6. Drizzle the dressing over the salad and toss until well combined.

To serve, divide the salad between two plates.

ROASTED TURKEY BREAST WITH MUSHROOMS & BRUSSELS SPROUTS

Nutrition: Cal 210;Fat 9 g; Carb 6 g;Protein 27 g
Serving 4; Cook time 50 min

Ingredients
- 2 tbsp olive oil
- 1 tsp salt
- 1 tsp black pepper
- 1 tsp garlic powder
- 1 pound turkey breast raw, cut into 1 inch cubes
- 1/2 pound brussels sprouts cleaned, cut in half
- 1 cups mushrooms cleaned

Instructions
1. Preheat the oven to 350 degrees Fahrenheit.
2. In a small mixing bowl, combine olive oil, salt, black pepper, and garlic powder.
3. In a 9 x 6-inch casserole dish, combine turkey, Brussels sprouts, and mushrooms. Pour the olive oil mixture over the top.
4. Cover the dish with foil and bake for 45 minutes or until the turkey is cooked through and is no longer pink. Ensure that the internal temperature of the turkey reaches 165 degrees Fahrenheit for food safety.

BEEF AND LAMB

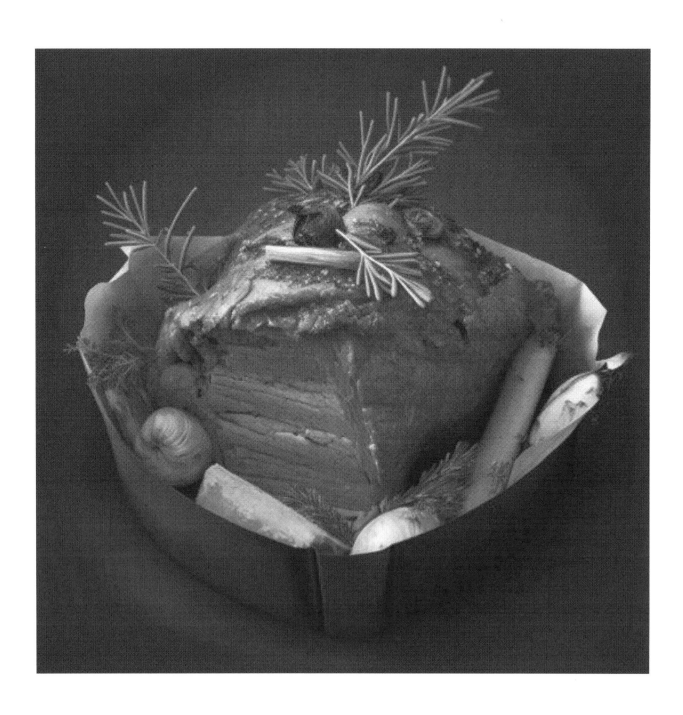

BLUE CHEESE BACON BURGERS

Nutrition: Cal 772;Fat 54 g;Carb 6 g;Protein 61 g
Serving 4; Cook time 20 min

Ingredients
- 1½ pounds ground beef
- 4 slices Perfectly Cooked Bacon , crumbled
- ½ cup crumbled blue cheese
- 1 tablespoon Worcestershire sauce
- 2 large eggs
- Salt
- Freshly ground black pepper
- 1 romaine lettuce head, chopped
- 1 avocado, chopped
- 1 cup grape tomatoes

Instructions
1. In a large mixing bowl, combine the beef, bacon, blue cheese, Worcestershire sauce, and eggs. Season with salt and pepper. Shape 4 patties using your hands. Cover with plastic wrap and refrigerate for 30 minutes to 2 hours.
2. Preheat the grill or broiler on high heat. Cook the patties for 4 to 5 minutes on each side, or until they reach your desired level of doneness. Remove from the grill and allow them to cool.
3. Divide the lettuce, avocado, and tomatoes among 4 storage containers. Place a burger patty on top of each.

BACON CHEESEBURGER SKILLET

Nutrition: Cal 518;Fat 38 g;Carb 1 g;Protein 39 g
Serving 2; Cook time 15 min

Ingredients
- 1/2 pound ground beef
- 4 strips of bacon, chopped
- 1/2 cup shredded cheddar cheese
- Salt and pepper, to taste

Instructions
1. Heat a large skillet over medium-high heat.
2. Add the chopped bacon to the skillet and cook until crispy.
3. Remove the bacon with a slotted spoon and set aside.
4. In the same skillet, add the ground beef and cook until browned and cooked through.
5. Drain any excess grease from the skillet.
6. Add the cooked bacon back to the skillet and stir to combine.

7. Sprinkle the shredded cheddar cheese over the top of the beef mixture.
8. Cover the skillet and cook until the cheese is melted and bubbly, about 2-3 minutes.
9. Season with salt and pepper, to taste.
10. Serve immediately.

BACON MUSHROOM SWISS STEAK

Nutrition: Cal 527;Fat 34 g;Carb 2 g;Protein 50 g
Serving 2; Cook time 20 min

Ingredients
- 2 beef sirloin steaks (about 6-8 ounces each)
- 4 strips of bacon, chopped
- 4 ounces sliced mushrooms
- 1/4 cup shredded Swiss cheese
- Salt and pepper, to taste

Instructions
1. Preheat the oven to 375°F.
2. Season the beef steaks with salt and pepper.
3. In a large oven-safe skillet, cook the chopped bacon over medium-high heat until crispy.
4. Remove the bacon with a slotted spoon and set aside.
5. In the same skillet, add the sliced mushrooms and cook until they release their moisture and are browned.
6. Remove the mushrooms from the skillet and set aside.
7. In the same skillet, add the seasoned beef steaks and sear for 2-3 minutes on each side until browned.
8. Top each steak with the cooked bacon and mushrooms, and sprinkle with shredded Swiss cheese.
9. Place the skillet in the preheated oven and bake for 10-12 minutes, or until the cheese is melted and bubbly and the beef is cooked to your liking.
10. Serve immediately.

BACON BEEF SKILLET WITH CHEESY GREEN BEANS

Nutrition: Cal 425;Fat 24 g;Carb 9 g;Protein 44 g
Serving 2; Cook time 20 min

Ingredients
- 1/2 pound beef sirloin, sliced into thin strips
- 4 strips of bacon, chopped
- 4 ounces sliced champignon mushrooms
- 8 ounces fresh green beans, trimmed

- 1/2 cup shredded cheddar cheese
- Salt and pepper, to taste

Instructions

1. Heat a large skillet over medium-high heat.
2. Add the chopped bacon to the skillet and cook until crispy.
3. Remove the bacon with a slotted spoon and set aside.
4. In the same skillet, add the sliced beef and cook until browned and cooked through.
5. Remove the beef from the skillet and set aside.
6. In the same skillet, add the sliced champignon mushrooms and cook until they release their moisture and are browned.
7. Remove the mushrooms from the skillet and set aside.
8. In the same skillet, add the trimmed green beans and cook until they are tender-crisp.
9. Add the cooked beef, bacon, and mushrooms back to the skillet and stir to combine.
10. Sprinkle the shredded cheddar cheese over the top of the beef and vegetable mixture.
11. Cover the skillet and cook until the cheese is melted and bubbly, about 2-3 minutes.
12. Season with salt and pepper, to taste.

BEEF AND VEGETABLE SKILLET WITH YOGURT SAUCE

Nutrition: Cal 403;Fat 22 g;Carb 14 g;Protein 41 g
Serving 2; Cook time 20 min

Ingredients

- 1/2 pound beef sirloin, sliced into thin strips
- 4 strips of bacon, chopped
- 4 ounces sliced champignon mushrooms
- 8 ounces fresh green beans, trimmed
- 1 red bell pepper, seeded and sliced
- 1/2 cup plain Greek yogurt
- Salt and pepper, to taste

Instructions

1. Heat a large skillet over medium-high heat.
2. Add the chopped bacon to the skillet and cook until crispy.
3. Remove the bacon with a slotted spoon and set aside.
4. In the same skillet, add the sliced beef and cook until browned and cooked through.
5. Remove the beef from the skillet and set aside.
6. In the same skillet, add the sliced champignon mushrooms and cook until they release their moisture and are browned.

7. Remove the mushrooms from the skillet and set aside.
8. In the same skillet, add the trimmed green beans and sliced bell pepper, and cook until they are tender-crisp.
9. Add the cooked beef, bacon, and mushrooms back to the skillet and stir to combine.
10. In a small bowl, whisk together the Greek yogurt with salt and pepper to taste.
Serve the beef and vegetable mixture with a dollop of the yogurt sauce on top.

CREAMY BEEF AND SPINACH SKILLET

Nutrition: Cal 516;Fat 41 g;Carb 5 g;Protein 30 g
Serving 2; Cook time 20 min

Ingredients

- 1/2 pound beef sirloin, sliced into thin strips
- 1/2 cup heavy cream
- 2 cups fresh spinach leaves
- 2 ounces Dor Blue cheese, crumbled
- 4 ounces sliced mushrooms
- Salt and pepper, to taste

Instructions

1. Preheat a large skillet over medium-high heat.
2. Add the sliced beef and cook until it is thoroughly browned and cooked through.
3. Remove the beef from the skillet and set it aside.
4. In the same skillet, add the sliced mushrooms and cook until they release their moisture and are nicely browned.
5. Incorporate the fresh spinach leaves into the skillet and cook until they are wilted.
6. Return the cooked beef to the skillet and stir to combine.
7. Pour the heavy cream over the beef and vegetable mixture, and stir to ensure even distribution.
8. Bring the mixture to a simmer and let it cook until the cream has slightly thickened.
9. Stir in the crumbled Dor Blue cheese until it is melted and fully combined.
10. Season with salt and pepper according to taste.
11. Serve the hot beef and spinach skillet, optionally garnished with additional crumbled Dor Blue cheese if desired.

BACON-WRAPPED BEEF ROLLS

Nutrition: Cal 481;Fat 37 g;Carb 9 g;Protein 27 g
Serving 2; Cook time 35 min

Ingredients
- 1/2 pound beef top sirloin, sliced into 4 thin pieces
- 4 slices of bacon
- 4 pitted prunes, chopped
- 1/4 cup chopped walnuts
- Salt and pepper, to taste
- Toothpicks

FOR THE CREAMY PEPPER SAUCE:
- 1/4 cup heavy cream
- 1 tablespoon butter
- 1/2 teaspoon black pepper
- Salt, to taste

Instructions
1. Preheat the oven to 375°F (190°C).
2. Arrange the beef slices and season each one with salt and pepper.
3. In a small bowl, combine the chopped prunes and walnuts.
4. Spoon the prune and walnut mixture onto each beef slice.
5. Roll up each slice of beef tightly, securing the rolls with toothpicks.
6. Wrap a slice of bacon around each beef roll, securing it with toothpicks as needed.
7. Place the beef rolls on a baking sheet and bake for 20-25 minutes, or until the bacon is crispy and the beef is cooked through.
8. While the beef rolls are baking, prepare the creamy pepper sauce by gently heating the heavy cream and butter in a small saucepan over low heat.
9. Season the sauce with black pepper and salt to taste, stirring until well combined.
   Serve the bacon-wrapped beef rolls hot, drizzled with the creamy pepper sauce.

SESAME-CRUSTED BEEF ROLLS

Nutrition: Cal 430;Fat 31 g;Carb 6 g;Protein 31 g
Serving 2; Cook time 25 min

Ingredients
- 1/2 pound beef top sirloin, sliced into 4 thin pieces
- Salt and pepper, to taste
- 1/4 cup almond flour
- 1/4 cup sesame seeds
- 1 egg, beaten
- 1 tablespoon coconut oil
- 1 tablespoon soy sauce
- 1 tablespoon rice vinegar
- 1 tablespoon sesame oil
- 1/2 teaspoon garlic powder
- 1/4 teaspoon ginger powder
- Sliced green onions, for garnish

Instructions
1. Preheat your oven to 375°F (190°C).
2. Arrange the beef slices and season each one with salt and pepper.
3. In a shallow dish, combine almond flour and sesame seeds.
4. Dip each beef slice into the beaten egg, then coat it in the almond flour and sesame seed mixture.
5. Heat coconut oil in a skillet over medium-high heat.
6. Add the beef rolls and cook for 2-3 minutes on each side, until they turn golden brown and crispy.
7. Transfer the beef rolls to a baking sheet and bake for 10-12 minutes, or until cooked to your desired level of doneness.
8. While the beef rolls are baking, prepare the sauce by mixing together soy sauce, rice vinegar, sesame oil, garlic powder, and ginger powder.
9. Serve the hot beef rolls, drizzled with the sauce and garnished with sliced green onions.

BEEF AND VEGETABLE STIR-FRY

Nutrition: Cal 323;Fat 21 g;Carb 8 g;Protein 26 g
Serving 2; Cook time 20 min

Ingredients
- 1/2 pound beef sirloin, thinly sliced
- 1 tablespoon coconut oil
- 1 small zucchini, sliced
- 1 small onion, sliced
- 1 small bell pepper, sliced
- 1 small tomato, chopped
- Salt and pepper, to taste
- 1 tablespoon sesame seeds

Instructions
1. Heat the coconut oil in a large skillet over high heat.
2. Add the beef slices and cook for 2-3 minutes until browned.
3. Add the zucchini, onion, and bell pepper to the skillet and cook for another 2-3 minutes until the vegetables are tender-crisp.

4. Add the chopped tomato to the skillet and season with salt and pepper.
5. Stir everything together and cook for another 1-2 minutes until the tomato is heated through.
6. Sprinkle sesame seeds over the top of the stir-fry.

CREAMY GARLIC BEEF AND BRUSSELS SPROUTS SKILLET

Nutrition: Cal 490;Fat 39 g;Carb 8 g;Protein 28 g
Serving 2; Cook time 20 min

Ingredients
- 1/2 pound ground beef
- 1 cup Brussels sprouts, trimmed and halved
- 2 cloves garlic, minced
- 2 ounces cream cheese
- Salt and pepper, to taste
- 1 tablespoon olive oil

Instructions
1. Heat the olive oil in a large skillet over medium-high heat.
2. Add the ground beef and garlic to the skillet and cook until browned, stirring occasionally.
3. Introduce the Brussels sprouts to the skillet and cook until they become tender and develop a slight browning.
4. Reduce the heat to low and incorporate the cream cheese into the skillet, stirring until it is fully melted and combined with the beef and Brussels sprouts.
5. Season with salt and pepper according to taste.

VITELLO TONNATO

Nutrition: Cal 357;Fat 27 g;Carb 1 g;Protein 26 g
Serving 4; Cook time 20 min

Ingredients
- 1/2 pound cooked veal, thinly sliced
- 1/4 cup canned tuna, drained
- 1 tablespoon capers, drained
- 1/4 cup mayonnaise
- 1 tablespoon lemon juice
- Salt and pepper, to taste
- Romaine lettuce leaves, for serving

Instructions
1. In a blender or food processor, combine the canned tuna, capers, mayonnaise, lemon juice, and a pinch of salt and pepper.
2. Blend until the mixture achieves a smooth and creamy consistency.
3. Arrange the veal slices on a serving plate.

4. Spoon the tuna sauce over the veal slices, ensuring they are completely covered.
5. Serve the dish chilled and accompany it with Romaine lettuce leaves for a refreshing and crunchy side.

KETO BEEF WELLINGTON

Nutrition: Cal 506;Fat 36 g;Carb 7 g;Protein 40 g
Serving 2; Cook time 20 min

Ingredients
- 1 pound beef tenderloin
- Salt and pepper, to taste
- 2 tablespoons olive oil
- 2 tablespoons Dijon mustard
- 2 cloves garlic, minced
- 1 tablespoon chopped fresh thyme
- 1/2 cup almond flour
- 1/2 cup finely chopped mushrooms
- 1/4 cup finely chopped onion
- 1 egg, beaten

Instructions
1. Preheat the oven to 400°F.
2. Season the beef tenderloin with salt and pepper.
3. Heat the olive oil in a skillet over medium-high heat. Add the beef tenderloin and sear for 2-3 minutes on each side until browned.
4. Remove the beef tenderloin from the skillet and let it cool for a few minutes.
5. Spread Dijon mustard over the beef tenderloin.
6. In a small bowl, mix together minced garlic, chopped thyme, and almond flour. Spread this mixture over the mustard-coated beef tenderloin.
7. In the same skillet, sauté the chopped mushrooms and onions until they are softened.
8. Place the sautéed mushrooms and onions over the almond flour mixture.
9. Roll out a piece of parchment paper and place the beaten egg on it. Place the beef tenderloin in the center and use the parchment paper to wrap the beef tenderloin into a cylinder shape, pressing the egg-washed sides together.
10. Bake in the preheated oven for 20-25 minutes or until the beef reaches your desired level of doneness.
11. Let the beef Wellington rest for 5-10 minutes before slicing and serving.

AVOCADO WITH GROUND BEEF AND CHEESE

Nutrition: Cal 428;Fat 36 g;Carb 6 g;Protein 19 g
Serving 4; Cook time 20 min

Ingredients
- 2 ripe avocados
- 1/2 pound ground beef
- 1/4 cup shredded cheese
- Salt and pepper to taste
- Optional: chopped cilantro and lime wedges for serving

Instructions
1. Preheat the oven to 375°F (190°C).
2. Cut the avocados in half and remove the pits.
3. In a skillet, cook the ground beef over medium heat until browned. Season with salt and pepper to taste.
4. Spoon the cooked ground beef into the avocado halves, dividing it evenly.
5. Sprinkle shredded cheese over the top of the ground beef.
6. Bake the stuffed avocados in the preheated oven for 10-15 minutes or until the cheese is melted and bubbly.
7. Garnish with chopped cilantro and serve with lime wedges on the side, if desired.

KETO BEEF NACHOS

Nutrition: Cal 496;Fat 37 g;Carb 7 g;Protein 26 g
Serving 2; Cook time 20 min

Ingredients
- 1/2 lb ground beef
- 1/2 cup chopped onion
- 1/2 cup diced bell pepper
- 1 tsp chili powder
- 1/2 tsp ground cumin
- 1/2 tsp garlic powder
- 1/4 tsp salt
- 1/4 tsp black pepper
- 1/4 cup water
- 1 medium avocado
- 1/4 cup sour cream
- 1 tbsp lime juice
- 1/4 tsp salt
- 1/2 cup sliced cucumber
- 1/2 cup sliced zucchini
- 1/2 cup sliced bell pepper

Instructions

1. Preheat the oven to 375°F. Arrange vegetable chips on a baking sheet and set aside.
2. In a skillet, cook the ground beef over medium-high heat until browned. Add the chopped onion and diced bell pepper, and continue to cook until the vegetables are tender.
3. Add the chili powder, ground cumin, garlic powder, salt, black pepper, and water to the skillet. Stir until well combined.
4. Spoon the beef mixture over the vegetable chips.
5. Bake the beef nachos in the oven for 10-12 minutes or until the cheese is melted and bubbly.
6. Meanwhile, in a blender or food processor, combine the avocado, sour cream, lime juice, and salt. Blend until smooth.
7. Serve the beef nachos with the avocado sauce on top.

CHINESE CABBAGE BEEF ROLLS

Nutrition: Cal 383;Fat 28 g;Carb 10 g;Protein 25 g
Serving 4; Cook time 20 min

Ingredients
- 4 large Chinese cabbage leaves
- 300g ground beef
- 1 small onion, chopped
- 1 clove garlic, minced
- 1 tsp ginger, grated
- 2 tbsp coconut aminos
- 2 tbsp sesame oil
- 1/4 tsp red pepper flakes
- Salt and black pepper, to taste
- 1/2 cup smoked sour cream sauce (recipe below)

FOR THE SMOKED SOUR CREAM SAUCE:
- 1/2 cup sour cream
- 1 tbsp smoked paprika
- 1 tbsp lemon juice
- Salt and black pepper, to taste

Instructions
1. Preheat the oven to 350°F (180°C).
2. Trim the tough part of the cabbage leaves and blanch them in boiling water for 3 minutes. Drain and set aside.
3. In a large bowl, combine ground beef, onion, garlic, ginger, coconut aminos, sesame oil, red pepper flakes, salt, and black pepper.
4. Lay the cabbage leaves flat and distribute the beef mixture equally among them. Roll up the cabbage leaves and secure with toothpicks.

5. Place the cabbage rolls in a baking dish and bake for 25-30 minutes or until the beef is cooked through.
6. While the cabbage rolls are baking, prepare the smoked sour cream sauce by whisking together sour cream, smoked paprika, lemon juice, salt, and black pepper in a small bowl.
7. Serve the cabbage rolls hot, topped with the smoked sour cream sauce. Enjoy!

KETO EGG-STUFFED BEEF CUTLETS WITH MUSHROOMS

Nutrition: Cal 570;Fat 45 g;Carb 3 g;Protein 36 g
Serving 2; Cook time 25 min

Ingredients
- 1/2 lb ground beef
- 1/4 cup pork lard
- 2 large eggs, hard-boiled and chopped
- 1/4 cup onion, finely chopped
- 1/2 cup mushrooms, finely chopped
- Salt and pepper, to taste

Instructions
1. In a mixing bowl, combine ground beef, salt, and pepper.
2. Divide the meat mixture into 4 portions and flatten each portion to create thin cutlets.
3. In a separate bowl, mix together chopped eggs, onion, and mushrooms.
4. Place a spoonful of the egg mixture onto each cutlet, then roll up the cutlets and secure with toothpicks.
5. In a frying pan, heat the lard over medium heat. Fry the cutlets until browned on all sides and cooked through, about 10-12 minutes.
6. Serve hot with your favorite low-carb vegetables.

CREAMY BEEF LIVER WITH CARAMELIZED ONIONS

Nutrition: Cal 307;Fat 22 g;Carb 6 g;Protein 20 g
Serving 2; Cook time 25 min

Ingredients
- 300g beef liver, sliced
- 1 large onion, sliced
- 2 tbsp butter
- 1/4 cup sour cream
- Salt and pepper to taste

Instructions

1. Heat a large skillet over medium-high heat and add the butter, allowing it to melt.
2. Add the sliced onions to the skillet and cook, stirring occasionally, until caramelized for about 10 minutes.
3. Remove the onions from the skillet and set them aside.
4. In the same skillet, add the sliced beef liver and cook until browned on both sides, approximately 2-3 minutes per side.
5. Return the caramelized onions to the skillet with the beef liver.
6. Pour in the sour cream and stir to combine it with the beef liver and onions.
7. Reduce the heat to low and let the mixture simmer for 5 minutes, stirring occasionally.

BEEF LIVER PATE

Nutrition: Cal 502;Fat 46 g;Carb 6 g;Protein 15 g
Serving 2; Cook time 60 min

Ingredients
- 1/2 pound beef liver
- 1/4 cup butter, softened
- 1/4 cup heavy cream
- 1/2 onion, chopped
- 1 clove garlic, minced
- 1 teaspoon dried thyme
- 1/4 teaspoon salt
- 1/8 teaspoon black pepper

Instructions
1. Begin by rinsing the beef liver with cold water and then patting it dry using paper towels. Proceed to cut the liver into small pieces.
2. Heat 2 tablespoons of butter in a frying pan over medium heat. Add the onion and garlic to the pan and cook until they become softened, which typically takes around 5 minutes.
3. Introduce the liver to the pan and continue cooking until it is browned on both sides, usually around 5 minutes per side.
4. Add the thyme, salt, and black pepper to the pan, stirring well to combine the flavors.
5. Remove the pan from the heat and allow it to cool for a few minutes.
6. Transfer the liver mixture, along with the remaining butter and heavy cream, to a food processor or blender. Blend the ingredients until you achieve a smooth consistency.
7. Transfer the prepared pate to a bowl and refrigerate it for at least 1 hour before serving.

CREAMY BEEF LIVER AND VEGETABLES

Nutrition: Cal 420;Fat 31 g;Carb 8 g;Protein 24 g
Serving 2; Cook time 25 min

Ingredients

- 1 pound beef liver, sliced
- Salt and pepper to taste
- 2 tablespoons olive oil
- 1 onion, sliced
- 1 bell pepper, sliced
- 2 cloves garlic, minced
- 1 cup heavy cream
- 1/4 cup grated parmesan cheese
- 1/4 cup chopped fresh parsley

Instructions

1. Begin by seasoning the beef liver with an appropriate amount of salt and pepper.
2. Heat olive oil in a large skillet over medium-high heat. Add the beef liver to the skillet and cook for approximately 2-3 minutes per side, or until it develops a desirable brown color. Proceed to remove the beef liver from the skillet and set it aside.
3. In the same skillet, incorporate the onion and bell pepper. Cook for about 3-4 minutes, or until they become softened.
4. Add the minced garlic to the skillet and cook for an additional minute.
5. Pour in the heavy cream, ensuring to stir the ingredients thoroughly for proper combination. Allow the sauce to cook for approximately 3-4 minutes, or until it reaches a desired thickened consistency.
6. Return the beef liver to the skillet and cook for an additional 2-3 minutes, or until the liver is thoroughly cooked.
7. Introduce the grated Parmesan cheese and chopped parsley into the skillet, gently stirring them into the mixture.
8. Serve the dish hot and savor its delightful flavors.

BEEF LIVER WITH VEGETABLES IN TOMATO SAUCE

Nutrition: Cal 389;Fat 16 g;Carb 17 g;Protein 38 g
Serving 2; Cook time 25 min

Ingredients

- 400g beef liver, sliced
- 1 onion, chopped
- 2 cloves garlic, minced
- 1 red bell pepper, sliced
- 1 zucchini, sliced
- 1 can (400g) diced tomatoes
- 1 tsp paprika powder
- Salt and pepper, to taste
- 2 tbsp olive oil

Instructions

1. Begin by heating olive oil in a pan over medium heat. Add onion and garlic, and sauté them until the onion turns soft and translucent.
2. Introduce the sliced beef liver to the pan and cook it for approximately 2-3 minutes on each side, ensuring it develops a pleasing brown color. Proceed by removing the liver from the pan and setting it aside.
3. Add sliced red bell pepper and zucchini to the pan, and cook them for about 5-7 minutes, or until the vegetables reach a tender consistency.
4. Incorporate canned diced tomatoes, paprika powder, salt, and pepper into the pan, ensuring they are well mixed.
5. Return the beef liver to the pan, spooning some of the tomato sauce over it.
6. Cover the pan and allow the dish to simmer for approximately 5-10 minutes, until the liver is thoroughly cooked and the sauce has thickened to a desired consistency.
7. Serve the dish hot, accompanied by a side of keto-friendly vegetables such as broccoli or cauliflower.

BEEF LIVER JAPANESE STYLE

Nutrition: Cal 292;Fat 14 g;Carb 5 g;Protein 29 g
Serving 2; Cook time 20 min

Ingredients

- 250g beef liver, sliced into thin pieces
- 1 tablespoon coconut oil
- 1 tablespoon grated ginger
- 2 cloves garlic, minced
- 1/4 cup soy sauce
- 2 tablespoons sake
- 1 tablespoon erythritol or any keto-friendly sweetener
- 1/2 teaspoon sesame oil
- 1/4 teaspoon black pepper
- 1 tablespoon green onion, chopped

Instructions

1. Combine soy sauce, sake, erythritol, sesame oil, and black pepper in a bowl. Set aside.

2. Heat coconut oil in a pan over medium-high heat.
3. Add sliced beef liver to the pan and cook for 1-2 minutes on each side until browned.
4. Add minced garlic and grated ginger to the pan and cook for another 1-2 minutes.
5. Pour in the sauce mixture and cook for 1-2 minutes until the sauce thickens.
6. Garnish with chopped green onions and serve hot.

KETO BEEF LIVER FRITTERS

Nutrition: Cal 329;Fat 24 g;Carb 7 g;Protein 20 g
Serving 2; Cook time 20 min

Ingredients
- 8 oz beef liver, chopped
- 2 tbsp almond flour
- 1 tbsp coconut flour
- 1 egg
- 1/4 cup chopped onion
- 1 clove garlic, minced
- 1/4 tsp salt
- 1/4 tsp black pepper
- 2 tbsp ghee or coconut oil

Instructions
1. In a bowl, combine the chopped beef liver, almond flour, coconut flour, egg, chopped onion, minced garlic, salt, and black pepper until thoroughly combined.
2. Heat ghee or coconut oil in a large skillet over medium heat.
3. Shape the beef liver mixture into 8 fritters and place them in the hot skillet.
4. Cook the fritters for approximately 3-4 minutes per side, or until they are browned and cooked through.
5. Serve the fritters with your choice of keto-friendly sauce or dip. Enjoy!

PANCAKES STUFFED WITH BEEF LIVER

Nutrition: Cal 486;Fat 37 g;Carb 9 g;Protein 37 g
Serving 2; Cook time 25 min

Ingredients
- 1/2 pound beef liver, chopped
- 1/2 onion, chopped
- 2 eggs, beaten
- Salt and pepper, to taste
- 1/2 cup almond flour
- 1/2 tsp baking powder
- 1/4 cup water
- 1 tbsp coconut oil

Instructions
1. In a skillet set over medium-high heat, cook the beef liver and onion until the liver is fully cooked and the onion is softened.
2. Add the beaten eggs to the skillet and scramble them until cooked through.
3. Season with salt and pepper to taste.
4. In a separate bowl, combine the almond flour, baking powder, and water, mixing until a smooth batter forms.
5. Heat coconut oil in a non-stick skillet over medium heat.
6. Pour 1/4 cup of the batter onto the skillet and spread it into a thin, round pancake shape.
7. Cook for 2-3 minutes, or until bubbles form on the surface and the edges begin to turn golden.
8. Flip the pancake and cook for an additional 1-2 minutes.
9. Repeat the process with the remaining batter to make a total of 4 pancakes.
10. Spoon the beef liver and egg mixture onto two of the pancakes.
11. Top with the remaining pancakes to create two stuffed pancakes.

BEEF LIVER GOULASH

Nutrition: Cal 297;Fat 14 g;Carb 7 g;Protein 28 g
Serving 2; Cook time 20 min

Ingredients
- 200g beef liver, sliced
- 1 onion, diced
- 1 red bell pepper, diced
- 1 tsp paprika
- 1/2 tsp caraway seeds
- 1/2 tsp garlic powder
- 1/2 cup beef broth
- 2 tbsp tomato paste
- 2 tbsp sour cream
- 1 tbsp olive oil
- Salt and pepper to taste

Instructions
1. Season the sliced beef liver with salt and pepper to your taste preference.
2. Heat a skillet over medium-high heat and add 1 tablespoon of olive oil.
3. Add the diced onion and red bell pepper to the skillet and sauté them until softened, which should take approximately 5 minutes.

4. Add the sliced beef liver to the skillet and continue sautéing for another 3-4 minutes or until the liver is browned.
5. Sprinkle paprika, caraway seeds, and garlic powder over the beef liver and vegetables in the skillet. Stir well to combine all the flavors.
6. Pour beef broth and add tomato paste to the skillet, bring the mixture to a simmer, and cook for about 5 minutes until the sauce has thickened slightly.
7. Remove the skillet from the heat, stir in sour cream to add a creamy touch to the dish, and it is ready to be served.

BEEF LIVER CASSEROLE

Nutrition: Cal 529;Fat 43 g;Carb 6 g;Protein 25 g
Serving 2; Cook time 30 min

Ingredients
- 200g beef liver, sliced
- 1 small zucchini, sliced
- 1 small yellow squash, sliced
- 1/2 cup chopped mushrooms
- 1/4 cup chopped onion
- 1/2 cup shredded cheddar cheese
- 2 tbsp butter
- 1/2 cup heavy cream
- 1 tsp garlic powder
- Salt and pepper to taste

Instructions
1. Preheat the oven to 375°F (190°C) to ensure it reaches the desired temperature for baking.
2. Season the sliced beef liver with salt and pepper according to your taste preferences.
3. Heat a skillet over medium-high heat and add 1 tablespoon of butter to melt and create a flavorful base.
4. Sauté the sliced beef liver in the skillet for approximately 3-4 minutes on each side or until nicely browned. Once done, set the beef liver aside.
5. Utilize the remaining butter in the skillet to sauté the zucchini, yellow squash, mushrooms, and onion until they become tender and have softened, which usually takes about 5 minutes.
6. Incorporate the garlic powder and heavy cream into the skillet, ensuring they are well combined with the sautéed vegetables.
7. Arrange the sliced beef liver on the bottom of a small casserole dish, creating a base for the dish.

8. Pour the sautéed vegetable mixture over the beef liver, evenly distributing it across the casserole dish. For an added touch of flavor, sprinkle shredded cheddar cheese on top.
9. Place the casserole dish in the preheated oven and bake for approximately 15-20 minutes or until the cheese has melted and turned beautifully bubbly.

BEEF LIVER WITH ZUCCHINI PANCAKES

Nutrition: Cal 482;Fat 35 g;Carb 6 g;Protein 28 g
Serving 2; Cook time 25 min

Ingredients
- 200g beef liver, sliced
- 1 small zucchini, grated
- 1 egg
- 1/4 cup almond flour
- 1/4 cup grated parmesan cheese
- 2 tbsp chopped fresh parsley
- 2 tbsp olive oil
- Salt and pepper to taste

Instructions
1. Season the sliced beef liver with salt and pepper to your desired taste.
2. Heat a skillet over medium-high heat and add 1 tablespoon of olive oil, allowing it to heat up.
3. Add the sliced beef liver to the skillet and sauté for approximately 3-4 minutes on each side, or until the liver is nicely browned. Once done, set the beef liver aside.
4. In a medium bowl, combine the grated zucchini, egg, almond flour, Parmesan cheese, parsley, and salt and pepper to taste, mixing all the ingredients thoroughly.
5. Heat another skillet over medium heat and add 1 tablespoon of olive oil to it.
6. Spoon the zucchini mixture into the skillet to form small pancakes. Cook the pancakes for about 2-3 minutes on each side or until they turn a golden brown color.
7. Serve the cooked beef liver slices alongside the zucchini pancakes, creating a delicious and nutritious meal.

VIETNAMESE BEEF LIVER

Nutrition: Cal 215;Fat 11 g;Carb 3 g;Protein 26 g
Serving 2; Cook time 20 min

Ingredients

- 200g beef liver, sliced
- 2 cloves garlic, minced
- 1 small red chili pepper, thinly sliced
- 2 tbsp fish sauce
- 2 tbsp lime juice
- 1 tsp coconut sugar
- 1 tbsp olive oil
- Salt and pepper to taste
- Fresh cilantro leaves for garnish

Instructions

1. Season the sliced beef liver with salt and pepper according to your taste preferences.
2. Heat a skillet over medium-high heat and add 1 tablespoon of olive oil, allowing it to heat up.
3. Add the sliced beef liver to the skillet and sauté for approximately 3-4 minutes on each side or until it is nicely browned. Once done, set the beef liver aside.
4. In a small bowl, whisk together minced garlic, thinly sliced chili pepper, fish sauce, lime juice, and coconut sugar, ensuring all the ingredients are well combined.
5. Pour the sauce mixture over the beef liver slices and toss them gently to coat them evenly with the flavorful sauce.
6. Serve the beef liver slices, and for an added touch, garnish them with fresh cilantro leaves to enhance their presentation and add a burst of freshness to the dish.

BEEF LIVER WITH MIXED VEGETABLES SAUTEED

Nutrition: Cal 315;Fat 18 g;Carb 28 g;Protein 10 g
Serving 2; Cook time 20 min

Ingredients

- 200g beef liver, sliced
- 1/2 head of broccoli, cut into small florets
- 2 medium carrots, peeled and sliced
- 1 small onion, chopped
- 1/2 cup green beans, trimmed
- 2 tbsp butter
- Salt and pepper to taste

Instructions

1. Begin by seasoning the sliced beef liver with salt and pepper to your preferred taste.

2. Heat a skillet over medium-high heat and add 1 tablespoon of butter, allowing it to melt and heat up.
3. Add the seasoned beef liver slices to the skillet and sauté them for approximately 3-4 minutes on each side, or until they are nicely browned. Once done, set them aside.
4. In the same skillet, add the remaining 1 tablespoon of butter and sauté the broccoli florets, sliced carrots, chopped onion, and green beans for 5-7 minutes, or until they become tender.
5. Return the sautéed beef liver slices to the skillet and heat them through with the mixed vegetables, allowing the flavors to meld together.
6. Serve the dish hot and savor the delicious combination of beef liver and vegetables. Enjoy your meal!

KETO BAKED BEEF WITH MIXED VEGETABLES

Nutrition: Cal 407;Fat 27 g;Carb 9 g;Protein 33 g
Serving 2; Cook time 35 min

Ingredients

- 300g beef (sirloin, ribeye, or other cut), sliced into 2 pieces
- 1 small yellow squash, sliced
- 1 small zucchini, sliced
- 1 small onion, sliced
- 1 small red bell pepper, sliced
- 2 cloves garlic, minced
- 2 tbsp olive oil
- Salt and pepper to taste

Instructions

1. Preheat your oven to 400°F (200°C) to ensure it reaches the desired temperature for cooking.
2. Place the sliced beef on a baking sheet, ensuring it is evenly spread out, and season it with salt and pepper according to your taste preferences.
3. In a separate bowl, combine the sliced zucchini, yellow squash, onion, red bell pepper, minced garlic, and olive oil. Mix them well together and season with salt and pepper to enhance the flavors.
4. Arrange the mixed vegetables around the beef slices on the same baking sheet, ensuring they are spread out evenly.

5. Transfer the baking sheet to the preheated oven and bake for approximately 15-20 minutes. Keep an eye on the beef to ensure it is cooked to your desired level of doneness, and check the tenderness of the vegetables. Cooking times may vary, so adjust accordingly.
6. Once cooked, remove from the oven and serve the dish hot. The combination of flavorful beef and tender vegetables will make for a delicious and satisfying meal. Enjoy!

PARMESAN-CRUSTED BEEF LIVER CUTLETS

Nutrition: Cal 368;Fat 26 g;Carb 4 g;Protein 26 g
Serving 2; Cook time 30 min

Ingredients
- 200g beef liver, sliced into cutlets
- 1/4 cup almond flour
- 1/4 cup grated parmesan cheese
- 1 tsp garlic powder
- 1 tsp dried thyme
- 1/2 tsp paprika
- 1 egg, beaten
- 2 tbsp butter
- Salt and pepper to taste
- Lemon wedges for serving

Instructions
1. In a shallow dish, combine almond flour, grated Parmesan cheese, garlic powder, dried thyme, paprika, salt, and pepper, ensuring all the ingredients are well mixed.
2. Dip each beef liver cutlet into the beaten egg, making sure to coat it thoroughly, and then coat it with the almond flour mixture, pressing gently to adhere the coating to the cutlet.
3. Heat a skillet over medium-high heat and add 2 tablespoons of butter, allowing it to melt and heat up.
4. Add the coated beef liver cutlets to the skillet and cook for approximately 2-3 minutes on each side, or until they turn a golden brown color and are cooked through.
5. Once done, serve the beef liver cutlets, accompanied by lemon wedges on the side. The tanginess of the lemon adds a refreshing touch to complement the flavors of the dish.

BEEF LIVER WITH CAULIFLOWER DEMIGLACE

Nutrition: Cal 354;Fat 23 g;Carb 8 g;Protein 28 g
Serving 2; Cook time 25 min

Ingredients
- 200g beef liver, sliced
- 1/2 head of cauliflower, cut into small florets
- 1/2 cup beef broth
- 2 tbsp butter
- 2 tbsp heavy cream
- 1 tsp arrowroot powder
- Salt and pepper to taste
- Fresh parsley for garnish

Instructions
1. Begin by seasoning the sliced beef liver with salt and pepper to your preferred taste.
2. Heat a skillet over medium-high heat and add 1 tablespoon of butter, allowing it to melt and heat up.
3. Add the seasoned beef liver slices to the skillet and sauté them for approximately 3-4 minutes on each side, or until they are nicely browned. Once done, set them aside.
4. In a separate skillet, combine the cauliflower florets and beef broth. Bring the mixture to a boil, then reduce the heat and let it simmer for 5-7 minutes until the cauliflower becomes tender.
5. Using a blender or food processor, blend the cooked cauliflower with the remaining 1 tablespoon of butter, heavy cream, and arrowroot powder until you achieve a smooth consistency.
6. Return to the same skillet used for the beef liver and add the cauliflower puree. Allow it to simmer for an additional 2-3 minutes, or until the sauce has thickened to your liking.
7. Serve the sautéed beef liver slices alongside the cauliflower demi-glace sauce, and garnish with fresh parsley for added flavor and presentation. Enjoy your dish!

KETO LEMON-ROSEMARY BEEF BAKE

Nutrition: Cal 355;Fat 23 g;Carb 4 g;Protein 32 g
Serving 2; Cook time 30 min

Ingredients

- 300g beef (sirloin, ribeye, or other cut), sliced into 2 pieces
- 2 cloves garlic, minced
- 1 lemon, juiced and zested
- 2 tbsp Dijon mustard
- 1 tbsp fresh rosemary, chopped
- 2 tbsp olive oil
- Salt and pepper to taste

Instructions

1. Preheat your oven to 400°F (200°C) to ensure it reaches the desired temperature for cooking.
2. In a small bowl, combine minced garlic, lemon juice and zest, Dijon mustard, chopped rosemary, olive oil, and salt and pepper according to your taste preferences. Mix the ingredients well to create a flavorful mustard mixture.
3. Place the sliced beef on a baking sheet, ensuring it is spread out evenly. Use a brush or spoon to spread the mustard mixture over both sides of the beef, ensuring it is coated evenly.
4. Transfer the baking sheet to the preheated oven and bake for approximately 15-20 minutes. Monitor the beef closely and adjust the cooking time according to your desired level of doneness. Cooking times may vary depending on the thickness of the beef slices.
5. Once the beef is cooked to your liking, remove it from the oven and allow it to rest for a few minutes. This resting period helps the juices redistribute and enhances the tenderness and flavor of the beef.
6. Serve the beef hot, either as individual slices or as part of a larger meal. The mustard and herb flavors will complement the beef, creating a delicious and satisfying dish. Enjoy!

KETO BEEF LIVER QUENELLE VEGETABLE SOUP

Nutrition: Cal 279;Fat 21 g;Carb 6 g;Protein 16 g
Serving 2; Cook time 30 min

Ingredients

- 400ml beef broth
- 1 small onion, chopped
- 2 garlic cloves, minced
- 1 small zucchini, chopped
- 1 small yellow squash, chopped
- 1 small carrot, chopped
- 1/2 cup green beans, chopped
- 2 tbsp olive oil
- Salt and pepper to taste

FOR THE BEEF LIVER QUENELLES:

- 100g beef liver, minced
- 1 egg
- 2 tbsp almond flour
- 1 tbsp chopped parsley
- Salt and pepper to taste

Instructions

1. In a large pot, heat the olive oil over medium heat. Add the chopped onion and garlic, and cook until softened, about 3-4 minutes. Stir occasionally to prevent burning.
2. Add the chopped zucchini, yellow squash, carrot, and green beans to the pot. Season with salt and pepper to taste, and cook for another 3-4 minutes. Stir the vegetables occasionally to ensure even cooking.
3. Pour the beef broth into the pot and bring it to a boil. Once boiling, reduce the heat to a simmer and let it cook for about 15 minutes, or until the vegetables are tender. The simmering will allow the flavors to meld together.
4. While the soup is simmering, prepare the beef liver quenelles. In a mixing bowl, combine the minced beef liver, egg, almond flour, chopped parsley, salt, and pepper. Mix everything together until well combined.
5. Using a teaspoon, shape small quenelles or meatballs from the beef liver mixture. Set them aside on a plate or cutting board.
6. Once the vegetables are tender, gently drop the beef liver quenelles into the soup. Cook for an additional 5-7 minutes, or until the quenelles are cooked through. They will float to the surface once they're done.
7. Serve the soup hot, making sure to include some vegetables and beef liver quenelles in each bowl. Enjoy the flavors and warmth of the soup!

KETO BEEF RAGOUT WITH RED WINE AND MUSHROOMS

Nutrition: Cal 388;Fat 27 g;Carb 4 g;Protein 22 g
Serving 2; Cook time 30 min

Ingredients
- 250g beef chuck, cut into bite-sized pieces
- 1 small onion, chopped
- 2 garlic cloves, minced
- 2 tbsp olive oil
- 1/2 cup red wine
- 1/2 cup beef broth
- 1/2 cup chopped mushrooms
- 1 tsp dried thyme
- Salt and pepper to taste

Instructions
1. In a large Dutch oven or heavy pot, heat the olive oil over medium-high heat. Add the chopped onion and garlic, and cook until softened, about 3-4 minutes.
2. Add the beef chuck to the pot. Season with salt and pepper to taste, and cook for about 5-7 minutes, or until browned on all sides.
3. Pour in the red wine and beef broth, and stir to combine. Add the chopped mushrooms and dried thyme, and bring to a simmer.
4. Cover the pot and reduce the heat to low. Let simmer for about 1 hour, or until the beef is tender and the sauce has thickened.
5. Serve hot, garnished with fresh herbs if desired.

KETO BEEF AND CABBAGE SKILLET

Nutrition: Cal 412;Fat 27 g;Carb 14 g;Protein 29 g
Serving 2; Cook time 35 min

Ingredients
- 1 pound of beef, thinly sliced
- 1/2 head of cabbage, chopped
- 1 small onion, chopped
- 1 medium tomato, chopped
- 2 tablespoons of olive oil
- Salt and black pepper to taste

Instructions
1. Heat a skillet over medium-high heat and add the olive oil. Once the oil is hot, add the sliced beef and season it with salt and black pepper. Cook for about 5-6 minutes, stirring occasionally, until the beef is browned on all sides. Ensure that the beef is cooked to your desired level of doneness.
2. Add the chopped onion to the skillet and stir it for 2-3 minutes until it becomes translucent and slightly softened.
3. Incorporate the chopped cabbage into the skillet and stir it to combine with the beef and onion. Cook for approximately 10-12 minutes, stirring occasionally, until the cabbage is tender and slightly caramelized. The cabbage should retain some crispness while being cooked.
4. Add the chopped tomato to the skillet and stir it to combine with the beef and cabbage. Cook for an additional 2-3 minutes until the tomato is slightly softened and starts to release its juices.
5. Serve the Keto Beef and Cabbage Skillet hot as a hearty and flavorful dish. Enjoy the combination of tender beef, caramelized cabbage, and the freshness of the tomato. This dish is low-carb and suitable for a ketogenic diet.

BEEF AND CREAM CHEESE VEGGIE ROLLS.

Nutrition: Cal 562;Fat 38 g;Carb 5 g;Protein 50 g
Serving 2; Cook time 50 min

Ingredients
- 1 beef roll (such as London broil or flank steak), pounded to a thin, even thickness
- 4 oz. cream cheese, softened
- 1/2 cup mixed vegetables (such as bell peppers, onions, and mushrooms), diced
- Salt and pepper to taste

Instructions
1. Preheat the oven to 375°F (190°C).
2. Lay the pounded beef roll flat on a work surface.
3. Spread the softened cream cheese over the beef roll, leaving a 1-inch border around the edges.
4. Sprinkle the mixed vegetables evenly over the cream cheese.
5. Season with salt and pepper to taste.
6. Starting at one end, tightly roll up the beef, tucking in the ends as you go.
7. Secure the roll with toothpicks.
8. Place the beef roll on a baking sheet and bake for 30-40 minutes, until cooked through.
9. Let the beef roll rest for 5-10 minutes before slicing and serving.

BEEF AND MUSHROOM COCONUT SOUP

Nutrition: Cal 675;Fat 54 g;Carb 14 g;Protein 35 g
Serving 2; Cook time 60 min

Ingredients

- 1 lb. beef stew meat
- 4 cups beef broth
- 1 can (14 oz.) full-fat coconut cream
- 8 oz. mushrooms, sliced
- 1/2 onion, chopped
- 2 garlic cloves, minced
- 1 can (14 oz.) diced tomatoes
- 2 tablespoons lime juice
- 2 tablespoons coconut oil
- Salt and pepper to taste

Instructions

1. In a large pot, heat the coconut oil over medium-high heat. Add the beef stew meat to the pot and cook it, stirring occasionally, until it is browned on all sides. This step helps to develop flavor and texture in the meat.
2. Add the chopped onion and garlic to the pot. Sauté them for about 2-3 minutes, until the onion becomes translucent and the garlic becomes fragrant. Stir them occasionally to prevent burning.
3. Pour in the beef broth, covering the meat and onions. Bring the mixture to a boil.
4. Reduce the heat to low and let the soup simmer for 30-40 minutes. This allows the beef to become tender and infuses the flavors of the broth and aromatics.
5. Add the sliced mushrooms to the pot and cook for an additional 5-7 minutes, or until the mushrooms are tender. Stir them occasionally as they cook.
6. Stir in the diced tomatoes and lime juice, and cook for an additional 5-10 minutes, until heated through. This adds brightness and acidity to the soup.
7. Finally, stir in the coconut cream and cook for an additional 5-10 minutes, until heated through. The coconut cream adds richness and a creamy texture to the soup.
8. Taste the soup and season with salt and pepper to your liking. Adjust the seasoning as needed.
9. Divide the soup into two bowls and serve it hot. Enjoy the flavorful and comforting beef stew with the added richness of coconut cream.

GROUND BEEF AND CABBAGE STIR-FRY

Nutrition: Cal 550;Fat 33 g;Carb 13 g;Protein 49 g
Serving 4; Cook time 35 min

Ingredients

- 1 tablespoon coconut oil
- 1½ pounds ground beef
- 2 garlic cloves, minced
- 1 green cabbage head, cored and chopped
- 2 tablespoons coconut aminos
- 2 tablespoons apple cider vinegar
- Salt
- Freshly ground black pepper
- 4 scallions, both white and green parts, chopped
- Sesame seeds (optional)
- Sriracha (optional)
- Toasted sesame oil (optional)

Instructions

1. In a large skillet, heat the oil over medium heat. Add the beef and garlic to the skillet and cook, stirring occasionally, until the beef is browned. This usually takes about 5 to 7 minutes.
2. Add the cabbage to the skillet with the beef and continue to cook. Stir the mixture occasionally and cook until the cabbage becomes slightly wilted. This usually takes about 8 to 10 minutes.
3. Once the cabbage is wilted, add the coconut aminos and vinegar to the skillet. Season with salt and pepper to taste. Stir everything together to combine the flavors and allow the ingredients to simmer for a few more minutes.
4. Taste the dish and adjust the seasonings as needed. You can add more salt, pepper, or any other desired seasonings to enhance the flavor.
5. Remove the skillet from the heat and transfer the beef and cabbage mixture to a serving dish.
6. Serve hot and enjoy your flavorful beef and cabbage dish!

BACON CHEESEBURGER SOUP

Nutrition: Cal 315;Fat 20 g;Carb 6 g;Protein 27 g
Serving 4; Cook time 25 min

Ingredients:

- 4 slices uncooked bacon
- 8 ounces ground beef (80% lean)
- 1 medium yellow onion, chopped
- 1 clove garlic, minced
- 3 cups beef broth
- 2 tablespoons tomato paste

- 2 teaspoons Dijon mustard
- Salt and pepper
- 1 cup shredded lettuce
- ½ cup shredded cheddar cheese

Instructions:

1. Cook the bacon in a saucepan until crisp. Drain the bacon on paper towels and chop it into small pieces.
2. Reheat the bacon fat in the saucepan and add the beef. Cook the beef until it is browned.
3. Drain away half of the fat from the saucepan.
4. Reheat the saucepan and add the onion and garlic. Cook for about 6 minutes until the onion becomes translucent.
5. Stir in the broth, tomato paste, and mustard. Season with salt and pepper to taste.
6. Add the beef back into the saucepan and simmer on medium-low heat for 15 minutes, covered.
7. Spoon the beef mixture into bowls and top with shredded lettuce, cheddar cheese, and the cooked bacon.

BRAISED LAMB SHANKS

Nutrition: Cal 365;Fat 21 g;Carb 6 g;Protein 35 g
Serving 4; Cook time 3 hours 20 min

Ingredients:

- 4 lamb shanks (1.6 кg/ 3.5 кg) - will yield about 60% meat
- 1 tsp sea salt
- 1/2 tsp black pepper
- 2 tbsp virgin avocado oil (30 ml)
- 1 medium red onion, diced (85 g/ 3 oz)
- 4 cloves garlic, minced
- 1 medium carrot, sliced (60 g/ 2.1 oz)
- 3 celery stalks, sliced (120 g/ 4.2 oz)
- 2 cups dry red wine (480 ml/ 16 fl oz)
- 2 cups chicken stock (480 ml/ 16 fl oz)
- 2 cinnamon sticks or 1/2 tsp cinnamon
- 2 bay leaves
- 4 sprigs rosemary

Instructions:

1. Preheat the oven to 160 °C/320 °F (fan assisted) or 180 °C/355 °F (conventional). Season the lamb shanks with salt and pepper.
2. Peel and dice the onion, mince the garlic, peel and slice the carrot, and chop the celery.
3. Grease a large casserole dish with avocado oil or ghee. Add the lamb shanks and cook on high heat from all sides for a few minutes until browned.
4. Once browned, transfer the lamb to a plate. Browning the lamb will add fantastic flavor! (Note: If you're planning to make these in a slow cooker, check the recipe tips in the post above.)
5. Add the onion and cook for about 3 to 5 minutes, frequently scraping the bottom of the pan to combine with the browned juices from the lamb. Add the garlic, carrot, and celery, stir again, and cook for a minute.
6. Pour in the wine and stock. Add the cinnamon (you can use 2 cinnamon sticks or 1/2 tsp ground cinnamon), bay leaves, and rosemary.
7. Place in the oven and cook for 2 1/2 to 3 hours. Once baked, remove from the oven, remove the lid, and let it cool down for a few minutes.
8. This braised lamb is best served with cauliflower mash. Try it with Keto Creamy Cauliflower Mash, Cauliflower Mash with Roasted Garlic & Thyme, or Keto Celeriac Cauli-Mash.
9. To store, let it cool down and refrigerate for up to 4 days. The cooked meat can also be frozen in a sealed container for up to 3 months.

KETO LAMB CURRY WITH SPINACH

Nutrition: Cal 497;Fat 18 g;Carb 8 g;Protein 62 g
Serving 2; Cook time 4 hours

Ingredients:

- 1 medium Red onion (quartered and sliced)
- 2 clove(s) Garlic
- 2 tbsp minced Ginger root
- 2 tsp Cardamom, ground
- 6 clove Cloves (whole)
- 2 tsp Coriander, ground (ground)
- 1 tsp Turmeric, powder
- 1/2 tsp Chili powder
- 1 tsp Garam masala
- 2 tsp Cumin
- 500 gm Lamb, cubed for stew, lean
- 1 can(s) (14oz) Diced tomatoes, canned
- 500 gm Spinach (fresh)

Instructions:

1. Place all the ingredients in the slow cooker (except for the spinach) and stir.

2. Cook on HIGH for 4-5 hours or LOW for 8 hours.
3. Mix in the spinach right before serving, allowing the heat to wilt it.

KETO LAMB ROAST WITH CHIMICHURRI SAUCE

Nutrition: Cal 573;Fat 46 g;Carb 2 g;Protein 32 g
Serving 2; Cook time 4 hours

Ingredients:
- 1 medium Red onion (quartered and sliced)
- 2 clove(s) Garlic
- 2 tbsp minced Ginger root
- 2 tsp Cardamom, ground
- 6 clove Cloves (whole)
- 2 tsp Coriander, ground (ground)
- 1 tsp Turmeric, powder
- 1/2 tsp Chili powder
- 1 tsp Garam masala
- 2 tsp Cumin
- 500 gm Lamb, cubed for stew, lean
- 1 can(s) (14oz) Diced tomatoes, canned
- 500 gm Spinach (fresh)

CHIMICHURRI SAUCE
- 2 cups fresh parsley leaves and tender stems
- 2 Tbsp fresh oregano leaves
- 1 medium jalapeño, halved and seeded
- 1/2 tsp crushed red pepper flakes
- 1 garlic clove
- 3/4 cup extra-virgin olive oil
- ~ sea salt and freshly ground black pepper
- 2 Tbsp red wine vinegar

Instructions:
1. In a small bowl, combine the rosemary, garlic powder, salt, and pepper. Add the butter and mix to make a paste. Thoroughly coat the lamb with the garlic-herb paste, rubbing it into the meat with your hands to completely coat. Place the roast in a zip-lock bag and chill for 2 hours or overnight.
2. Heat the oven to 375°F (190°C). Put the lamb on a rack in a roasting pan and roast until an instant-read thermometer registers 130°F (55°C) for rare or 140°F (60°C) for medium-rare, for about 1 3/4 to 2 hours. Tent the lamb with foil for the last hour of cooking to prevent it from getting too brown. Let the meat rest for 20 minutes (or up to 45 minutes) before slicing.

3. Slice the lamb thinly and serve it with a side of chimichurri sauce.

KETO LAMB ROAST WITH CHIMICHURRI SAUCE

Nutrition: Cal 573;Fat 46 g;Carb 2 g;Protein 32 g
Serving 2; Cook time 4 hours

Ingredients:
- 1 medium Red onion (quartered and sliced)
- 2 clove(s) Garlic
- 2 tbsp minced Ginger root
- 2 tsp Cardamom, ground
- 6 clove Cloves (whole)
- 2 tsp Coriander, ground (ground)
- 1 tsp Turmeric, powder
- 1/2 tsp Chili powder
- 1 tsp Garam masala
- 2 tsp Cumin
- 500 gm Lamb, cubed for stew, lean
- 1 can(s) (14oz) Diced tomatoes, canned
- 500 gm Spinach (fresh)

CHIMICHURRI SAUCE
- 2 cups fresh parsley leaves and tender stems
- 2 Tbsp fresh oregano leaves
- 1 medium jalapeño, halved and seeded
- 1/2 tsp crushed red pepper flakes
- 1 garlic clove
- 3/4 cup extra-virgin olive oil
- ~ sea salt and freshly ground black pepper
- 2 Tbsp red wine vinegar

Instructions:
4. In a small bowl, combine the rosemary, garlic powder, salt, and pepper. Add the butter and mix to make a paste. Thoroughly coat the lamb with the garlic-herb paste, rubbing it into the meat with your hands to completely coat. Place the roast in a zip-lock bag and chill for 2 hours or overnight.
5. Heat the oven to 375°F (190°C). Put the lamb on a rack in a roasting pan and roast until an instant-read thermometer registers 130°F (55°C) for rare or 140°F (60°C) for medium-rare, for about 1 3/4 to 2 hours. Tent the lamb with foil for the last hour of cooking to prevent it from getting too brown. Let the meat rest for 20 minutes (or up to 45 minutes) before slicing.
6. Slice the lamb thinly and serve it with a side of chimichurri sauce.

BEEF AND PEPPER KEBABS

Nutrition: Cal 365;Fat 21 g;Carb 6 g;Protein 35 g
Serving 2; Cook time 40 min

Ingredients:
- 2 tablespoons olive oil
- 1 ½ tablespoons balsamic vinegar
- 2 teaspoons Dijon mustard
- Salt and pepper
- 8 ounces beef sirloin, cut into 2-inch pieces
- 1 small red pepper, cut into chunks
- 1 small green pepper, cut into chunks

Instructions:
1. Whisk together the olive oil, balsamic vinegar, and mustard in a shallow dish to make the marinade.
2. Season the steak with salt and pepper, then toss it in the marinade.
3. Let the steak marinate for 30 minutes, allowing the flavors to infuse. Then, slide the steak onto skewers with the peppers.
4. Preheat a grill pan to high heat and grease it with cooking spray.
5. Cook the kebabs for 2 to 3 minutes on each side until the beef reaches your desired doneness.

SLOW-COOKER BEEF CHILI

Nutrition: Cal 395; Fat 20 g; Carb 12 g; Protein 42 g
Serving 4; Cook time 6 hours

Ingredients:
- 1 tablespoon coconut oil
- 1 medium yellow onion, chopped
- 3 cloves garlic, minced
- 1 pound ground beef (80% lean)
- 1 small red pepper, chopped
- 1 small green pepper, chopped
- 1 cup diced tomatoes
- 1 cup low-carb tomato sauce
- 1 tablespoon chili powder
- 2 teaspoons dried oregano
- 1 ½ teaspoons dried basil
- Salt and pepper
- ¾ cup shredded cheddar cheese
- ½ cup diced red onion

Instructions:
1. Heat the oil in a skillet over medium-high heat.
2. Add the onions and sauté for 4 minutes, then stir in the garlic and cook for an additional minute.
3. Stir in the beef and cook until it is browned. Drain some of the fat if desired.
4. Spoon the mixture into a slow cooker and add the spices.
5. Cover and cook on low heat for 5 to 6 hours, allowing the flavors to meld together.
6. Spoon the chili into bowls and serve with shredded cheddar cheese and diced red onion as desired.

KETO MONGOLIAN BEEF

Nutrition: Cal 350;Fat 14 g; Carb 17 g;Protein 30 g
Serving 4; Cook time 25 min

Ingredients
- 1 Tablespoon avocado oil
- 2 teaspoons Minced ginger
- 1 Tablespoon Minced garlic
- 1/2 Cup Soy sauce or Coconut aminos
- 1/2 cup Water
- 3/4 cup Granulated sweetener
- 1 1/2 pounds Flank steak or Flatiron steak
- 1/4 teaspoon Red pepper flakes
- 5 Stems Green onions-cut diagonal into 2 inch pieces
- 1/4 teaspoon xanthan gum

Instructions
MAKING THE SAUCE:
1. Heat 1 tablespoon Avocado Oil in a medium saucepan over medium heat.
2. Add ginger, garlic, red pepper flakes and stir for 30 seconds.
3. Add soy sauce, water and sweetener. Bring to a boil and simmer until thickened. Should take about 5 minutes.
4. Remove from skillet to a bowl and set aside.

FOR THE STEAK:
1. Slice flank steak against the grain into 1/4 inch slices with the knife held at a 45 degree angle. Some of the really long pieces I cut in half to make them more bite-sized.
2. Heat avocado oil in skillet over medium-high heat.
3. Add beef (may need to cook in 2 batches) and cook 2-3 minutes, until brown, flipping pieces over to cook both sides.
4. Add the sauce to the pan along with the xantham gum and cook over medium heat for a few minute, Stirring to coat meat.
5. Add green onions and remove from heat.

GROUND BEEF AND CABBAGE STIR-FRY

Nutrition: Cal 550;Fat 33 g;Carb 13 g;Protein 49 g
Serving 4; Cook time 35 min

Ingredients
- 1 tablespoon coconut oil
- 1½ pounds ground beef
- 2 garlic cloves, minced
- 1 green cabbage head, cored and chopped
- 2 tablespoons coconut aminos
- 2 tablespoons apple cider vinegar
- Salt
- Freshly ground black pepper
- 4 scallions, both white and green parts, chopped
- Sesame seeds (optional)
- Sriracha (optional)
- Toasted sesame oil (optional)

Instructions
1. In a large skillet, heat the oil over medium heat.
2. Cook the beef and garlic in the skillet until the beef is browned, which usually takes around 5 to 7 minutes.
3. Add the cabbage to the skillet and continue cooking until the cabbage becomes slightly wilted. This usually takes around 8 to 10 minutes.
4. Stir in the coconut aminos and vinegar, and season with salt and pepper according to your taste.

KETO BACON CHEESEBURGER WRAPS

Nutrition: Cal 267;Fat 20 g; Carb 4 g;Protein 19 g
Serving 4; Cook time 30 min

Ingredients
- 7 oz. bacon
- 4 oz. mushrooms, sliced
- 1½ lbs ground beef or ground turkey
- ½ tsp salt
- ¼ tsp pepper
- 1 cup (4 oz.) shredded cheddar cheese
- 1 butterhead lettuce, leaves separated and washed
- 8 (5 oz.) cherry tomatoes, sliced

Instructions
1. Heat a large skillet over medium heat and add the bacon. Cook the bacon for about 15 minutes, or until it becomes crispy. Once crispy, remove the bacon from the pan and set it aside.

2. In the same skillet, with the bacon fat still present, increase the heat to medium-high. Add the mushrooms and sauté them for about 5 to 7 minutes, or until they are browned and tender. Set the mushrooms aside.
3. Add the ground beef, salt, and pepper to the skillet. Sauté the beef, using the back of a wooden spoon to break up any chunks, for about 10 minutes, or until it is evenly browned.
4. To serve, spoon the ground beef onto the lettuce leaves and layer the cheddar cheese, bacon, mushrooms, and tomatoes on top.

MEATBALLS IN TOMATO SAUCE

Nutrition: Cal 388;Fat 27 g; Carb 11 g;Protein 23 g
Serving 8; Cook time 25 min

Ingredients
FOR MEATBALLS
- Ground beef (2 lbs)
- Eggs (2)
- Garlic (3 cloves)
- Oregano (dry, 2 teaspoons)
- Salt (1 along with a half teaspoon)
- Pepper (1 teaspoon)
- Onion powder (2 teaspoons)

FOR THE TOMATO SAUCE
- Coconut oil (2 teaspoons)
- Garlic (2 cloves)
- Tomatoes (grated or blended, around 30 oz.)
- Onion (1, chopped)
- Water (¼ cup)
- Tomato paste (2 tbsp)
- Salt (2 teaspoons)

Instructions
1. Start by mixing the ingredients for the meatballs together in a bowl. Make sure they are well combined.
2. Take portions of the meat mixture and roll them into small balls. Set them aside.
3. Set your pressure cooker to the "Sauté" function and add coconut oil (or avocado oil) to the pot.
4. Add the garlic and onion to the pot and sauté for about 5 minutes, stirring occasionally, until the onion becomes tender.
5. Press the "Cancel" button on the pressure cooker. Add the broth, grated tomatoes, tomato paste, and salt to the pot. Place the meatballs into the sauce, ensuring they are well covered.
6. Close the pressure cooker and seal the pressure valve. Set it to the "Manual" setting and cook the meatballs for 7 minutes.

7. Once the cooking time is complete, allow the pressure to release naturally for 10 minutes.
8. Serve the meatballs with pasta, vegetables, or enjoy them on their own.

POMEGRANATE MOLASSES ROASTED CHUCK

Nutrition: Cal 466 ;Fat 32 g; Carb 3 g;Protein 37 g
Serving 10; Cook time 55 min

Ingredients
- 3 lbs chuck steak, boneless
- 2 tsp salt
- 1 ½ tsp freshly grounded black pepper
- 1 ¼ tsp garlic powder
- 1 tbsp pomegranate molasses
- 2 tbsp balsamic vinegar
- 1 onion, finely chopped
- 2 cups regular water
- ½ tsp xanthan gum (it is possible to use 1 tsp of Agar Agar if unavailable)
- 1/3 cup fresh parsley, finely chopped

Instructions
1. Begin by slicing the meat in half on a cutting board. Season each half with salt, pepper, and garlic powder.
2. Place the Instant Pot on the stovetop and select the "Sauté" mode.
3. Add the seasoned meat to the pot and cook until it is browned on both sides.
4. Once the meat has browned, add the remaining ingredients, including pomegranate molasses, balsamic vinegar, onion, and half of the water.
5. Cover the pot and set the timer for 35 minutes.
6. After the cooking time has elapsed, manually release the pressure by pressing the "venting" function.
7. Remove the lid once all the pressure has been released. Transfer the meat to a cutting board and remove any excess fat or debris. Slice the meat into large pieces.
8. Simmer the sauce that remains in the pot by setting the pot to "sauté" mode. Allow it to simmer for 10 minutes or until the liquid has reduced.
9. Stir in the xanthan gum to thicken the sauce, then return the meat to the pot and stir to coat it in the sauce.
10. Turn off the heat and transfer the meat to a serving plate. Drizzle the sauce over the meat and garnish with parsley. Serve hot.

SPICY MINCED LAMB WITH PEAS AND TOMATO SAUCE

Nutrition: Cal 242 ;Fat 12 g; Carb 10 g;Protein 24 g
Serving 6; Cook time 55 min

Ingredients
- 2 lbs ground lamb
- 3 tbsp ghee
- 1 onion, finely chopped
- 5 cloves garlic, crushed
- 1 tsp ground ginger
- 1 Serrano pepper, chopped
- 2 tsp ground coriander
- 1 tsp red pepper flakes
- 1 tsp Kosher salt
- ½ tsp turmeric powder
- ¾ tsp freshly ground black pepper
- ½ tsp chat masala
- ¾ tsp ground cumin
- ¼ tsp cayenne powder
- 2 cardamom pods, shell removed
- 1 can diced tomatoes
- 1 can peas
- Fresh cilantro, finely chopped

Instructions
1. Place the Instant Pot over medium heat and select the "Sauté" function. Add the ghee and onion to the pot. Stir until the onion becomes tender.
2. Stir in the ginger, garlic, and spices. Cook for 3 minutes, then add the minced meat to the pot.
3. Stir the meat until it is browned and well coated with the spices.
4. Add the tomatoes and peas to the pot. Cover the pot and set it to "Keep Warm" mode. Choose the "Bean/Chili" option.
5. When the cooking time is complete, release the pressure from the pot. Set the pot back to "Sauté" mode and allow the liquid to simmer for ten minutes until reduced.
6. Transfer the meat to a serving bowl, sprinkle fresh cilantro on top, and serve hot.

ROASTED LAMB SHANKS WITH VEGETABLES

Nutrition: Cal 422 ;Fat 20 g; Carb 35 g;Protein 48 g
Serving 4; Cook time 65 min

Ingredients
•4 lbs lamb shanks
•2 tsp salt
•1 tsp freshly ground black pepper
•3 tbsp ghee
•3 carrots, diced
•3 celery stalks, sliced
•1 large onion, diced
•2 tbsp tomato paste
•4 cloves garlic, minced
•1 can diced tomatoes
•1 1/3 cup bone broth
•2 tsp fish sauce (optional)
•1 ½ tbsp balsamic vinegar
•½ cup fresh parsley, finely chopped

Instructions
1. Season the lamb with salt and pepper on both sides.
2. Place the Instant Pot over medium heat and select the "Sauté" mode. Add the ghee to the pot and stir until melted. Add the lamb and brown it for a few minutes.
3. Transfer the browned lamb to a plate. Add the vegetables to the pot and sauté them for a few minutes. Season with salt and pepper.
4. Stir in the tomato paste and garlic for a minute. Return the lamb to the pot and add the diced tomatoes.
5. Pour in the broth, fish sauce, and vinegar.
6. Cover the pot, press "Cancel/Keep Warm," and manually set the timer for 45 minutes. Lower the temperature after the first 5 minutes.
7. When the cooking time ends, release the pressure.
8. Transfer the cooked lamb to a serving platter and pour the remaining sauce over the meat. Garnish with fresh parsley and serve hot.

BARACOA-STYLE SHREDDED BEEF

Nutrition: Cal 435 ;Fat 31 g; Carb 4.5 g;Protein 31 g
Serving 12; Cook time 75 min

Ingredients
•3 lbs minced beef
•2 cups bread crumbs
•4 eggs
•1 tsp salt
•1 tsp freshly ground black pepper
•1 tsp garlic powder
•4 oz mozzarella cheese, sliced
•¼ cup fresh basil, finely chopped
•1 cup beef broth
•¼ cup light brown sugar
•½ cup ketchup
•2 tbsp Dijon mustard
•1 tbsp Worcestershire sauce

Instructions
1. Trim any excess body fat from the meat and cut it into 4 large pieces. Season both sides of the meat with salt and pepper.
2. Place the Instant Pot over medium heat and add one tablespoon of olive oil. Cook the meat in two batches until browned, for a couple of minutes per side.
3. Meanwhile, in a food processor, blend together the onion, vinegar, lime juice, garlic, peppers, broth, cumin, cloves, and tomato paste until smooth and free of lumps.
4. Pour the blended mixture into the Instant Pot with the meat and add the bay leaves.
5. Cover the pot and set it to the "Beef/Stew" setting for one hour.
6. Once the cooking time is complete, manually release the pressure and uncover the pot.
7. Transfer the meat to a cutting board and use two forks to shred it.
8. Discard the bay leaves and return the shredded meat to the pot. Cover the pot and allow the meat to sit for 10 minutes.
9. Serve the shredded meat as a filling for tortilla wraps, tacos, or sandwiches, and enjoy it with your favorite sauce.

AVOCADO BEEF CHILI WITH COCONUT YOGURT

Nutrition: Cal 366 ;Fat 8.5 g; Carb 90 g;Protein 55 g
Serving 8; Cook time 25 min

Ingredients
- 2 tbsp avocado oil
- 1 onion, finely chopped
- 1 red bell pepper, diced
- 1 tsp salt
- 3 tbsp tomato paste
- 5 garlic cloves, crushed
- 3 lbs ground beef
- 4 tsp chili powder
- 2 tsp dried oregano
- 2 tsp ground cumin
- ½ tsp red pepper flakes
- 1 can roasted diced tomatoes
- 1/3 cup bone broth
- 1 tbsp fish sauce
- 2 tsp apple cider vinegar
- 1 ripe avocado, cubed
- 2 scallion, sliced
- 1/3 cup fresh parsley
- ½ cup coconut yogurt
- 1 lime, cut into wedges

Instructions
1. Place the Instant Pot over medium heat and set it on "Sauté". Heat the avocado oil and stir in the onions and peppers. Season with salt and sauté for a couple of minutes until tender.
2. Add the tomato paste and crushed garlic to the pot.
3. Stir in the ground beef, season with more salt, and mix using a wooden spoon for 6 minutes.
4. Season the meat with chili powder, oregano, cumin, and red pepper flakes.
5. Drain the tomatoes and stir them into the meat. Pour in the broth, fish sauce, and vinegar.
6. Cover the pot and set it to "Pressure Cook". Manually set the time for 15 minutes.
7. Once the time is up, manually release the pressure and remove the lid.
8. To serve, transfer the chili to serving bowls, top with avocado, scallions, and a dollop of coconut yogurt. Garnish with fresh parsley and serve with lime wedges.

SPARE RIBS WITH CURRY SAUCE

Nutrition: Cal 522 ;Fat 23 g; Carb 15 g;Protein 71 g
Serving 4; Cook time 45 min

Ingredients
- 3 lbs lamb spare ribs
- 2 tbsp salt, divided
- 2 tbsp freshly ground black pepper
- 2 tbsp curry powder, divided
- 3 tsp coconut oil
- 1 onion, pureed
- 4 ripe tomatoes, pureed
- 5 cloves garlic, crushed
- Juice of 1 lemon
- 1 bunch fresh cilantro, finely chopped
- 5 scallion, finely chopped

Instructions
1. Start by seasoning the ribs with one tablespoon of salt, pepper, and curry powder.
2. Place the ribs in a shallow dish and cover them. Refrigerate overnight.
3. To cook the ribs, put the Instant Pot over medium heat. Melt the oil in the pot and add in half of the ribs. You want to prepare them in batches so that they're cooked evenly.
4. Once the ribs have browned on each side, transfer them to a plate and repeat with the remaining half.
5. When the next batch of ribs is browned, transfer them to a plate and stir in the crushed garlic. Stir for half a minute. Add the pureed tomato and onion. Add the remaining salt and pepper, lemon juice, and half of the cilantro.
6. Bring the sauce to a boil and add the ribs back into the pot. Cover the pot and turn down the heat. Set the timer for 20 minutes. Once the time is up, allow the pressure to be released naturally.
7. To serve, transfer the ribs onto a serving platter and garnish with scallion and cilantro. Serve hot.

RED PEPPER FLAKES BEEF RIBS WITH RICE

Nutrition: Cal 537 ;Fat 24 g; Carb 7g;Protein 67 g
Serving 6; Cook time 45 min

Ingredients
- 3 lbs beef short ribs, boneless
- 2 tbsp red pepper flakes
- 2 tsp salt
- 2 tbsp butter
- 1 onion, finely chopped
- 2 tbsp tomato paste
- 5 garlic cloves, minced
- 2/3 cup roasted tomato salsa (accessible in supermarkets)
- 2/3 cup beef broth
- 1 tsp fish sauce
- ½ tsp freshly ground black pepper
- 1 small bunch fresh cilantro, finely chopped

Instructions
1. On a cutting board, cut the meat into cubes or slices. Place the meat into a bowl and add the red pepper flakes and salt.
2. Place the Instant Pot over medium heat, set on "Sauté," and melt the butter. Stir in the onion and keep stirring until it becomes translucent.
3. Add the tomato paste, garlic, and salsa. Stir for a minute.
4. Drop the meat into the pot and pour in the broth and fish sauce. Stir to combine.
5. Cover the pot and set it on "Keep Warm" and "Meat/Stew" mode. Let it cook for about half an hour.
6. Once the time is up, allow the pressure to be released naturally.
7. Meanwhile, cook the rice according to the instructions on the package.
8. To serve, put the rice into a serving bowl and top it with the meat. Drizzle with the meat sauce and garnish with fresh cilantro.

BEEF AND PASTA CASSEROLE

Nutrition: Cal 182 ;Fat 5.3 g; Carb 28 g;Protein 14 g
Serving 4; Cook time 30 min

Ingredients
- 17 ounces pasta
- 1 pound beef, ground
- 13 ounces mozzarella cheese, shredded
- 16 ounces tomato puree
- 1 celery stalk, chopped
- 1 yellow onion, chopped
- 1 carrot, chopped
- 1 tbsp dark wine
- 2 tbsp butter
- Salt and black pepper to taste

Instructions
1. Set your Instant Pot to the Sauté mode and add the butter, allowing it to melt.
2. Add carrots, onions, and celery to the pot and sauté for 5 minutes.
3. Incorporate the beef, salt, and pepper, and continue cooking for an additional 10 minutes.
4. Pour in the wine while stirring the ingredients, and cook for another minute.
5. Add pasta, tomato puree, and enough water to cover the pasta. Stir the mixture, cover the Instant Pot, and set it to cook on High pressure for 6 minutes.
6. Safely release the pressure, uncover the pot, and add cheese. Stir well to melt the cheese into the dish. Serve and enjoy.

KOREAN HOT BEEF SALAD

Nutrition: Cal 310 ;Fat 9 g; Carb 18 g;Protein 35 g
Serving 4 Cook time 35 min

Ingredients
- ¼ cup Korean soybean paste
- 1 cup chicken stock
- 2 pounds beef steak, cut into thin strips
- ¼ tsp red pepper flakes
- Salt and black pepper to taste
- 1 yellow onion, thinly sliced
- 1 zucchini, cubed
- 1 ounce shiitake mushroom caps, cut into quarters
- 12 ounces extra firm tofu, cubed
- 1 chili pepper, sliced
- 1 scallion, chopped

Instructions
1. Set your Instant Pot to the Sauté mode and add stock and soybean paste. Stir and simmer for two minutes.
2. Add beef, salt, pepper, and pepper flakes. Stir the ingredients, cover the Instant Pot, and cook on High pressure for fifteen minutes.

3. Quickly release the pressure, then add tofu, onion, zucchini, and mushrooms. Stir the mixture, bring it to a boil, cover the Instant Pot again, and cook on High pressure for an additional 4 minutes.

4. Release the pressure once more, adjust the salt and pepper to taste, and add chili and scallions. Stir everything together well. Ladle the dish into bowls and serve.

BEEF BOURGUIGNON

Nutrition: Cal 442 ;Fat 17 g; Carb 16 g;Protein 39 g
Serving 6; Cook time 45 min

Ingredients
- 5 pounds round steak, cut into small cubes
- 2 carrots, sliced
- ½ cup beef stock
- 1 cup dry burgandy or merlot wine
- 3 bacon slices, chopped
- 8 ounces mushrooms, cut into quarters
- 2 tbsp white flour
- 12 pearl onions
- 2 garlic cloves, minced
- ¼ tsp basil, dried
- Salt and black pepper to taste

Instructions
1. Set your Instant Pot to the Sauté mode and add bacon, allowing it to brown for 2 minutes.
2. Incorporate the beef pieces and stir, ensuring they brown evenly for 5 minutes.
3. Introduce flour into the mixture, stirring thoroughly to combine.
4. Season with salt, pepper, wine, stock, onions, garlic, and basil. Stir the ingredients together, cover the Instant Pot, and set it to cook on High pressure for a duration of 20 minutes.
5. Safely release the pressure, uncover the pot, and add mushrooms and carrots. Recover the pot and continue cooking on High pressure for an additional 5 minutes.
6. Once again, release the pressure, and carefully transfer the flavorful beef bourguignon onto plates using a spoon. Serve and enjoy.

CHINESE BEEF AND BROCCOLI

Nutrition: Cal 310 ;Fat 9 g; Carb 18 g;Protein 35 g
Serving 4 Cook time 20 min

Ingredients
- 3 pounds chuck roast, cut into thin strips
- 1 tbsp peanut oil
- 1 yellow onion, chopped
- ½ cup beef stock
- 1 pound broccoli florets
- 2 tsp toasted sesame oil
- 2 tbsp potato starch

For the marinade:
- ½ cup soy sauce
- ½ cup black soy sauce
- 1 tbsp sesame oil
- 2 tbsp fish sauce
- 5 garlic cloves, minced
- 3 red peppers, dried and crushed
- ½ tsp Chinese five spice
- White rice, already cooked for servings
- Toasted sesame seeds for serving

Instructions
1. In a bowl, combine black soy sauce, soy sauce, fish sauce, 1 tablespoon of sesame oil, 5 garlic cloves, five spice, and crushed red peppers. Stir the ingredients together until well mixed.
2. Add beef strips to the bowl and toss them to coat them evenly with the marinade. Let the beef marinate for ten minutes.
3. Set your Instant Pot to the Sauté mode and add peanut oil. Heat the oil in the pot.
4. Add onions to the pot, stir, and fry them for 4 minutes.
5. Add the marinated beef and its marinade to the pot. Stir the mixture and cook for 2 minutes.
6. Pour in the stock, stir everything together, cover the Instant Pot, and cook on High pressure for 5 minutes.
7. Allow the pressure to release naturally for ten minutes. Then, uncover the Instant Pot and add a cornstarch paste made by mixing ¼ cup of liquid from the pot with cornstarch until smooth. Place broccoli in the steamer basket, cover the pot again, and cook for 3 minutes on High pressure.
8. Release the pressure again and serve the beef in bowls on top of rice. Add the broccoli on the side, drizzle toasted sesame oil over the contents of the bowls, sprinkle sesame seeds, and enjoy this delicious Chinese meal.

MERLOT LAMB SHANKS

Nutrition: Cal 430 ;Fat 17 g; Carb 11 g;Protein 50 g
Serving 4 Cook time 45 min

Ingredients
- 4 lamb shanks
- 2 tbsp extra virgin organic olive oil
- 2 tbsp white flour
- 1 yellow onion, finely chopped
- 3 carrots, roughly chopped
- 2 garlic cloves, minced
- 2 tbsp tomato paste
- 1 tsp oregano, dried
- 1 tomato, roughly chopped
- 2 tbsp water
- 4 ounces red Merlot wine
- Salt and black pepper to taste
- 1 beef bouillon cube

Instructions
1. In a bowl, combine flour with salt and pepper.
2. Add lamb shanks to the bowl and toss them to coat them with the flour mixture.
3. Set your Instant Pot to the Sauté mode, add oil, and heat it up.
4. Add the coated lamb shanks to the pot and brown them on all sides. Once browned, transfer the lamb shanks to a bowl.
5. Add onions, oregano, carrots, and garlic to the pot. Stir and cook for 5 minutes.
6. Add tomatoes, tomato paste, water, wine, and a bouillon cube to the pot. Stir everything together and bring it to a boil.
7. Return the lamb shanks to the pot, cover it, and cook on High pressure for 25 minutes.
8. Release the pressure and place one lamb shank on each plate. Pour the cooking sauce over the lamb shanks and serve with seasonal vegetables.

MOROCCAN LAMB

Nutrition: Cal 434 ;Fat 21 g; Carb 41 g;Protein 20 g
Serving 6 Cook time 35 min

Ingredients
- 2 ½ pounds lamb shoulder, chopped
- 3 tbsp honey
- 3 ounces almonds, peeled and chopped
- 9 ounces prunes, pitted
- 8 ounces vegetable stock
- 2 yellow onions, chopped
- 2 garlic cloves, minced
- 1 bay leaf
- Salt and black pepper to tastes
- 1 cinnamon stick
- 1 tsp cumin powder
- 1 tsp turmeric powder
- 1 tsp ginger powder
- 1 tsp cinnamon powder
- Sesame seeds for servings
- 3 tbsp extra virgin organic olive oil

Instructions
1. In a bowl, combine cinnamon powder, ginger, cumin, turmeric, garlic, and 2 tablespoons of extra virgin olive oil. Stir well to mix.
2. Add the meat to the bowl and toss to coat it with the spice mixture.
3. Place the prunes in a separate bowl, cover them with hot water, and set aside.
4. Set your Instant Pot to Sauté mode and add the remaining olive oil. Allow it to heat up.
5. Add the onions to the pot, stir, and cook for 3 minutes. Transfer the onions to the bowl and set aside.
6. Add the meat to the pot and brown it for 10 minutes.
7. Add the stock, cinnamon stick, bay leaf, and return the onions to the pot. Stir everything together, cover the pot, and cook on High pressure for 25 minutes.
8. Release the pressure naturally, uncover the pot, and add the drained prunes, salt, pepper, and honey. Stir well.
9. Set the pot to Simmer mode and cook the mixture for 5 minutes. Discard the bay leaf and cinnamon stick.
10. Divide the dish among plates and sprinkle almonds and sesame seeds on top.

LAMB RAGOUT

Nutrition: Cal 360 ;Fat 14 g; Carb 15 g;Protein 30 g
Serving 8 Cook time 75 min

Ingredients
- 1 ½ pounds mutton, bone-in
- 2 carrots, sliced
- ½ pound mushrooms, sliced
- 4 tomatoes, chopped
- 1 small yellow onion, chopped
- 6 garlic cloves, minced
- 2 tbsp tomato paste
- 1 tsp vegetable oil

- Salt and black pepper to taste
- 1 tsp oregano, dried
- A handful parsley, finely chopped

Instructions

1. Set your Instant Pot to Sauté mode and heat the oil.
2. Add the meat to the pot and brown it on all sides.
3. Add tomato paste, tomatoes, onion, garlic, mushrooms, oregano, carrots, and enough water to cover the ingredients.
4. Season with salt and pepper, stir everything together, cover the pot, and cook on High pressure for one hour.
5. Release the pressure, remove the meat from the pot, and discard any bones. Shred the meat.
6. Return the shredded meat to the pot, add parsley, and stir to combine.
7. Adjust the seasoning with more salt and pepper if needed, and serve immediately.

LAMB AND BARLEY BOWLS

Nutrition: Cal 484 ;Fat 19 g; Carb 21 g;Protein 44 g
Serving 4 Cook time 60 min

Ingredients

- 6 ounces barley
- 5 ounces peas
- 1 lamb leg, already cooked, boneless and chopped
- 3 yellow onions, chopped
- 5 carrots, chopped
- 6 ounces beef stock
- 12 ounces water
- Salt and black pepper to taste

Instructions

1. In your Instant Pot, combine stock, water, and barley. Cover the pot and cook on High pressure for 20 minutes.
2. Release the pressure, uncover the pot, and add onions, peas, and carrots. Stir everything together, cover the pot again, and cook on High pressure for another ten minutes.
3. Release the pressure once again, add the meat, and season with salt and pepper to taste. Stir everything together, then dish the mixture into bowls and serve.

LAMB AND VEGETABLE SKEWERS WITH YOGURT SAUCE

Nutrition: Cal 553 ;Fat 43 g; Carb 8 g;Protein 33 g
Serving 2 Cook time 50 min

Ingredients

- 1 lb. lamb, cut into bite-sized pieces
- 1 large tomato, chopped
- 1 bell pepper, chopped
- 2 garlic cloves, minced
- 1/2 onion, chopped
- 1/2 cup plain yogurt
- 2 tablespoons olive oil
- Salt and pepper to taste
- Skewers

Instructions

1. Begin by soaking the skewers in water for a minimum of 30 minutes.
2. Preheat your oven to 400°F (200°C).
3. In a bowl, combine the lamb, chopped tomato, chopped bell pepper, minced garlic, chopped onion, olive oil, salt, and pepper.
4. Thread the lamb and vegetables onto the soaked skewers.
5. Place the skewers on a baking sheet and bake in the preheated oven for 15-20 minutes, or until the lamb is cooked through.
6. In a small bowl, mix together the yogurt, minced garlic, and salt to prepare the yogurt sauce.
7. Serve the hot skewers with the yogurt sauce on the side.

LAMB CHOPS WITH LEMON AND GARLIC

Nutrition: Cal 450 ;Fat 35 g; Carb 2 g;Protein 30 g
Serving 2 Cook time 25 min

Ingredients

- 4 lamb chops
- 2 tablespoons olive oil
- 2 tablespoons lemon juice
- 2 garlic cloves, minced
- 1 teaspoon dried oregano
- Salt and pepper to taste

Instructions

1. Preheat a grill or grill pan to medium-high heat.
2. In a small bowl, combine olive oil, lemon juice, minced garlic, dried oregano, salt, and pepper.

3. Brush the marinade over both sides of the lamb chops.
4. Place the lamb chops on the grill and cook for 3-4 minutes per side, or until the desired level of doneness is reached.
5. Remove the lamb chops from the grill and let them rest for a few minutes before serving.

LAMB CASSOULET DE PROVENCE

Nutrition: Cal 390 ;Fat 22 g; Carb 10 g;Protein 35 g
Serving 2 Cook time 90 min

Ingredients
- 1 lb. lamb, cut into bite-sized pieces
- 2 cups chicken broth
- 1 can (14 oz.) diced tomatoes
- 1/2 onion, chopped
- 2 garlic cloves, minced
- 2 carrots, chopped
- 2 celery stalks, chopped
- 1/4 cup parsley, chopped
- 2 tablespoons olive oil
- Salt and pepper to taste

Instructions
1. Preheat the oven to 350°F.
2. Heat the olive oil in a large pot over medium-high heat.
3. Add the lamb and cook until it is evenly browned on all sides.
4. Incorporate the chopped onion and garlic, and sauté them for 2-3 minutes until the onion becomes translucent.
5. Pour in the chicken broth and diced tomatoes.
6. Introduce the chopped carrots and celery, stirring to combine all the ingredients.
7. Season with salt and pepper to enhance the flavors to your taste.
8. Bring the mixture to a gentle boil.
9. Cover the pot securely and transfer it to the preheated oven.
10. Bake for approximately 1-1.5 hours, or until the lamb reaches a tender consistency.
11. Remove the pot from the oven, and garnish the dish by sprinkling freshly chopped parsley over the top.
12. Serve the delicious lamb stew while it's still hot and enjoy.

KETO LAMB AND EGGPLANT LASAGNE

Nutrition: Cal 629 ;Fat 46 g; Carb 16 g;Protein 235 g
Serving 2 Cook time 60 min

Ingredients
- 1 pound lamb shoulder, cut into small pieces
- 1 medium eggplant, sliced lengthwise into thin strips
- 1 cup ricotta cheese
- 1/2 cup grated parmesan cheese
- 1 egg, beaten
- 1 can diced tomatoes (14.5 oz)
- 2 cloves garlic, minced
- 2 tablespoons olive oil
- Salt and black pepper to taste

Instructions
1. Preheat the oven to 375°F (190°C).
2. Heat a large skillet over medium-high heat and add the olive oil.
3. Add the lamb pieces to the skillet and cook them until they are browned on all sides, which should take about 5-7 minutes.
4. Stir in the minced garlic and cook for an additional minute.
5. Add the diced tomatoes to the skillet and simmer the mixture for 5-10 minutes until the sauce has thickened.
6. In a separate bowl, combine the ricotta cheese, Parmesan cheese, and beaten egg.
7. Grease a 9x9-inch baking dish and start layering the dish with strips of eggplant, followed by the lamb and tomato sauce, and then the ricotta mixture. Repeat the layering until all the ingredients are used up.
8. Cover the baking dish with aluminum foil and bake in the preheated oven for 45-50 minutes, or until the eggplant is fully cooked and the cheese is melted and bubbly.
9. Remove the dish from the oven and let it cool for 10 minutes before serving.

PROVENCAL LAMB STEW SAVOUR

Nutrition: Cal 420 ;Fat 26 g; Carb 10 g;Protein 31 g
Serving 4 Cook time 90 min

Ingredients
- 1 lb. lamb stew meat
- 1 tablespoon olive oil
- 1 onion, chopped
- 2 garlic cloves, minced
- 1 can (14 oz.) diced tomatoes
- 1/2 cup dry red wine
- 1/2 cup beef broth
- 1 tablespoon chopped fresh rosemary
- 1 tablespoon chopped fresh thyme
- 1 bay leaf
- Salt and pepper to taste

Instructions
1. In a large pot, heat the olive oil over medium-high heat and brown the lamb stew meat on all sides.
2. Add the chopped onion and garlic to the pot and sauté for 2-3 minutes, until the onion is translucent.
3. Pour in the diced tomatoes, red wine, and beef broth, and stir to combine.
4. Add the chopped fresh rosemary, chopped fresh thyme, bay leaf, salt, and pepper, and bring the mixture to a boil.
5. Reduce the heat to low and simmer for 1-1.5 hours, until the lamb is tender.
6. Discard the bay leaf and serve the stew hot.

KETO FRENCH-INSPIRED LAMB MEDALLIONS

Nutrition: Cal 498 ;Fat 33 g; Carb 6 g;Protein 36 g
Serving 2 Cook time 35 min

Ingredients
- 1 lb. lamb, cut into bite-sized pieces
- 1 tablespoon olive oil
- 2 tablespoons butter
- 1 onion, chopped
- 2 garlic cloves, minced
- 1/2 cup dry red wine
- 1/2 cup beef broth
- 1 tablespoon tomato paste
- 1 tablespoon chopped fresh parsley
- 1 tablespoon chopped fresh thyme
- Salt and pepper to taste

Instructions
1. In a large skillet, heat the olive oil and butter over medium-high heat.
2. Add the lamb and cook for 3-4 minutes per side, until browned.
3. Remove the lamb from the skillet and set it aside.
4. Add the chopped onion to the skillet and sauté for 2-3 minutes, until softened.
5. Add the minced garlic to the skillet and sauté for an additional 1-2 minutes.
6. Pour in the red wine and beef broth, and stir in the tomato paste.
7. Bring the mixture to a boil, then reduce the heat to low.
8. Add the lamb back into the skillet and stir in the chopped parsley and thyme.
9. Simmer the lamb for 15-20 minutes, until the sauce has thickened and the lamb is cooked through.
10. Season with salt and pepper to taste.

KETO LAMB AND VEGETABLE STEW

Nutrition: Cal 459 ;Fat 34 g; Carb 8 g;Protein 25 g
Serving 2 Cook time 50 min

Ingredients
- 1 pound lamb shoulder, cut into small pieces
- 2 medium sweet peppers, sliced
- 1 small eggplant, diced
- 1 medium leek, sliced
- 2 cloves garlic, minced
- 2 medium tomatoes, diced
- 1 teaspoon dried thyme
- 2 tablespoons olive oil
- Salt and black pepper to taste

Instructions
1. Heat a large pot over medium-high heat and add the olive oil.
2. Add the lamb pieces to the pot and cook until browned on all sides, about 5-7 minutes.
3. Add the sliced sweet peppers, diced eggplant, and sliced leek to the pot and cook until they are slightly softened, about 5 minutes.
4. Add the minced garlic, diced tomatoes, and dried thyme to the pot and stir to combine.
5. Cover the pot and simmer on low heat for 30-40 minutes until the lamb is tender and the vegetables are fully cooked.
6. Season the stew with salt and black pepper to taste.

KETO RUSSIAN-STYLE LAMB STEW

Nutrition: Cal 460 ;Fat 35 g; Carb 14 g;Protein 25 g
Serving 2 Cook time 70 min

Ingredients

- 1 pound lamb shoulder, cut into small pieces
- 2 tablespoons olive oil
- 1 small onion, diced
- 2 cloves garlic, minced
- 2 medium carrots, sliced
- 2 medium turnips, diced
- 1 cup beef broth
- 1 tablespoon tomato paste
- 1 teaspoon dried thyme
- Salt and black pepper to taste

Instructions

1. Heat a large pot over medium-high heat. Add the olive oil.
2. Add the lamb pieces to the pot and cook until browned on all sides, about 5-7 minutes.
3. Add the diced onion and minced garlic to the pot and cook until they are slightly softened, about 5 minutes.
4. Add the sliced carrots and diced turnips to the pot and stir to combine.
5. Pour in the beef broth, tomato paste, and dried thyme. Stir to combine.
6. Cover the pot and simmer on low heat for 45-60 minutes until the lamb is tender and the vegetables are fully cooked.
7. Season the stew with salt and black pepper to taste.

MEXICAN STYLE LAMB

Nutrition: Cal 324 ;Fat 9 g; Carb 19 g;Protein 15 g
Serving 4 Cook time 60 min

Ingredients

- 1 yellow onion, chopped
- 2 tbsp extra virgin olive oil
- Salt to taste
- ½ bunch cilantro, finely chopped
- 3 pounds lamb shoulder, cubed
- 19 ounces enchilada sauce
- 3 garlic cloves, minced
- Corn tortillas, warm for serving
- Lime wedges for serving
- Refried beans for serving

Instructions

1. Place enchilada sauce in a bowl and add lamb meat, allowing it to marinate for 24 hours.
2. Set your Instant Pot to Sauté mode and heat the oil.
3. Add onions and garlic, and sauté for 5 minutes.
4. Add the marinated lamb, salt, and the remaining marinade. Stir well, bring to a boil, cover, and cook on High for 45 minutes.
5. Release the pressure, transfer the cooked meat to a cutting board, and let it cool for a few minutes.
6. Shred the meat and place it in a bowl.
7. Pour the cooking sauce over the shredded meat and mix well.
8. Divide the meat onto tortillas, sprinkle cilantro on each, add beans, squeeze lime juice over them, roll them up, and serve.

GOAT AND TOMATO POT

Nutrition: Cal 340 ;Fat 4 g; Carb 12 g;Protein 12 g
Serving 4 Cook time 70 min

Ingredients

- 4 ounces tomato paste
- 1 yellow onion, chopped
- 3 garlic cloves, crushed
- A dash of sherry wine
- 17 ounces goat meat, cubed
- 1 carrot, chopped
- 1 celery rib, chopped
- ½ cup water
- Salt and black pepper to taste
- 1 cup chicken stock
- 2 tbsp extra virgin olive oil
- 1 tbsp cumin seeds, ground
- A pinch of rosemary, dried
- 2 roasted tomatoes, chopped

Instructions

1. Set your Instant Pot to Sauté mode, add 1 tablespoon of oil, and heat it.
2. Add goat meat, salt, and pepper, and brown it for a few minutes on both sides.
3. Stir in cumin seeds and rosemary, cook for just two minutes, and transfer to a bowl.
4. Add the remaining oil to the pot and heat it.
5. Stir in onions, garlic, salt, and pepper, and cook for 1 minute.
6. Add carrots and celery, stir, and cook for 2 minutes.

7. Add sherry wine, stock, water, goat meat, tomato paste, more salt, and pepper. Stir well, cover, and cook on High for 40 minutes.
8. Allow the pressure to release naturally, then uncover the pot, add tomatoes, stir, divide the dish among plates, and serve.

SPICY TACO MEAT

Nutrition: Cal 414 ;Fat 21 g; Carb 7 g;Protein 47 g
Serving 6 Cook time 45 min

Ingredients
- 2 lbs ground beef
- 1/2 tbsp chili powder
- 1/4 Tsp chipotle powder
- 1 tsp cayenne
- 1/2 Tsp cumin
- 1/2 Tsp smoked paprika
- 1/2 Tsp turmeric
- 2 tsp oregano
- 2 large sweet peppers, diced
- 1 large onion, diced
- 4 tbsp olive oil
- 3 garlic cloves, minced
- 1/4 Tsp black pepper
- 1 tsp salt

Instructions
1. Place all ingredients, except for the meat, into the Instant Pot.
2. Select the sauté function and stir-fry for 5 minutes.
3. Add the ground beef and stir until lightly browned.
4. Seal the pot with the lid and cook on HIGH pressure for 30 minutes.
5. Allow the steam to release naturally, then open the pot.
6. Select the sauté function again and stir for 10 minutes.
7. Garnish with freshly chopped cilantro and serve.

BEEF STROGANOFF

Nutrition: Cal 317 ;Fat 19 g; Carb 8 g;Protein 29 g
Serving 4 Cook time 40 min

Ingredients
- Beef (1 pound, chopped in cubes)
- Bacon (2 slices, cut in cubes)
- Beef stock (250 ml)
- Mushrooms (9 oz.)
- Onion (1, chopped)
- Tomato paste (3 tbsp)
- Smoked paprika (1 tbsp)
- Sour cream
- Garlic (2 cloves, chopped)

Instructions
1. Add oil to the pressure cooker dish and set it to "Sauté" mode. Add the onions, bacon, and garlic, and cook briefly until the onions are tender.
2. Place the beef in the cooker and continue cooking until the meat is browned on all sides.
3. Add the mushrooms, beef broth, tomato paste, and paprika, and stir well. Close the lid and set it to high-pressure cooking for 30 minutes.
4. Use the quick-release method to release the pressure.
5. Serve the dish while hot and top it with sour cream.

KETO BEEF AND BROCCOLI

Nutrition: Cal 294;Fat 14 g; Carb 13 g;Protein 29 g
Serving 4; Cook time 35 min

Ingredients
- 1 pound flank steak sliced into 1/4 inch thick strips
- 5 cups small broccoli florets about 7 ounces
- 1 tablespoon avocado oil
- For the sauce:
- 1 yellow onion sliced
- 1 Tbs butter
- ½ tbs olive oil
- 1/3 cup low-sodium soy sauce
- ⅓ cup beef stock
- 1 tablespoon fresh ginger minced
- 2 cloves garlic minced

Instructions
1. Heat avocado oil in a pan over medium heat for a few minutes or until hot.
2. Add sliced beef and cook until it browns, less than 5 minutes. Avoid stirring too much to allow it to brown. Transfer to a plate and set aside.
3. In the same skillet, add onions with butter and olive oil. Cook for 20 minutes until the onions are caramelized and tender.
4. Add all the other sauce ingredients to the skillet and stir together over medium-low heat until it starts to simmer, about 5 minutes.
5. Use an immersion blender to blend the sauce until smooth.

6. Keep the sauce warm over low heat and add broccoli to the skillet.
7. Return the beef to the pan and toss with broccoli and sauce on top. Stir until everything is coated with the sauce.
8. Bring to a simmer and cook for another few minutes until the broccoli is tender.
9. Season with salt and pepper to taste, if needed.
10. Serve immediately, optionally pairing it with cooked cauliflower rice.

MEATLOAF RECIPE

Nutrition: Cal 575;Fat 44 g; Carb 10 g;Protein 35 g
Serving 4; Cook time 70 min

Ingredients

- 1 tablespoon tallow
- 1 small onion finely chopped
- 2 cloves garlic crushed
- 2 pounds ground beef
- 2 large eggs
- 2 tablespoons oregano dried
- 1 1/2 teaspoon salt
- 1/4 teaspoon pepper ground
- 1/3 cup low carb marinara sauce
- 1/3 cup almond flour
- 2 tablespoons low carb marinara sauce extra

Instructions

1. Preheat the oven to 160°C/320°F and prepare a loaf tin by lining it with baking paper.
2. Place a non-stick frying pan over high heat and sauté the onion and garlic in the tallow until the onion turns translucent. Set it aside to cool slightly.
3. In a large mixing bowl, combine the warm onion mixture with all the remaining ingredients, except for the extra marinara sauce.
4. Mix the ingredients thoroughly using clean hands or wearing disposable gloves.
5. Press the mixture firmly into the base of the prepared loaf tin, ensuring there are no air bubbles and the top is smooth.
6. Bake for 50 minutes.
7. Drain off some of the juices and spread the extra marinara sauce on top of the meatloaf.
8. Bake for another 10 minutes.
9. Allow the meatloaf to rest for 10 minutes before slicing and serving.

LOW CARB BEEF BOLOGNESE SAUCE

Nutrition: Cal 279;Fat 21 g; Carb 5 g;Protein 17 g
Serving 6; Cook time 75 min

Ingredients

- 4 cups of Beef Stock or Broth
- 2 ounces of Tallow
- 1 medium Onion, diced
- 6 cloves of Garlic, crushed
- 1 tablespoon of Marjoram, dried
- 1 teaspoon of Salt
- 3 pounds of Ground Beef
- 24 ounces of Tomato Puree
- 2 tablespoons of Basil, chopped
- 2 tablespoons of Oregano, chopped
- 1 tablespoon of Parsley, chopped
- 1 teaspoon of Pepper

Instructions

1. Place the beef stock in a small saucepan and simmer over medium-high heat until it reduces to 1 cup of liquid.
2. In a large saucepan over high heat, melt the tallow and allow it to heat up.
3. Add the diced onion, garlic, marjoram, and salt. Sauté for 5 minutes until the onions have softened and turned translucent.
4. Add the ground beef and sauté until browned. Reduce the heat to low.
5. Pour in the tomato puree and reduced beef stock. Simmer uncovered, stirring occasionally, for 30-60 minutes until the liquid is mostly absorbed, resulting in a thick and rich sauce.
6. Add the remaining ingredients, check the seasoning, and add more salt or pepper if desired.
7. Remove from the heat, serve, and enjoy.

KETO LAMB CHOPS ON THE GRILL

Nutrition: Cal 446;Fat 27 g; Carb 4 g;Protein 22 g
Serving 8; Cook time 30 min

Ingredients

- 3 lbs of lamb loin chops (I had 8 6oz chops)
- 1/4 cup of white wine vinegar
- 1/2 cup of olive oil
- 1 teaspoon of oregano
- 1/2 teaspoon of salt
- 1/4 teaspoon of pepper
- 2 cloves of garlic, crushed
- zest of 1 lemon
- juice of 2 lemons (approx. 6 tablespoons)

Instructions

1. Whisk together all of the marinade ingredients. Place the lamb chops in a large resealable bag and pour the marinade over them.
2. Seal the bag and use your hands to thoroughly coat the chops with the marinade. Place the bag in the refrigerator and let the chops marinate for 8 hours or overnight.
3. When ready to cook, remove the lamb chops from the refrigerator and let them sit at room temperature for 15 minutes. Transfer them to a plate and discard the marinade.
4. Grill the lamb chops for approximately 5-6 minutes per side, depending on their size and thickness. For chops that are about 1-1.5 inches thick, grilling for 6 minutes on each side should result in a medium-rare doneness. Adjust the cooking time accordingly based on your preference for doneness.

ROSEMARY DIJON ROASTED LAMB CHOPS

Nutrition: Cal 446;Fat 40 g; Carb 2 g;Protein 18 g
Serving 4; Cook time 17 min

Ingredients
- 1 tbsp Dijon mustard
- 2 cloves garlic minced
- 3 tbsp olive oil
- 2 tsp fresh rosemary finely chopped
- 1/2 tsp salt
- 1/4 tsp pepper
- 4 lamb loin chops aprrox 2 lbs with bone-in

Instructions

1. In a bowl, whisk together Dijon mustard, garlic, olive oil, rosemary, salt, and pepper until well combined. Place the lamb chops in a large zip-top bag or airtight container. Coat the lamb chops on both sides with the Dijon mixture. Allow the lamb to marinate in the refrigerator for at least 30 minutes, or up to 24 hours.
2. Position an oven rack to the highest position and line a broiler pan with aluminum foil.
3. Remove the lamb chops from the marinade and place them onto the prepared pan. Preheat the oven to the broil setting on high and place the pan into the oven.

4. Cook the lamb chops for approximately 8 minutes, until they are nicely browned. Flip the chops and continue cooking for an additional 3-5 minutes, depending on your desired level of doneness (3 minutes for medium rare, 4 minutes for medium, 5 minutes for well done).

KETO LAMB KOFTAS

Nutrition: Cal 330;Fat 26 g; Carb 3 g;Protein 22 g
Serving 4; Cook time 20 min

Ingredients
- 500 g minced (ground) lamb (1.1 lb)
- 1 garlic clove, minced
- 1/2 medium yellow onion, diced (50 g/ 1.8 oz)
- 1 tsp dried oregano
- 2 tbsp chopped fresh parsley
- 1/2 tsp sea salt
- 1/4 tsp ground black pepper
- 1 tbsp extra virgin olive oil (15 ml)

Instructions

1. Prior to starting, place your skewers in cold water for at least 30 minutes to soak. Alternatively, if you are using stainless steel skewers, they do not require soaking.
2. In a large mixing bowl, combine minced lamb, diced onions, chopped garlic, finely chopped parsley, and the herbs and seasonings. Make sure to retain the olive oil.
3. Thoroughly mix the ingredients together using your hands until well combined.
4. Divide the mixture into eight portions and shape each portion around a skewer. Gently squeeze and press the mixture around the skewer until you are satisfied with the result. If your skewers fit in a pan, heat it on the stovetop. Alternatively, you can cook them on a barbecue if the skewers are too big for a pan.
5. Before placing the koftas on the hot pan or barbecue, brush the surface with the retained olive oil.
6. Once cooked, you can store the koftas covered in the refrigerator for up to four days.

LAMB MEATBALLS WITH MINT GREMOLATA

Nutrition: Cal 306;Fat 17 g; Carb 4 g;Protein 34 g
Serving 4; Cook time 20 min

Ingredients
FOR THE MEATBALLS:
- 2 lbs ground lamb
- 2 eggs
- 1/2 cup superfine almond flour
- 1/4 cup fresh parsley, chopped
- 1 clove garlic, minced
- 1 1/2 Tbsp Za'atar seasoning
- 1 tsp kosher salt
- 3 Tbsp water
- 2 Tbsp olive oil for frying

FOR THE GREMOLATA:
- 2 Tbsp chopped fresh parsley
- 2 Tbsp chopped fresh mint
- 1 Tbsp lime zest
- 2 cloves garlic, minced

Instructions
FOR THE MEATBALLS:
1. Combine the meatball ingredients (except olive oil) in a medium bowl and mix well.
2. Form into 24 one and a half inch (approximately) meatballs.
3. Heat the olive oil in a nonstick saute pan over medium heat.
4. Cook the meatballs in batches until brown on both sides and cooked through – about 2-3 minutes per side.
5. Remove cooked meatballs and place on a paper towel lined plate until ready to serve.
6. Serve warm, sprinkled generously with gremolata.

FOR THE GREMOLATA:
7. Combine the ingredients in a small bowl and mix well.

SWISS CHEESE BEEF ZUCCHINI CASSEROLE

Nutrition: Cal 454;Fat 30 g; Carb 13 g;Protein 30 g
Serving 4; Cook time 2 hours

Ingredients
- 1 pound extra-lean ground beef
- 4 cups zucchini, sliced
- 10 ounces cream of mushroom soup
- 1/2 cup onion, chopped
- 1/4 tsp ground black pepper
- 1 cup Swiss cheese, shredded

Instructions
1. Heat a skillet over medium-high heat and brown the ground beef with onions and peppers until it is no longer pink. Drain any excess fat.
2. In an Instant Pot, layer the zucchini and beef mixture alternately.
3. Spread soup over the top layer and sprinkle with cheese.
4. Cover the Instant Pot and turn the steam release handle to the venting position.
5. Select the slow cooker setting and set it to medium heat.
6. Cook the dish for 120 minutes, allowing the flavors to meld together and the zucchini to become tender.

BEEF AND BROCCOLI STIR-FRY

Nutrition: Cal 588;Fat 38 g; Carb 6 g;Protein 54 g
Serving 4; Cook time 25 min

Ingredients
- 6 tablespoons coconut aminos
- ¼ cup avocado oil
- 2 tablespoons toasted sesame oil
- 1 teaspoon garlic powder
- 1 teaspoon onion powder
- Salt
- Freshly ground black pepper
- 1½ pounds sirloin steak, cut into ¼-inch-thick slices

FOR THE BEEF AND BROCCOLI
- 1 teaspoon salt, plus more for seasoning
- 2 broccoli crowns, florets separated and trimmed
- 2 tablespoons avocado oil
- 3 garlic cloves, minced
- 1 tablespoon finely minced ginger or ½ tablespoon ground ginger
- ¼ cup coconut aminos
- ¼ cup toasted sesame oil
- Freshly ground black pepper

Instructions
TO MAKE THE MARINADE
1. In a bowl, combine the coconut aminos, avocado oil, sesame oil, garlic powder, onion powder, salt, and pepper. Add the steak and toss to coat. Marinate for at least 30 minutes or up to 24 hours in the refrigerator.

TO MAKE THE BEEF AND BROCCOLI
1. Fill a large pot halfway with water and add 1 teaspoon of salt. Bring to a boil.

2. Add the broccoli and blanch for 1 to 3 minutes; drain in a colander. Rinse with cold water to prevent further cooking. Set aside.
3. Heat a large skillet over medium-high heat and combine the avocado oil, garlic, and ginger and cook for 30 seconds.
4. Add the sliced beef, discarding the marinade, and cook, stirring constantly, for 2 to 3 minutes. Add the broccoli, coconut aminos, and sesame oil to the skillet and season with salt and pepper. Continue to cook until the beef has reached your desired doneness (about 5 to 7 minutes for medium).
5. Divide the stir-fry evenly between 4 storage containers.

HEARTY BEEF AND BACON CASSEROLE

Nutrition: Cal 410;Fat 26 g; Carb 8 g;Protein 37 g
Serving 8; Cook time 55 min

Ingredients
- 8 slices uncooked bacon
- 1 medium head cauliflower, chopped
- ¼ cup canned coconut milk
- Salt and pepper
- 2 pounds ground beef (80% lean)
- 8 ounces mushrooms, sliced
- 1 large yellow onion, chopped
- 2 cloves garlic, minced

Instructions
1. Preheat the oven to 375°F.
2. Cook the bacon in a skillet until crisp, then drain on paper towels and chop.
3. Bring a pot of salted water to boil, then add the cauliflower.
4. Boil for 6 to 8 minutes until tender, then drain and add to a food processor with the coconut milk.
5. Blend the mixture until smooth, then season with salt and pepper.
6. Cook the beef in a skillet until browned, then drain the fat.
7. Stir in the mushrooms, onion, and garlic, then transfer to a baking dish.
8. Spread the cauliflower mixture over top and bake for 30 minutes.
9. Broil on high heat for 5 minutes, then sprinkle with bacon to serve.

SLOW COOKER BEEF BOURGUIGNON

Nutrition: Cal 335;Fat 12 g; Carb 6 g;Protein 37 g
Serving 8; Cook time 4 hours 55 min

Ingredients
- 2 tablespoons olive oil
- 2 pounds boneless beef chuck roast, cut into chunks
- Salt and pepper
- ¼ cup almond flour
- ½ cup beef broth
- 2 cups red wine (dry)
- 2 tablespoons tomato paste
- 1 pound mushrooms, sliced
- 1 large yellow onion, cut into chunks

Instructions
1. Heat the oil in a large skillet over medium-high heat.
2. Season the beef with salt and pepper, then coat it with almond flour.
3. Add the beef to the skillet and cook until browned on all sides, then transfer it to a slow cooker.
4. Reheat the skillet over medium-high heat, then pour in the broth.
5. Scrape up the browned bits, then whisk in the wine and tomato paste.
6. Bring the mixture to a boil, then pour it into the slow cooker.
7. Add the mushrooms and onion, then stir everything together.
8. Cover and cook on low heat for 4 hours until the meat is very tender. Serve hot.

PEPPER GRILLED RIBEYE WITH ASPARAGUS

Nutrition: Cal 380;Fat 25 g; Carb 4.5 g;Protein 35 g
Serving 4; Cook time 20 min

Ingredients
- 1 pound asparagus, trimmed
- 2 tablespoons olive oil
- Salt and pepper
- 1 pound ribeye steak
- 1 tablespoon coconut oil

Instructions
1. Preheat the oven to 400°F and line a small baking sheet with foil.
2. Toss the asparagus with olive oil and spread it out on the baking sheet.

3. Season the asparagus with salt and pepper, then place it in the oven.
4. Rub the steak with pepper and season it with salt.
5. Melt the coconut oil in a cast-iron skillet and heat it over high heat.
6. Add the steak to the skillet and cook for 2 minutes, then flip it.
7. Transfer the skillet to the oven and cook for 5 minutes or until the steak reaches the desired level of doneness.
8. Slice the steak and serve it with the roasted asparagus.

STEAK KEBABS WITH PEPPERS AND ONIONS

Nutrition: Cal 350;Fat 20 g; Carb 6,5 g;Protein 35 g
Serving 4; Cook time 40 min

Ingredients
- 1 pound beef sirloin, cut into 1-inch cubes
- ¼ cup olive oil
- 2 tablespoons balsamic vinegar
- Salt and pepper
- 1 medium yellow onion, cut into chunks
- 1 medium red pepper, cut into chunks
- 1 medium green pepper, cut into chunks

Instructions
1. Coat the steak cubes with olive oil, balsamic vinegar, salt, and pepper.
2. Thread the cubes onto skewers along with the peppers and onions.
3. Preheat the grill to high heat and grease the grates.
4. Grill the kebabs for 2 to 3 minutes on each side or until cooked to your desired level of doneness.

SEARED LAMB CHOPS WITH ASPARAGUS

Nutrition: Cal 380;Fat 18.5 g; Carb 4,5 g;Protein 48 g
Serving 4; Cook time 20 min

Ingredients
- 8 bone-in lamb chops
- Salt and pepper
- 1 tablespoon fresh chopped rosemary
- 1 tablespoon olive oil
- 1 tablespoon butter
- 16 spears asparagus, cut into 2-inch chunks

Instructions

1. Season the lamb with salt and pepper then sprinkle with rosemary.
2. Heat the oil in a large skillet over medium-high heat.
3. Add the lamb chops and cook for 2 to 3 minutes on each side until seared.
4. Remove the lamb chops to rest and reheat the skillet with the butter.
5. Add the asparagus and turn to coat then cover the skillet.
6. Cook for 4 to 6 minutes until tender-crisp and serve with the lamb.

ROSEMARY-GARLIC LAMB RACKS

Nutrition: Cal 354;Fat 30 g; Carb 1 g;Protein 21 g
Serving 4; Cook time 1 hours 35 min

Ingredients
- 4 tablespoons extra-virgin olive oil
- 2 tablespoons finely chopped
- fresh rosemary
- 2 teaspoons minced garlic
- Pinch sea salt
- 2 (1-pound) racks French-cut
- lamb chops (8 bones each)

Instructions
1. In a small bowl, whisk together the olive oil, rosemary, garlic, and salt.
2. Place the racks in a sealable freezer bag and pour the olive oil mixture into the bag. Massage the meat through the bag to ensure it is thoroughly coated with the marinade. Press the air out of the bag and seal it.
3. Marinate the lamb racks in the refrigerator for 1 to 2 hours.
4. Preheat the oven to 450°F.
5. Place a large ovenproof skillet over medium-high heat. Remove the lamb racks from the bag and sear them in the skillet on all sides, approximately 5 minutes in total.
6. Arrange the racks upright in the skillet, with the bones interlaced, and roast them in the oven until they reach your desired doneness, about 20 minutes for medium-rare or until the internal temperature reaches 125°F.
7. Let the lamb rest for 10 minutes, then cut the racks into chops.
8. Serve 4 chops per person.

LAMB LEG WITH SUN-DRIED TOMATO PESTO

Nutrition: Cal 352;Fat 29 g; Carb 5 g;Protein 17 g
Serving 8; Cook time 85 min

Ingredients
FOR THE PESTO
- 1 cup sun-dried tomatoes packed
- in oil, drained
- ¼ cup pine nuts
- 2 tablespoons extra-virgin olive oil
- 2 tablespoons chopped fresh basil
- 2 teaspoons minced garlic

FOR THE LAMB LEG
- 1 (2-pound) lamb leg
- Sea salt
- Freshly ground black pepper
- 2 tablespoons olive oil

Instructions
TO MAKE THE PESTO
1. Place the sun-dried tomatoes, pine nuts, olive oil, basil, and garlic in a blender or food processor; process until smooth.
2. Set aside until needed.

TO MAKE THE LAMB LEG
1. Preheat the oven to 400°F.
2. Season the lamb leg all over with salt and pepper.
3. Place a large ovenproof skillet over medium-high heat and add the olive oil.
4. Sear the lamb on all sides until nicely browned, about 6 minutes in total.
5. Spread the sun-dried tomato pesto all over the lamb and place the lamb on a baking sheet. Roast until the meat reaches your desired doneness, about 1 hour for medium.
6. Let the lamb rest for 10 minutes before slicing and serving.

BACON-WRAPPED BEEF TENDERLOIN

Nutrition: Cal 565;Fat 49 g; Carb 2 g;Protein 28 g
Serving 4; Cook time 25 min

Ingredients
- 4 (4-ounce) beef tenderloin steaks
- Sea salt
- Freshly ground black pepper
- 8 bacon slices
- 1 tablespoon extra-virgin olive oil

Instructions

1. Preheat the oven to 450°F.
2. Season the steaks with salt and pepper.
3. Wrap each steak snugly around the edges with 2 slices of bacon and secure the bacon with toothpicks.
4. Place a large skillet over medium-high heat and add the olive oil.
5. Pan-sear the steaks for 4 minutes per side and transfer them to a baking sheet.
6. Roast the steaks until they reach your desired doneness, about 6 minutes for medium.
7. Remove the steaks from the oven and let them rest for 10 minutes.
8. Remove the toothpicks and serve.

CHEESEBURGER CASSEROLE

Nutrition: Cal 410;Fat 33 g; Carb 3g;Protein 20 g
Serving 6; Cook time 40 min

Ingredients
- 1 pound 75% lean ground beef
- ½ cup chopped sweet onion
- 2 teaspoons minced garlic
- 1&½ cups shredded aged Cheddar, divided
- ½ cup heavy (whipping) cream
- 1 large tomato, chopped
- 1 teaspoon minced fresh basil
- ¼ teaspoon sea salt
- ⅛ teaspoon freshly ground black pepper

Instructions
1. Preheat the oven to 350°F.
2. Place a large skillet over medium-high heat and add the ground beef.
3. Brown the beef until cooked through, about 6 minutes, and spoon off any excess fat.
4. Stir in the onion and garlic and cook until the vegetables are tender, about 4 minutes.
5. Transfer the beef and vegetables to an 8-by-8-inch casserole dish.
6. In a medium bowl, stir together 1 cup of shredded cheese and the heavy cream, tomato, basil, salt, and pepper until well combined.
7. Pour the cream mixture over the beef mixture and top the casserole with the remaining ½ cup of shredded cheese.
8. Bake until the casserole is bubbly and the cheese is melted and lightly browned, about 30 minutes.

PORK AND HAM

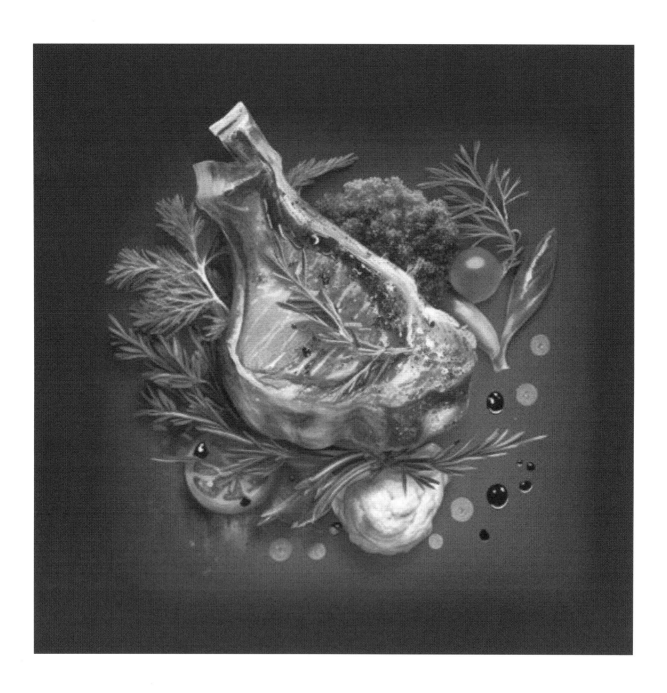

THREE MEAT AND CHEESE SANDWICH

Nutrition: Cal 610;Fat 48 g;Carb 3 g;Protein 40 g
Serving 1; Cook time35 min

Ingredients:
- 1 large egg, separated
- Pinch cream of tartar
- Pinch salt
- 1 ounce cream cheese, softened
- 1 ounce sliced ham
- 1 ounce sliced hard salami
- 1 ounce sliced turkey
- 2 slices cheddar cheese

Instructions:
1. Preheat the oven to 300°F and line a baking sheet with parchment paper.
2. In a mixing bowl, beat the egg whites with the cream of tartar and salt until soft peaks form.
3. In another bowl, whisk the cream cheese and egg yolks until smooth and pale yellow.
4. Gently fold in the beaten egg whites, a little at a time, until the mixture is smooth and well combined.
5. Spoon the batter onto the prepared baking sheet, forming two even circles.
6. Bake for 25 minutes, or until the bread is firm and lightly browned.
7. To assemble the sandwich, layer the sliced meats and cheeses between the two bread circles.
8. Grease a skillet with cooking spray and heat it over medium heat.
9. Place the sandwich in the skillet and cook until the bottom is browned, then flip and cook until the cheese is just melted.

HAM AND PROVOLONE SANDWICH

Nutrition: Cal 425;Fat 31 g;Carb 5 g;Protein 31 g
Serving 1; Cook time 35 min

Ingredients:
- 1 large egg, separated
- Pinch cream of tartar
- Pinch salt
- 1 ounce cream cheese, softened
- ¼ cup shredded provolone cheese
- 3 ounces sliced ham

Instructions:

1. To prepare the bread, preheat the oven to 300°F and line a baking sheet with parchment paper.
2. In a mixing bowl, beat the egg whites with cream of tartar and salt until soft peaks form.
3. In a separate bowl, whisk the cream cheese and egg yolks until smooth and pale yellow.
4. Gradually fold in the egg whites into the cream cheese mixture until smooth and well combined.
5. Spoon the batter onto the baking sheet, forming two even circles.
6. Bake for 25 minutes until the bread is firm and lightly browned.
7. Spread butter on one side of each bread circle, then place one circle in a preheated skillet over medium heat.
8. Sprinkle with cheese and add the sliced ham, then top with the other bread circle, butter-side-up.
9. Cook the sandwich for a minute or two, then carefully flip it over.
10. Allow it to cook until the cheese is melted, then serve.

HAM, EGG, AND CHEESE SANDWICH

Nutrition: Cal 365;Fat 21 g;Carb 6.5 g;Protein 35.5 g
Serving 1; Cook time35 min

Ingredients:
- 1 large egg, separated
- Pinch cream of tartar
- Pinch salt
- 1 ounce cream cheese, softened
- 1 large egg
- 1 teaspoon butter
- 3 ounces sliced ham
- 1 slice cheddar cheese

Instructions:
1. Preheat the oven to 300°F and line a baking sheet with parchment paper.
2. In a mixing bowl, beat the egg whites with the cream of tartar and salt until soft peaks form.
3. In another bowl, whisk the cream cheese and egg yolks until smooth and pale yellow.
4. Gently fold in the beaten egg whites, a little at a time, until the mixture is smooth and well combined.
5. Spoon the batter onto the prepared baking sheet, forming two even circles.
6. Bake for 25 minutes, or until the bread is firm and lightly browned.

7. To complete the sandwich, fry the egg in butter in a skillet until it reaches your desired doneness.
8. Arrange the sliced ham on top of one bread circle.
9. Top with the fried egg and sliced cheese, and then place the second bread circle on top.
10. Serve immediately, or cook the sandwich in a greased skillet to melt the cheese before serving.

CHOPPED KALE SALAD WITH BACON DRESSING

Nutrition: Cal 230;Fat 12 g;Carb 14 g;Protein 16 g
Serving 2; Cook time 15 min

Ingredients:
- 6 slices uncooked bacon
- 2 tablespoons apple cider vinegar
- 1 teaspoon Dijon mustard
- Liquid stevia, to taste
- Salt and pepper
- 4 cups fresh chopped kale
- ¼ cup thinly sliced red onion

Instructions:
1. Cook the bacon in a skillet until crispy, then remove it to a paper towel-lined plate and chop it.
2. In the same skillet, reserve ¼ cup of the bacon grease and warm it over low heat.
3. Whisk in the apple cider vinegar, mustard, and stevia, and season with salt and pepper.
4. Add the kale to the skillet and cook for 1 minute, tossing it in the dressing.
5. Divide the dressed kale between two plates.
6. Top the salads with red onion and chopped bacon.
7. Serve the salads immediately.

SKINNY OVEN FRIED PORK CHOPS

Nutrition: Cal 380;Fat 21 g;Carb 7 g;Protein 40 g
Serving 6; Cook time 25 min

Ingredients:
- 2 lbs pork loin chops (6 pork chops approx.)
- 1 cup buttermilk
- 1 cup almond flour/meal
- 1 tablespoon unflavored whey protein isolate powder
- 1 teaspoon kosher salt
- 1 teaspoons garlic powder
- 2 teaspoons Italian seasoning
- 1 tablespoon grated parmesan cheese (optional)
- Parsley or cilantro for garnishing (optional)
- Avocado and tomato salad to serve (optional)

Instructions:
1. Trim any excess fat from the pork chops, if necessary.
2. In a large bowl, pour the buttermilk over the pork chops, making sure they are fully covered. Refrigerate the pork chops for at least 2 hours or overnight. Remove them from the fridge 30 minutes before cooking.
3. Preheat the oven to 425°F. Line a large baking sheet with non-stick aluminum foil or lightly spray a large non-stick baking sheet with oil.
4. In a large shallow bowl, combine almond flour/meal, tapioca, salt, garlic, Italian seasoning, and Parmesan cheese if desired.
5. Take a pork chop from the buttermilk, allowing any excess milk to drip off. Coat the pork chop in the crumb mixture, making sure it is fully coated. Place it on the prepared baking sheet.
6. Lightly spray a little more oil on top of the pork chops.
7. Bake the pork chops uncovered for 20 to 25 minutes, or until the pork is cooked to an internal temperature of 145°F.

CREAMY HONEY & MUSTARD PORK RIBS

Nutrition: Cal 385 ;Fat 17 g; Carb 16 g;Protein 39 g
Serving 6 Cook time 4 hours

Ingredients
- 3 1/2 pounds country style pork ribs
- 1/2 cup honey mustard
- 1 cup BBQ sauce
- 2 tsp Salt-Free Seasoning Blend

Instructions
1. Place the ribs in the Instant Pot.
2. In a small bowl, stir together barbecue sauce, honey mustard, and seasoning blend.
3. Pour the sauce mixture over the ribs in the Instant Pot, stirring to coat them evenly.
4. Cover the Instant Pot and turn the steam release handle to the venting position.
5. Select the slow cooker setting and set it to high. Cook the ribs for 4 hours.
6. Once cooked, transfer the ribs to a serving platter.

7. Strain the sauce from the Instant Pot into a bowl and skim off any excess fat.
8. Drizzle some of the sauce over the ribs and serve the remaining sauce on the table for additional dipping or drizzling.

TENDER AND JUICY SHREDDED PORK

Nutrition: Cal 550 ;Fat41 g; Carb 2 g;Protein 38 g
Serving 8 Cook time 8 hours

Ingredients
- 4 pounds pork shoulder roast
- 4 ounces green chilies, diced
- 1 cup using apple cider vinegar
- 1 1/2 tsp garlic, minced
- 1 cup onion, finely chopped
- 1 tsp ground black pepper
- 1 tsp salt

Instructions
1. Place the roast in the Instant Pot.
2. Combine the remaining ingredients and pour them over the roast.
3. Cover the Instant Pot and turn the steam release handle towards the venting position.
4. Select the slow cooker setting and set it to medium.
5. Cook the roast for 8 hours.
6. Remove the roast to a chopping board and shred it using two forks, discarding any fat and bones.

SESAME SHEET PAN PORK FAJITAS

Nutrition: Cal 323 ;Fat 18 g; Carb 2 g;Protein 34 g
Serving 8 Cook time 1 hour 30 min

Ingredients
- 2 lbs boneless pork chops
- 1 tsp avocado or olive oil
- Peppers, sliced optional
- onions, sliced optional
- Amazing Garlic Sauce
- 1 cup cilantro
- 1 tbsp ginger
- 4 cloves garlic
- 1 jalapeno, seeded {optional}
- 1/3 cup avocado oil
- 2 tsp sesame oil
- 1 tbsp apple cider vinegar
- 3 tbsp coconut aminos
- 2 tbsp lime juice

Instructions
1. Combine all the ingredients for the marinade in a food processor and pulse multiple times until the mixture is chopped with some liquid. The marinade should include 1 cup cilantro, 1 tbsp ginger, 4 cloves garlic, 1 jalapeno (seeded), 1/3 cup avocado oil, 2 tsp sesame oil, 1 tbsp apple cider vinegar, 3 tbsp coconut aminos, and 2 tbsp lime juice.
2. Slice the boneless pork chops into thin, uniform pieces against the grain. Add half of the marinade (reserving the other half) and stir to combine. Refrigerate for 30 minutes, up to 24 hours.
3. Slice onions and peppers, then toss them with 1 tsp of avocado or olive oil and a pinch of kosher salt.
4. Preheat the oven to 400 degrees F and place the oven rack on the middle rung.
5. Arrange the marinated pork and the pepper/onion mixture on a rimmed baking sheet.
6. Bake for 10 minutes, then switch the broiler to HIGH for an additional 4 minutes. Be sure to watch it closely to prevent burning.
7. Serve the pork with the peppers and onions on leaf lettuce for a gluten-free/Whole30 fajita option.

BRIGHT SALSA PORK CHOPS

Nutrition: Cal 460 ;Fat 22 g; Carb 8 g;Protein 25 g
Serving 2 Cook time 8 hours 20 min

Ingredients
- 2 x Pork Loins
- 75g Salsa
- 3 Tablespoon Lime Juice
- ½ tsp. Ground Cumin
- ½ tsp. Garlic Powder
- ½ tsp. Salt
- ½ tsp. Ground Black Pepper
- Calorie Free Cooking Spray

Instructions
1. In a small bowl, combine cumin, garlic powder, salt, and pepper. Rub the spice mixture into the pork chops, ensuring they are evenly coated.

2. Heat a skillet over medium heat and brown the pork chops for about 5 minutes on each side. This will help enhance the flavor and texture of the meat.
3. Spray the inside of your slow cooker with cooking spray to prevent sticking. Place the browned pork chops in the slow cooker.
4. Add salsa and a mixture of lime juice to the slow cooker. The salsa will provide a tangy and flavorful base for the dish, while the lime juice adds a refreshing citrus note.
5. Set your slow cooker to the low heat setting and cook the pork chops for 8 hours. This slow cooking process will ensure that the meat becomes tender and absorbs the flavors of the spices and salsa.

LOADED CAULIFLOWER

Nutrition: Cal 200;Fat 17 g; Carb 8 g;Protein 12 g
Serving 6; Cook time 20 min

Ingredients

- 1 pound cauliflower florettes
- 4 ounces sour cream
- 1 cup grated cheddar cheese
- 2 slices cooked bacon, crumbled
- 2 tablespoons snipped chives
- 3 tablespoons butter
- 1/4 teaspoon garlic powder
- Salt and pepper, to taste

Instructions

1. Cut the cauliflower into florettes and place them in a microwave-safe bowl. Add 2 tablespoons of water and cover the bowl with cling film. Microwave for 5-8 minutes until the cauliflower is completely cooked and tender. Drain any excess water and let it sit uncovered for a minute or two. Alternatively, you can steam the cauliflower using a conventional method. You may need to squeeze out any excess water from the cauliflower after cooking.

2. Transfer the cooked cauliflower to a food processor and process until it becomes fluffy. Add butter, garlic powder, and sour cream to the food processor and continue processing until it reaches a mashed potato-like consistency. Transfer the mashed cauliflower to a bowl and add most of the chives, reserving some to sprinkle on top later. Mix in half of the shredded cheddar cheese by hand. Season with salt and pepper.

3. Top the loaded cauliflower with the remaining cheese, chives, and bacon. Place it back in the microwave to melt the cheese, or you can place the cauliflower under the broiler for a few minutes until the cheese is melted and bubbly.

4. Divide the cauliflower into six portions visually. Each serving size is approximately 1/3 to 1/2 cup. Enjoy!

PAN-SEARED PORK TENDERLOIN MEDALLIONS

Nutrition: Cal 150;Fat 7 g; Carb 3 g;Protein 18 g
Serving 4; Cook time 18 min

Ingredients
- 1 tablespoon canola oil 1 (1-lb.)
- pork tenderloin, trimmed and cut crosswise into 12 medallions
- 1/2 teaspoon kosher salt
- 1/4 teaspoon garlic powder
- 1/4 teaspoon black pepper Fresh thyme leaves (optional)

Instructions
1. Heat oil in a 12-inch skillet over medium-high heat. Meanwhile, place the pork medallions on a work surface and gently press each one with the palm of your hand to flatten them to an even thickness.

2. In a small bowl, combine salt, garlic powder, and pepper. Sprinkle the seasoning mixture evenly over both sides of the pork medallions. Place the seasoned pork in the skillet in a single layer. Cook for about 3 minutes per side, or until the pork is cooked through and no longer pink in the center.

3. Remove the skillet from the heat and let the pork medallions stand for 5 minutes before serving. If desired, garnish with fresh thyme leaves for added flavor and presentation. Enjoy your deliciously cooked pork medallions!

COCONUT PORK CURRY

Nutrition: Cal 260;Fat 16 g; Carb 10 g;Protein 18 g
Serving 4; Cook time 60 min

Ingredients
- 1 teaspoon ground cumin
- 1 teaspoon ground coriander
- 1/2 teaspoon ground cinnamon
- 1/4 teaspoon ground chilli powder
- 800g diced pork
- 1 tablespoon vegetable oil
- 1 large (200g) brown onion, chopped
- 2 cloves garlic, chopped
- 4cm piece (20g) fresh ginger, grated
- 1 tablespoon water
- 400ml can coconut cream or coconut milk
- 2 tablespoons brown sugar
- 1 teaspoon salt
- 1 tablespoon lemon juice
- 1/4 cup fresh coriander leaves

Instructions
1. In a medium bowl, combine the spices. Add the pork to the bowl and toss to coat the pork evenly with the spice mixture.
2. Heat half of the oil in a large frying pan over medium heat. Cook the pork in two batches, using the remaining oil for the second batch, until it is browned on all sides. Once browned, remove the pork from the pan and set it aside.
3. In the same pan, add the onion, garlic, ginger, and water. Cook over medium heat, stirring occasionally, until the onion is softened. Return the pork to the pan and add the coconut cream, sugar, and salt. Simmer the mixture, covered, stirring occasionally, for about 1 to 1 1/2 hours, or until the pork is tender and the sauce has thickened.
4. Stir in the juice and season to taste with salt and pepper. Sprinkle the dish with chopped coriander before serving. Enjoy your flavorful and tender pork dish!

PORK SKEWERS WITH CHIMICHURRI

Nutrition: Cal 450;Fat 36 g; Carb 6 g;Protein 30 g
Serving 2; Cook time 20 min

Ingredients
- 1/2 pound boneless pork shoulder
- 1/4 teaspoon ground cumin
- 1/4 teaspoon paprika
- 1 tablespoon coconut oil
- 1/4 cup olive oil
- 1/4 cup diced green peppers
- 3 tablespoons fresh chopped parsley
- 1 tablespoon fresh chopped cilantro
- 1 1/2 tablespoons fresh lemon juice
- 1 garlic clove (minced)

Instructions
1. Begin by cutting the pork into approximately 1-inch thick slices, ensuring uniformity in size.
2. Season the pork slices with a well-balanced combination of salt, pepper, cumin, and paprika, evenly coating each piece.
3. Carefully thread the seasoned pork slices onto sturdy wooden skewers, preparing them for cooking.
4. In a skillet, heat a suitable amount of coconut oil over medium-high heat until it reaches the desired temperature.
5. Place the pork skewers in the heated skillet, ensuring they are arranged in a single layer, and allow them to cook until both sides are beautifully browned and the meat is thoroughly cooked.
6. Meanwhile, gather the remaining ingredients and combine them in a food processor.
7. Utilize the pulse function of the food processor to chop the ingredients, followed by blending until a smooth consistency is achieved.
8. To serve, generously spoon the flavorful chimichurri sauce over the cooked pork skewers, allowing the vibrant flavors to enhance the dish.
9. Present the dish with an appealing and professional plating, ensuring the pork skewers are the focal point, accompanied by any desired garnishes.

APRICOT GLAZED PORK

Nutrition: Cal 315;Fat 10 g; Carb 20 g;Protein 35 g
Serving 12; Cook time 4 hours

Ingredients
- 4 pounds boneless pork loin roast
- 1 cup onion, chopped
- 2 tbsp Dijon mustard
- 2 cups beef broth
- 1 cup apricot preserves

Instructions
1. Mix broth, preserves, onion, and mustard in instant pot.
2. Cut pork to match. Add to instant pot.

3. Cover and turn the steam release handle towards the venting position.
4. Select the slow cooker setting and set to high.
5. Cook for 4 hours.

PORK AND CAULIFLOWER GRATIN

Nutrition: Cal 430;Fat 32 g; Carb 6 g;Protein 27 g
Serving 2; Cook time 40 min

Ingredients
- 1/2 lb pork ham, diced
- 1 small head of cauliflower, cut into small florets
- 1/2 cup heavy cream
- 1/2 cup shredded cheese
- 2 garlic cloves, minced
- 1/4 tsp ground nutmeg
- Salt and pepper to taste

Instructions
1. Preheat your oven to 375°F (190°C) and prepare a baking dish by greasing it with cooking spray, ensuring even coverage.
2. Heat a skillet over medium-high heat and cook the diced pork ham until it is nicely browned and fully cooked.
3. In a large pot filled with salted water, blanch the cauliflower florets for approximately 3-4 minutes, or until they reach a slightly tender consistency. Drain the cauliflower thoroughly and transfer it to the greased baking dish, creating an even layer.
4. In a saucepan set over medium heat, combine the heavy cream, shredded cheese, minced garlic, ground nutmeg, salt, and pepper. Stir the mixture continuously until the cheese has completely melted, and the sauce appears smooth and well combined.
5. Pour the garlic cream sauce evenly over the cauliflower in the baking dish, ensuring each floret is coated.
6. Sprinkle the cooked pork ham over the cauliflower and sauce, evenly distributing it across the dish.
7. Place the baking dish in the preheated oven and bake for approximately 25-30 minutes, or until the top becomes golden brown and the sauce is bubbling.
8. Once done, remove the gratin from the oven and allow it to cool slightly before serving. The dish is now ready to be enjoyed as a delicious and comforting meal.

EASY BBQ HAM

Nutrition: Cal 315;Fat 15 g; Carb 2 g;Protein 35 g
Serving 24; Cook time 14 hours

Ingredients
- 3 pounds ham, boneless
- 2 cups water
- 2 cups onions, sliced
- 6 whole cloves
- 2 cups BBQ sauce

Instructions
1. Place half of the onions at the bottom of the Instant Pot.
2. Insert cloves into the ham and carefully position it on top of the onions in the Instant Pot.
3. Layer the remaining onions on top of the ham. Pour in the appropriate amount of water.
4. Securely close the Instant Pot lid and set the steam release handle to the venting position.
5. Select the slow cooker setting and adjust it to medium heat.
6. Allow the ham and onions to cook for approximately 10 hours.
7. Once cooked, shred or cut up the meat and onions to your desired consistency.
8. Return the shredded or cut-up ham and onions to the Instant Pot.
9. Add the desired amount of barbecue sauce and continue cooking for an additional 4 hours.

KETO PORK AND HAM SKEWERS

Nutrition: Cal 405;Fat 25 g; Carb 5 g;Protein 38 g
Serving 2; Cook time 25 min

Ingredients
- 1/2 lb pork, cut into cubes
- 1/2 lb ham, cut into cubes
- 1 medium tomato, diced
- 1 medium bell pepper, diced
- Salt and pepper to taste
- Wooden skewers, soaked in water for 30 minutes

Instructions
1. Preheat the grill to medium-high heat.
2. Thread the pork and ham cubes onto the wooden skewers, alternating between pork and ham.
3. Season the skewers with salt and pepper.
4. Grill the skewers for 10-12 minutes, turning occasionally, until the pork and ham are cooked through.
5. In a medium bowl, combine the diced tomato and bell pepper.

6. Season the salad with salt and pepper to taste.
7. Serve the pork and ham skewers hot, accompanied by the tomato and bell pepper salad.

ASPARAGUS WRAPPED IN PROSCIUTTO

Nutrition: Cal 555;Fat 45 g; Carb 6.7 g;Protein 33 g
Serving 3; Cook time 25 min

Ingredients
- Mushrooms (3 cups)
- Rice (1 ½ cups)
- Chicken stock (4 cups)
- Olive oil (1/4 cup)
- Onion (1 cup, chopped)
- Butter (unsalted, ¼ cup)
- White wine (3/4 cup)
- Rosemary
- Parmesan (half cup, grated)
- Salt and pepper

Instructions
1. Set the Pressure Cooker to "Sauté" mode. Add the olive oil and butter, allowing them to melt for a few minutes. Add the mushrooms and cook them for about 3 minutes.
2. Add the onion, stir, and cook for a couple more minutes. Then add the rosemary and cook for an additional minute.
3. Add the rice and stir until it is coated with the butter and olive oil mixture. Stir for a couple of minutes, then pour in the wine. Let it simmer for three more minutes.
4. Pour in the chicken stock and stir for a minute.
5. Now, close and secure the lid of the pressure cooker. Select the "High Pressure" setting and set the timer for 6 minutes.
6. Allow the pressure to release naturally for 5 minutes.
7. Open the lid and stir the risotto until it becomes creamy. Remove the rosemary (if using sprigs) or strain it out if it's chopped.
8. Season with salt, pepper, and Parmesan cheese. Stir until the cheese melts.

BRATWURSTS AND SAUERKRAUT

Nutrition: Cal 525;Fat 42 g; Carb 12 g;Protein 24 g
Serving 4; Cook time 50 min

Ingredients
- 2 tablespoons avocado oil
- 1 yellow onion, thinly sliced
- 1 pound bratwurst
- 1 (16-ounce) jar sauerkraut, drained
- 1½ cups chicken broth
- 1 teaspoon garlic powder
- Freshly ground black pepper

Instructions
1. In a large cast-iron skillet over medium heat, heat the oil. Add the onion and bratwurst and cook for 6 to 8 minutes, or until they start to develop some color.
2. Stir in the sauerkraut, broth, garlic powder, salt, and pepper. Simmer the mixture for 30 to 40 minutes, or until the sausages are fully cooked.
3. Divide 1 cup of sauerkraut and 1 bratwurst into each of the 4 storage containers.

SALAD WITH BROCCOLI, CAULIFLOWER AND BACON

Nutrition: Cal 164;Fat 14 g; Carb 8 g;Protein 5 g
Serving 4; Cook time 15 min

Ingredients
- Broccoli (3/4 cups, chopped)
- Cauliflower (3/4 cups, chopped)
- Bacon (3 slices, chopped)
- Onion (1, chopped)
- Vinegar (1 teaspoon)
- Sour cream (3/4 cups)

Instructions
1. Place the cauliflower and broccoli in the pressure cooker and set it to "Steam" for a few minutes, making sure not to overcook them. Remove the vegetables from the boiling water and set them aside.
2. Fry the bacon until it turns brown, then set it aside and let it cool.
3. In a mixing bowl, combine the onion (you can use spring onion as well), vinegar, salt, pepper, and sour cream.
4. Mix the sauce with the broccoli and cauliflower, and garnish with additional bacon pieces for decoration.

ROSEMARY ROASTED PORK WITH CAULIFLOWER

Nutrition: Cal 300;Fat 17 g; Carb 3 g;Protein 37 g
Serving 4; Cook time 30 min

Ingredients

- 1 ½ pounds boneless pork tenderloin
- 1 tablespoon coconut oil
- 1 tablespoon fresh chopped rosemary
- Salt and pepper
- 1 tablespoon olive oil
- 2 cups cauliflower florets

Instructions

1. Begin by rubbing the pork with coconut oil, ensuring all sides are coated. Then, season the pork with rosemary, salt, and pepper, evenly distributing the seasonings.
2. Heat the olive oil in a large skillet over medium-high heat until it shimmers.
3. Carefully add the seasoned pork to the skillet and cook for approximately 2 to 3 minutes on each side, or until the pork develops a browned crust.
4. Sprinkle the cauliflower florets around the pork in the skillet, distributing them evenly.
5. Reduce the heat to low, cover the skillet with a lid, and allow the pork and cauliflower to cook for approximately 8 to 10 minutes, or until the pork is thoroughly cooked.
6. Once cooked, remove the pork from the skillet and let it rest for a few minutes before slicing it. Serve the sliced pork alongside the cooked cauliflower.

SAUSAGE STUFFED BELL PEPPERS

Nutrition: Cal 355;Fat 23,5 g; Carb 16,5 g;Protein 19 g
Serving 4; Cook time 55 min

Ingredients

- 1 medium head cauliflower, chopped
- 1 tablespoon olive oil
- 12 ounces ground Italian sausage
- 1 small yellow onion, chopped
- 1 teaspoon dried oregano
- Salt and pepper
- 4 medium bell peppers

Instructions

1. Begin by preheating the oven to 350°F (175°C).
2. Using a food processor, pulse the cauliflower until it reaches a rice-like consistency, resembling grains.
3. Heat the oil in a skillet over medium heat and add the cauliflower rice. Cook for approximately 6 to 8 minutes, stirring occasionally, until the cauliflower becomes tender.
4. Transfer the cooked cauliflower rice to a bowl and set it aside. Reheat the skillet.
5. Add the sausage to the skillet and cook it until it browns. Once done, drain any excess fat from the skillet.
6. Stir the cooked sausage into the cauliflower rice. Then, add the onion, oregano, salt, and pepper, combining all the ingredients thoroughly.
7. Slice the tops off the peppers, removing the seeds and pith from the inside. Spoon the sausage mixture into each pepper, filling them up.
8. Place the peppers upright in a baking dish and cover the dish with foil.
9. Bake the stuffed peppers for 30 minutes. Then, remove the foil and bake for an additional 15 minutes, allowing the peppers to become tender and the flavors to meld. Serve the stuffed peppers hot.

BACON-WRAPPED PORK TENDERLOIN WITH CAULIFLOWER

Nutrition: Cal 330;Fat 18,5 g; Carb 3 g;Protein 38 g
Serving 4; Cook time 35 min

Ingredients

- 1 ¼ pounds boneless pork tenderloin
- Salt and pepper
- 8 slices uncooked bacon
- 1 tablespoon olive oil
- 2 cups cauliflower florets

Instructions

1. Preheat the oven to 425°F (220°C) and season the pork with salt and pepper to taste.
2. Wrap the seasoned pork with bacon slices and place it on a foil-lined roasting pan, ensuring that the bacon is securely wrapped around the pork.
3. Roast the pork in the preheated oven for approximately 25 minutes or until the internal temperature reaches 155°F (68°C). Use a meat thermometer to ensure accurate measurement.

4. Meanwhile, heat the oil in a skillet over medium heat on the stovetop.
5. Add the cauliflower to the skillet and sauté it for about 8 to 10 minutes, or until it reaches a tender-crisp consistency. Stir occasionally to ensure even cooking.
6. Turn on the broiler setting in your oven. Carefully move the cooked pork under the broiler for a few minutes to crisp up the bacon wrapping. Keep a close eye on it to prevent burning.
7. Once the pork is nicely browned and the bacon is crispy, remove it from the oven. Let it rest for a few minutes before slicing it into serving portions.
8. Serve the sliced pork with the sautéed cauliflower as a delicious and satisfying meal. Enjoy!

KETO BAKED PORK CHOPS WITH MUSHROOMS

Nutrition: Cal 370;Fat 23 g; Carb 5 g;Protein 34 g
Serving 2; Cook time 40 min

Ingredients
- 2 bone-in pork chops (about 1 inch thick)
- 1/2 cup sliced mushrooms
- 1/2 cup sliced onions
- 2 tbsp mayonnaise
- 1/4 cup shredded mozzarella cheese
- Salt and pepper to taste

Instructions
1. Preheat the oven to 375°F (190°C) and prepare a baking dish by lining it with parchment paper.
2. Season both sides of the pork chops with salt and pepper according to your taste preferences.
3. Heat a skillet over medium-high heat and sauté the sliced mushrooms and onions until they become tender and lightly browned, which should take approximately 5-7 minutes.
4. Spread a layer of mayonnaise on top of each pork chop, then place the sautéed mushrooms and onions on top of the mayonnaise layer.
5. Sprinkle shredded mozzarella cheese over the vegetables, ensuring an even distribution.
6. Transfer the prepared pork chops to the lined baking dish and bake them in the preheated oven for about 25-30 minutes, or until the pork chops are fully cooked and the cheese is melted and bubbly.

7. Once done, remove the baking dish from the oven and serve the hot and delicious pork chops.

KETO GRILLED PORK RIBS

Nutrition: Cal 584;Fat 48 g; Carb 3 g;Protein 33 g
Serving 2; Cook time 35 min

Ingredients
- 1 pound pork ribs
- 2 cloves garlic, minced
- 1 tablespoon smoked paprika
- 1 tablespoon ground cumin
- 1 tablespoon dried oregano
- 1 teaspoon onion powder
- Salt and black pepper to taste
- 2 tablespoons olive oil

Instructions
1. Preheat the grill to medium-high heat.
2. In a small bowl, combine the garlic, smoked paprika, cumin, oregano, onion powder, salt, black pepper, and olive oil to create a marinade.
3. Apply the marinade to the pork ribs, ensuring they are well coated on both sides.
4. Grill the pork ribs for approximately 10-15 minutes on each side, or until they are fully cooked and have achieved desirable grill marks.
5. Serve the grilled pork ribs hot and enjoy!

PORK RIBS WITH SPICE RUB

Nutrition: Cal 658;Fat 55 g; Carb 3 g;Protein 36 g
Serving 2; Cook time 2 hours 10 min

Ingredients
- 1 pound pork ribs
- 1 tablespoon smoked paprika
- 1 teaspoon garlic powder
- 1 teaspoon onion powder
- 1 teaspoon dried thyme
- 1 teaspoon dried oregano
- 1/2 teaspoon cumin
- Salt and black pepper to taste

Instructions
1. Preheat the oven to 300°F (150°C).
2. In a small bowl, mix together the smoked paprika, garlic powder, onion powder, dried thyme, dried oregano, cumin, salt, and black pepper.

3. Rub the spice mixture onto the pork ribs, making sure to cover all sides.
4. Place the ribs onto a baking sheet lined with aluminum foil.
5. Bake in the oven for 2-3 hours, until the meat is tender and falls off the bone.
6. Remove from the oven and let cool for 5-10 minutes before serving.

PORK RIBS WITH ROASTED VEGETABLES

Nutrition: Cal 515;Fat 35 g; Carb 10 g;Protein 32 g
Serving 2; Cook time 80 min

Ingredients
- 1 pound pork ribs
- 1 medium zucchini, sliced into rounds
- 1 medium red bell pepper, sliced into strips
- 1 medium yellow onion, sliced into wedges
- 2 cloves garlic, minced
- 2 tablespoons olive oil
- Salt and black pepper to taste

Instructions
1. Preheat the oven to 375°F (190°C).
2. In a large mixing bowl, combine the sliced zucchini, red bell pepper, and onion with minced garlic and olive oil. Toss them together until the vegetables are coated.
3. Season the pork ribs with salt and black pepper.
4. Place the pork ribs on a baking sheet lined with aluminum foil.
5. Arrange the seasoned vegetables around the pork ribs on the baking sheet.
6. Roast the pork ribs and vegetables in the oven for 40-45 minutes, or until the pork is cooked through and the vegetables are tender.
7. Remove from the oven and let it cool for a few minutes before serving. Enjoy your delicious roasted pork ribs and vegetables!

PORK ROLS WITH WALNUT, PRUNE, AND CHEESE

Nutrition: Cal 475;Fat 34 g; Carb 8 g;Protein 32 g
Serving 2; Cook time 35 min

Ingredients
- 4 thin pork cutlets
- 1/2 cup chopped walnuts
- 1/2 cup chopped pitted prunes
- 1/2 cup shredded cheese (such as Gouda or Cheddar)
- Salt and black pepper to taste
- 2 tablespoons olive oil

Instructions
1. Preheat the oven to 375°F (190°C).
2. Lay the pork cutlets flat on a work surface and sprinkle them with salt and black pepper.
3. In a small mixing bowl, combine the chopped walnuts, prunes, and shredded cheese.
4. Spoon the walnut, prune, and cheese mixture onto the center of each pork cutlet.
5. Roll up the pork cutlets, securing them with toothpicks to hold the filling inside.
6. Heat olive oil in a large skillet over medium-high heat.
7. Brown the pork rolls on all sides in the skillet, cooking them until they are nicely browned.
8. Transfer the browned pork rolls to a baking dish and bake in the preheated oven for 20-25 minutes, or until the pork is cooked through.
9. Remove the toothpicks from the pork rolls before serving. Enjoy your delicious stuffed pork rolls!

PORK ROLLS WITH MOZZARELLA

Nutrition: Cal 455;Fat 33 g; Carb 2 g;Protein 33 g
Serving 2; Cook time 45 min

Ingredients
- 4 thin pork cutlets
- 1/2 cup shredded mozzarella cheese
- 1 tablespoon chopped fresh thyme
- Salt and black pepper to taste
- 2 tablespoons olive oil
- 1/4 cup heavy cream
- 1/4 cup chicken broth
- 1 tablespoon Dijon mustard

Instructions
1. Preheat the oven to 375°F (190°C).
2. Lay the pork cutlets flat on a work surface and sprinkle them with salt and black pepper.
3. In a small mixing bowl, combine the shredded mozzarella cheese and chopped thyme.
4. Spoon the cheese and thyme mixture onto the center of each pork cutlet.
5. Roll up the pork cutlets, securing them with toothpicks to hold the filling inside.
6. Heat olive oil in a large skillet over medium-high heat.
7. Brown the pork rolls on all sides in the skillet, cooking them until they are nicely browned.

8. Transfer the browned pork rolls to a baking dish and bake in the preheated oven for 20-25 minutes, or until the pork is cooked through.
9. In the same skillet used to brown the pork rolls, add the heavy cream and chicken broth.
10. Cook over medium heat until the sauce thickens, stirring occasionally.
11. Whisk in the Dijon mustard and season with salt and black pepper to taste.
12. Remove the toothpicks from the pork rolls and serve them with the creamy mustard sauce. Enjoy your delicious stuffed pork rolls with creamy mustard sauce!

PORK ROLLS WITH BLUE CHEESE AND WALNUT

Nutrition: Cal 515;Fat 42 g; Carb 5 g;Protein 28 g
Serving 2; Cook time 40 min

Ingredients
- 4 thin pork cutlets
- 1/2 cup crumbled blue cheese
- 1/2 cup chopped walnuts
- Salt and black pepper to taste
- 2 tablespoons olive oil
- 1/4 cup heavy cream
- 1/4 cup chicken broth
- 1 tablespoon chopped fresh parsley

Instructions
1. Preheat the oven to 375°F (190°C).
2. Lay the pork cutlets flat on a work surface and sprinkle them with salt and black pepper.
3. In a small mixing bowl, combine the crumbled blue cheese and chopped walnuts.
4. Spoon the blue cheese and walnut mixture onto the center of each pork cutlet.
5. Roll up the pork cutlets, securing them with toothpicks to hold the filling inside.
6. Heat olive oil in a large skillet over medium-high heat.
7. Brown the pork rolls on all sides in the skillet, cooking them until they are nicely browned.
8. Transfer the browned pork rolls to a baking dish and bake in the preheated oven for 20-25 minutes, or until the pork is cooked through.
9. In the same skillet used to brown the pork rolls, add the heavy cream and chicken broth.
10. Cook over medium heat until the sauce thickens, stirring occasionally.
11. Remove the toothpicks from the pork rolls and serve them with the creamy sauce, garnished

with chopped fresh parsley. Enjoy your delicious stuffed pork rolls with creamy sauce!

PORK MEATBALLS WITH CREAMY MUSHROOM SAUCE

Nutrition: Cal 521;Fat 43 g; Carb 5 g;Protein 26 g
Serving 2; Cook time 40 min

Ingredients
- 1 pound ground pork
- 1/2 cup almond flour
- 1/4 cup grated Parmesan cheese
- 1 egg
- 1/2 teaspoon garlic powder
- Salt and black pepper to taste
- 2 tablespoons olive oil
- 8 oz mushrooms, sliced
- 1/2 cup heavy cream
- 1/4 cup chicken broth
- 1/4 cup grated Parmesan cheese
- Chopped fresh parsley for garnish

Instructions
1. Preheat the oven to 400°F (200°C).
2. In a large mixing bowl, combine the ground pork, almond flour, grated Parmesan cheese, egg, garlic powder, salt, and black pepper. Mix well until all the ingredients are evenly incorporated.
3. Shape the mixture into meatballs, about 1-2 inches in size.
4. Heat olive oil in a large skillet over medium-high heat.
5. Brown the meatballs on all sides in the skillet, cooking them until they develop a nice golden crust.
6. Transfer the browned meatballs to a baking dish and bake in the preheated oven for 15-20 minutes, or until the pork is fully cooked.
7. In the same skillet used to brown the meatballs, add the sliced mushrooms and cook until they release their moisture and become tender.
8. Pour in the heavy cream and chicken broth, bringing the mixture to a simmer.
9. Stir in the grated Parmesan cheese and continue to simmer until the sauce thickens to your desired consistency.
10. Season the sauce with salt and black pepper to taste.

11. Serve the meatballs with the creamy mushroom sauce, spooning the sauce over the meatballs. Garnish with chopped fresh parsley for added freshness and flavor. Enjoy your delicious pork meatballs with creamy mushroom sauce!

PORK MEATBALLS WITH VEGETABLE MARINARA SAUCE

Nutrition: Cal 475;Fat 35 g; Carb 9 g;Protein 30 g
Serving 2; Cook time 35 min

Ingredients
FOR THE PORK MEATBALLS:
- 1 pound ground pork
- 1/4 cup almond flour
- 1 egg
- 2 cloves garlic, minced
- 1 tablespoon fresh parsley, chopped
- 1/2 teaspoon salt
- 1/4 teaspoon black pepper

FOR THE VEGETABLE SAUCE:
- 1/2 onion, chopped
- 1 red bell pepper, chopped
- 2 garlic cloves, minced
- 1 can diced tomatoes (14.5 ounces)
- 1/4 teaspoon dried basil
- 1/4 teaspoon dried oregano
- 1/2 teaspoon salt
- 1/4 teaspoon black pepper

Instructions
1. In a large bowl, combine the ground pork, almond flour, egg, garlic, parsley, salt, and pepper. Mix well until all the ingredients are thoroughly incorporated.
2. Shape the mixture into 12-14 meatballs, forming them into even-sized balls. Place the meatballs on a baking sheet lined with parchment paper.
3. Bake the meatballs in the preheated oven for 20-25 minutes, or until they are fully cooked and browned.
4. While the meatballs are cooking, prepare the vegetable sauce. Heat a large skillet over medium heat and add the onion, bell pepper, and garlic. Cook for 5-7 minutes, or until the vegetables are soft and fragrant.
5. Add the diced tomatoes, basil, oregano, salt, and pepper to the skillet. Stir well to combine and bring the sauce to a simmer.
6. Reduce the heat to low and let the sauce simmer for 10-15 minutes, allowing it to thicken slightly.

7. Once the meatballs are cooked, add them to the skillet with the vegetable sauce. Gently stir to coat the meatballs with the sauce.
8. Serve the meatballs and sauce hot, garnishing with additional chopped fresh parsley if desired. They can be enjoyed on their own, with pasta, rice, or crusty bread.

KETO PORK MEATBALLS WITH BLUE CHEESE SAUCE

Nutrition: Cal 560;Fat 46 g; Carb 3 g;Protein 35 g
Serving 2; Cook time 40 min

Ingredients
FOR THE MEATBALLS:
- 1 lb ground pork
- 1/4 cup almond flour
- 1 large egg
- 1 tsp garlic powder
- 1 tsp onion powder
- 1 tsp dried thyme
- 1/2 tsp salt
- 1/4 tsp black pepper

FOR THE BLUE CHEESE SAUCE:
- 1/2 cup heavy cream
- 2 oz blue cheese, crumbled
- 1 tbsp unsalted butter
- 1 tbsp chopped fresh parsley
- Salt and pepper to taste

Instructions
1. Preheat the oven to 400°F (200°C) and line a baking sheet with parchment paper.
2. In a large bowl, combine ground pork, almond flour, egg, garlic powder, onion powder, dried thyme, salt, and black pepper. Mix well until all the ingredients are thoroughly combined.
3. Use your hands to shape the mixture into 16 meatballs, each about 1 1/2 inches in diameter.
4. Place the meatballs on the prepared baking sheet and bake for 18-20 minutes, or until they are golden brown and cooked through.
5. While the meatballs are baking, prepare the blue cheese sauce. In a small saucepan, heat the heavy cream and butter over medium heat until the butter is melted.
6. Add the crumbled blue cheese to the saucepan and whisk until the cheese is melted and the sauce is smooth. If the sauce is too thick, add a splash of water to thin it out.

7. Season the sauce with salt and pepper to taste, then stir in the chopped parsley.
8. Serve the pork meatballs with the blue cheese sauce on top. They can be enjoyed as an appetizer, served with a side salad or vegetables, or as a main course with pasta or rice.

PORK CHOPS WITH CARAMELIZED ONION, TOMATO, MAYONNAISE, AND CHEESE

Nutrition: Cal 570;Fat 39 g; Carb 7 g;Protein 46 g
Serving 2; Cook time 60 min

Ingredients
- 2 bone-in pork chops (6-8 ounces each)
- Salt and black pepper
- 1 tablespoon olive oil
- 1 medium onion, sliced
- 1 medium tomato, sliced
- 2 tablespoons mayonnaise
- 1/4 cup shredded cheddar cheese

Instructions
1. Preheat the oven to 375°F (190°C).
2. Season the pork chops with salt and black pepper on both sides.
3. In a large skillet over medium heat, heat the olive oil. Once the oil is hot, add the sliced onions and cook for 10-15 minutes, stirring occasionally, until they are caramelized and soft.
4. While the onions are cooking, place the pork chops in a baking dish. Top each pork chop with sliced tomatoes.
5. Spread 1 tablespoon of mayonnaise on each pork chop, covering the tomatoes.
6. Sprinkle the caramelized onions over the mayonnaise, and then top each pork chop with 2 tablespoons of shredded cheddar cheese.
7. Bake the pork chops in the preheated oven for 25-30 minutes, or until the cheese is melted and bubbly, and the pork is cooked through.
8. Serve the pork chops hot, garnished with additional chopped fresh parsley if desired. These flavorful and cheesy pork chops can be accompanied by roasted vegetables, mashed potatoes, or a side salad. Enjoy!

BAKED PORK CHOPS WITH PINEAPPLE

Nutrition: Cal 410;Fat 28 g; Carb 6 g;Protein 34 g
Serving 2; Cook time 40 min

Ingredients
- 2 bone-in pork chops (about 1 inch thick)
- 1/2 cup diced pineapple
- 2 tbsp mayonnaise
- 1/4 cup shredded cheddar cheese
- Salt and pepper to taste

Instructions
1. Preheat the oven to 375°F (190°C) and line a baking dish with parchment paper.
2. Season the pork chops with salt and pepper on both sides.
3. In a small bowl, mix together the diced pineapple and mayonnaise until well combined.
4. Place the pork chops in the prepared baking dish and spoon the pineapple mixture on top of each chop.
5. Sprinkle the shredded cheddar cheese on top of the pineapple mixture.
6. Bake for 25-30 minutes, until the pork chops are cooked through and the cheese is melted and bubbly.
7. Serve the pork chops hot. The combination of sweet pineapple, creamy mayo, and melted cheese adds delicious flavor to the pork chops. Enjoy!

ROASTED PORK LOIN WITH GRAINY MUSTARD SAUCE

Nutrition: Cal 368;Fat 29 g; Carb 2 g;Protein 25 g
Serving 2; Cook time 45 min

Ingredients
- 1 (2-pound) boneless pork loin roast
- Sea salt
- Freshly ground black pepper
- 3 tablespoons olive oil
- 1&1/2 cups heavy (whipping) cream
- 3 tablespoons grainy mustard, such as Pommery

Instructions
1. Preheat the oven to 375°F (190°C) and line a baking dish with parchment paper.
2. Season the pork chops with salt and pepper on both sides.

3. In a small bowl, mix together the diced pineapple and mayonnaise until well combined.
4. Place the pork chops in the prepared baking dish and spoon the pineapple mixture on top of each chop.
5. Sprinkle the shredded cheddar cheese on top of the pineapple mixture.
6. Bake for 25-30 minutes, until the pork chops are cooked through and the cheese is melted and bubbly.
7. Serve the pork chops hot. The combination of sweet pineapple, creamy mayo, and melted cheese adds delicious flavor to the pork chops. Enjoy!

FISH AND SEAFOOD

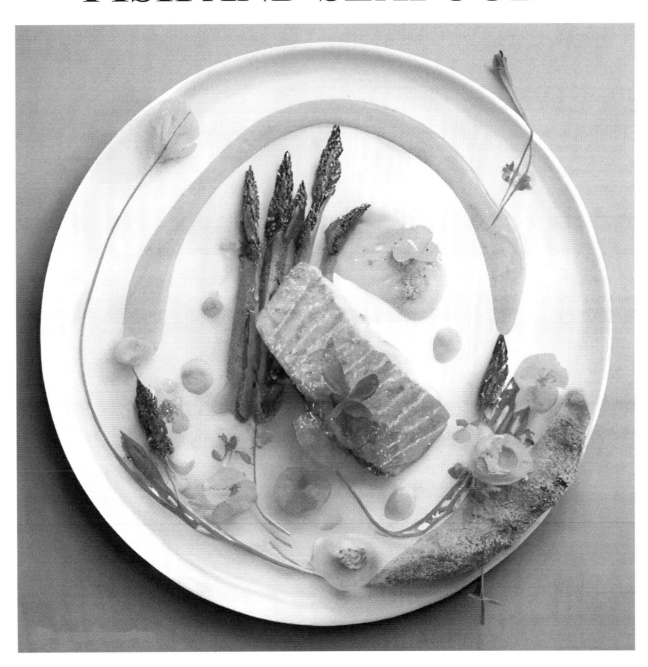

SALMON AND CREAM CHEESE SUSHI ROLLS

Nutrition: Cal 330;Fat 20 g;Carb 9 g;Protein 30 g
Serving 2; Cook time 15 min

Ingredients
- 4 sheets of nori seaweed
- 1/2 lb fresh salmon, sliced
- 4 oz cream cheese, softened
- 1 small cucumber, sliced into thin strips
- 2 tbsp rice vinegar
- 1 tsp Swerve (or other keto-friendly sweetener)
- 1 tsp salt
- Wasabi and soy sauce (optional)

Instructions
1. In a small bowl, mix the rice vinegar, Swerve (or any other sweetener of your choice), and salt together until the sweetener and salt are dissolved. This will create a sweet and tangy vinegar mixture that will be used for seasoning the sushi rice.
2. Lay a sheet of nori seaweed on a sushi mat or a piece of plastic wrap. This will serve as the base for rolling the sushi.
3. Spread a thin layer of cream cheese over the nori sheet, leaving a 1-inch border at the top. The cream cheese adds a creamy and tangy flavor to the sushi roll.
4. Place a layer of sliced salmon on top of the cream cheese. Make sure to evenly distribute the salmon slices across the nori sheet.
5. Add a layer of sliced cucumber on top of the salmon. The cucumber adds a refreshing crunch to the sushi roll.
6. Roll the sushi tightly, using the sushi mat or plastic wrap to help you. Start from the bottom edge of the nori sheet and roll it up, applying gentle pressure to ensure the ingredients stick together. Repeat this process with the remaining nori sheets and ingredients.
7. Once the sushi rolls are tightly rolled, use a sharp knife to slice them into bite-sized pieces. Wetting the knife with water between each cut can help prevent sticking.
8. Serve the sushi rolls with optional wasabi and soy sauce. Wasabi adds a spicy kick, while soy sauce provides a savory and salty dipping option for the sushi rolls. Enjoy your homemade sushi!

SALMON AND CAULIFLOWER RICE SUSHI ROLLS

Nutrition: Cal 470;Fat 33 g;Carb 15 g;Protein 32 g
Serving 2; Cook time 25 min

Ingredients
- 2 sheets of nori seaweed
- 1/2 lb fresh salmon, sliced
- 4 oz cream cheese, softened
- 1 cup cauliflower rice, cooked
- 1 small cucumber, sliced into thin strips
- 1 small avocado, sliced
- 2 tbsp rice vinegar
- 1 tsp Swerve (or other keto-friendly sweetener)
- 1 tsp salt
- Wasabi and soy sauce (optional)

Instructions
1. In a small bowl, mix the rice vinegar, Swerve (or any other sweetener of your choice), and salt together until the sweetener and salt are dissolved. This will create a sweet and tangy vinegar mixture that will be used for seasoning the cauliflower rice.
2. Lay a sheet of nori seaweed on a flat surface, such as a cutting board or sushi mat.
3. Spread a thin layer of cream cheese over the nori sheet, leaving a 1-inch border at the top. The cream cheese adds a creamy and tangy flavor to the nori envelope.
4. Place a layer of sliced salmon on top of the cream cheese. Ensure that the salmon slices are evenly distributed across the nori sheet.
5. Add a layer of cooked cauliflower rice on top of the salmon. The cauliflower rice serves as a low-carb alternative to traditional sushi rice.
6. Add a layer of sliced cucumber and avocado on top of the cauliflower rice. The cucumber and avocado provide a refreshing and creamy texture to the nori envelope.
7. Roll the nori tightly, starting from the bottom edge and rolling it up towards the top. Use a little water to moisten the top edge of the nori sheet and seal the roll. Repeat this process with the remaining nori sheets and ingredients.
8. Once the nori rolls are tightly rolled, use a sharp knife to slice them into bite-sized pieces. Wetting the knife with water between each cut can help prevent sticking.
9. Serve the nori envelopes with optional wasabi and soy sauce. Wasabi adds a spicy kick, while

soy sauce provides a savory and salty dipping option for the nori envelopes. Enjoy your delicious low-carb sushi alternative!

KETO CRISPY SKIN SALMON IN WHITE WINE SAUCE

Nutrition: Cal 374;Fat 15 g;Carb 2 g;Protein 48 g
Serving 2; Cook time 25 min

Ingredients:
- 1 pound of Wild salmon fillets
- 2 tablespoons of butter
- 2 tablespoons of avocado oil
- salt to taste
- juice from a lemon

For sauce:
- 1/2 cup of white wine
- 1/2 teaspoon of garlic crushed
- juice from a quarter of a lemon
- dash of white pepper
- 1/8 teaspoon of salt
- 1/4 cup of heavy whipping cream
- 2 tablespoons of butter
- 2 teaspoons of capers

Instructions:
1. First dry your salmon with paper towels so that it won't stick to the pan.
2. Heat oil and butter in a skillet over a medium-high heat.
3. Glaze the skin with a little oil, as well, and rub it in. Then season the skin with some salt, too.
4. When butter and oil start to sizzle, add salmon, skin side down. Press with your spatula so that the skin will cook evenly.
5. Now you can season your salmon with salt and squeeze some lemon juice on top too.
6. Cook for 3 minutes.
7. Then flip and sear the top for 2 minutes more. If your salmon is thick, it may need another minute.
8. Transfer salmon to a plate and set aside.

FOR SAUCE:

1. Wipe the pan clean and make your sauce in the same pan.
2. First bring your wine to a simmer and reduce by half the volume. This will take about five minutes. Then add garlic, salt, pepper, and a squeeze of lemon juice.
3. Whisk in cream and add the cold butter, one tablespoon at a time. As soon as all the butter is whisked in, stir in your capers and turn off the flame.
4. Spoon sauce onto each plate and place salmon skin side up on top of the sauce. Serve and enjoy.

ALASKAN SALMON WITH BUTTER CREAM SAUCE AND AVOCADO

Nutrition: Cal 490;Fat 31 g;Carb 12 g;Protein 31 g
Serving 2; Cook time 20 min

Ingredients:
- 1 tablespoons butter
- 2 tablespoons shallot, finely chopped
- ¼ cup dry white wine
- ¼ cup heavy whipping cream
- 1 avocado, cube
- Pinch of salt
- Pinch of pepper

Instructions:
1. Start by melting butter in a saucepan over medium heat. Allow it to fully melt and become hot.
2. Stir in the shallot and let it cook for about a minute until it becomes fragrant and slightly translucent.
3. Pour in the white wine and let it simmer for a couple of minutes. This helps cook off some of the alcohol and infuse the sauce with flavor.
4. Add the cream to the saucepan while continuing to stir. This will help incorporate the butter and cream together, creating a smooth and creamy consistency. Turn off the heat.
5. Add the avocado to the sauce and season it with salt and pepper according to your taste preferences. Stir gently to combine all the ingredients.
6. Set the sauce aside to keep it warm until you are ready to serve it. The residual heat from the pan will help keep it at a suitable temperature.
7. You can now use this delicious avocado cream sauce to accompany your desired dish. Enjoy!

GRILLED SALMON WITH PESTO AND ROASTED ASPARAGUS

Nutrition: Cal 447;Fat 31 g;Carb 7 g;Protein 36 g
Serving 2; Cook time 20 min

Ingredients:
- 2 salmon fillets (about 6 oz. each)
- 2 tbsp. of pesto
- 12 asparagus spears
- 2 tbsp. of olive oil
- Salt and pepper to taste

Instructions:
1. Preheat your oven to 400°F (200°C).
2. Rinse the asparagus and pat them dry. Place them on a baking sheet lined with parchment paper. Drizzle with olive oil and season with salt and pepper. Roast in the oven for 15-20 minutes, or until tender.
3. While the asparagus is roasting, heat up a grill pan over medium-high heat. Brush the salmon fillets with olive oil and season them with salt and pepper.
4. Place the salmon fillets on the grill pan, skin side down. Grill for 3-4 minutes on each side or until cooked to your desired level of doneness.
5. Once the salmon is cooked, remove it from the heat and spread a tablespoon of pesto over each fillet.
6. Serve the salmon fillets with the roasted asparagus on the side.

KETO ASIAN GLAZED SALMON

Nutrition: Cal 220;Fat 35 g;Carb 8 g;Protein 38 g
Serving 6; Cook time 23 min

Ingredients:
- 6 pieces of fresh salmon, about 2" wide/4 ounce
- ½ cup Brown Swerve
- ½ cup Liquid Aminos
- 1 teaspoon Sambal, plain or garlic
- 2 tablespoons rice vinegar
- 2 teaspoons toasted sesame oil
- 2 teaspoons fresh ginger, grated
- 1 teaspoon fresh garlic, grated
- Juice of ½ lime

Instructions:
1. Preheat the oven to 400°F (200°C).
2. In a cup, mix all the ingredients and transfer them into a small saucepan over medium heat. Simmer until the mixture is reduced by about a third, reaching a thick and sticky consistency.
3. Place the salmon fillets on a wire baking rack sprayed with nonstick spray and lined with foil for easier cleanup. Brush the glaze onto the salmon, making sure to cover all sides, and bake for 10 minutes.
4. Remove the salmon from the oven and increase the temperature to 450°F (230°C). Brush some more of the glaze over the tops of the salmon fillets and bake for another 3-5 minutes on the top rack of your oven. Keep a close eye on it to prevent burning.
5. Enjoy your glazed salmon with its sticky and flavorful glaze!

BACON-WRAPPED SALMON WITH SPINACH SALAD

Nutrition: Cal 505;Fat 38 g;Carb 3 g;Protein 35 g
Serving 2; Cook time 30 min

Ingredients:
- 2 salmon fillets (about 6 oz. each)
- 4 slices of bacon
- 2 cups of fresh spinach
- 2 tbsp. of olive oil
- 2 tbsp. of balsamic vinegar
- Salt and pepper to taste

Instructions:
1. Preheat your oven to 400°F (200°C).
2. Rinse the spinach and pat it dry. Place it in a large mixing bowl.
3. In a small bowl, whisk together the olive oil and balsamic vinegar to make a dressing. Pour the dressing over the spinach and toss to combine.
4. Wrap 2 slices of bacon around each salmon fillet, securing them with toothpicks if necessary.
5. Place the bacon-wrapped salmon fillets on a baking sheet lined with parchment paper. Season with salt and pepper.
6. Bake in the oven for 15-20 minutes, or until the salmon is cooked to your desired level of doneness.
7. Serve the salmon fillets on top of the spinach salad.
8. Enjoy your delicious bacon-wrapped salmon with a fresh and tangy spinach salad!

SMOKED SALMON AND ASPARAGUS FRITTATA

Nutrition: Cal 385;Fat 29 g;Carb 4 g;Protein 25 g
Serving 2; Cook time 25 min

Ingredients:
- 4 slices of bacon
- 12 asparagus spears, trimmed and cut into bite-sized pieces
- 4 oz. of smoked salmon, chopped
- 4 eggs
- 1/4 cup of heavy cream
- Salt and pepper to taste
- 1 tbsp. of olive oil

Instructions:
1. Preheat your oven to 350°F (180°C).
2. In a large oven-safe skillet, cook the bacon over medium heat until crisp. Remove the bacon from the skillet and set it aside.
3. Add the asparagus to the skillet and cook for 3-4 minutes, or until tender. Remove the asparagus from the skillet and set it aside with the bacon.
4. In a mixing bowl, whisk together the eggs, heavy cream, salt, and pepper.
5. Add the olive oil to the skillet and heat it over medium-high heat. Once the skillet is hot, pour the egg mixture into the skillet and stir gently to distribute the ingredients.
6. Add the cooked bacon, asparagus, and smoked salmon to the skillet, distributing them evenly over the egg mixture.
7. Transfer the skillet to the preheated oven and bake for 10-15 minutes, or until the frittata is cooked through and golden brown on top.
8. Remove the skillet from the oven and let it cool for a few minutes before slicing and serving.
9. Enjoy your delicious frittata with bacon, asparagus, and smoked salmon!

PARMESAN CRUSTED FLOUNDER FISH

Nutrition: Cal 550;Fat 35 g;Carb 8 g;Protein 38 g
Serving 2; Cook time 10 min

Ingredients:
- 1 lb wild-caught Flounder Fish thawed if using frozen
- 2 tablespoon Blanched Almond Flour
- 2 tablespoon finely grated Parmesan Cheese the powdered kind
- 1/8 teaspoon garlic powder
- 1/8 teaspoon onion powder
- 2 tablespoon Mayonnaise
- 1/4 teaspoon salt
- 1/8 teaspoon black pepper

Instructions:
1. Preheat Oven to 400°F (200°C), and grease a baking sheet.
2. In a mixing bowl combine: almond flour, parmesan cheese, garlic powder & onion powder. Set aside.
3. Making the parmesan coating.
4. Rinse fish fillets and pat dry with a paper towel. Salt and pepper on both sides of the fish fillets and place on the prepared baking sheet.
5. Brush the top side of each fish fillet with mayonnaise.
6. Sprinkle the parmesan mixture over the top of each fish fillet.
7. Sprinkle with coating.
8. Bake for 15 mins or until fish is done and coating has started to turn golden brown. If the coating is not browning then broil on low for a minute or two if needed.
9. Remove from oven & serve

SIMPLE TUNA SALAD ON LETTUCE

Nutrition: Cal 550;Fat 35 g;Carb 8 g;Protein 38 g
Serving 2; Cook time 10 min

Ingredients:
- 1/4 cup mayonnaise
- 1 tablespoon fresh lemon juice
- 1 tablespoon pickle relish
- 2 (6-ounce) cans tuna in oil, drained and flaked
- 1/2 cup cherry tomatoes, halved
- 1/4 cup diced cucumber
- Salt and pepper
- 4 cups chopped romaine lettuce

Instructions:
1. Whisk together mayonnaise, lemon juice, and relish in a bowl.
2. Add flaked tuna, tomatoes, and cucumber to the bowl. Season with salt and pepper.
3. Spoon the mixture over chopped lettuce to serve.
4. Enjoy your tuna salad with a flavorful dressing and fresh vegetables!

FRIED TUNA AVOCADO BALLS

Nutrition: Cal 455;Fat 38 g;Carb 8 g;Protein 23 g

Serving 4; Cook time 20 min

Ingredients:
- ¼ cup canned coconut milk
- 1 teaspoon onion powder
- 1 clove garlic, minced
- Salt and pepper
- 10 ounces canned tuna, drained
- 1 medium avocado, diced finely
- ½ cup almond flour
- ¼ cup olive oil

Instructions:
1. Whisk together coconut milk, onion powder, garlic, salt, and pepper in a bowl.
2. Flake the tuna into the bowl and stir in the avocado.
3. Divide the mixture into 10 to 12 balls and roll them in almond flour.
4. Heat the oil in a large skillet over medium-high heat.
5. Add the tuna avocado balls to the skillet and fry them until golden brown. Then, drain them on paper towels.

CREAMY SMOKED SALMON ZUCCHINI SPAGHETTI

Nutrition: Cal 327;Fat 24 g;Carb 8 g;Protein 20 g
Serving 2; Cook time 20 min

Ingredients:
- 8 oz. zucchini spaghetti
- 4 oz. smoked salmon, chopped
- 1/4 cup heavy cream
- 1/4 cup shredded Parmesan cheese
- 1 tbsp. olive oil
- Salt and pepper to taste

Instructions:
1. Heat the olive oil in a large skillet over medium-high heat.
2. Add the zucchini spaghetti to the skillet and cook for 2-3 minutes or until it starts to soften.
3. Add the chopped smoked salmon to the skillet and cook for an additional 1-2 minutes.
4. Pour the heavy cream over the zucchini and salmon mixture and bring it to a simmer.
5. Reduce the heat to low and let the mixture simmer for 3-4 minutes or until the sauce has thickened slightly.
6. Stir in the shredded Parmesan cheese and cook until the cheese has melted and the sauce is creamy.
7. Season with salt and pepper to taste.

8. Divide the mixture into two bowls and serve hot.
9. Enjoy your creamy zucchini spaghetti with smoked salmon!

SHRIMP AVOCADO SALAD

Nutrition: Cal 340;Fat 33 g; Carb 12 g;Protein 24 g
Serving 2; Cook time 10 min

Ingredients
- 8 ounces shrimp peeled, deveined, patted dry
- 1 large avocado, diced
- 1 small beefsteak tomato, diced and drained
- 1/3 cup crumbled feta cheese
- 1/3 cup freshly chopped cilantro or parsley
- 2 tablespoons salted butter, melted
- 1 tablespoon lemon juice
- 1 tablespoon olive oil
- 1/4 teaspoon salt
- 1/4 teaspoon black pepper

Instructions
1. Toss the shrimp with melted butter in a bowl until well-coated.
2. Heat a pan over medium-high heat for a few minutes until hot. Add the shrimp to the pan in a single layer, searing for a minute or until it starts to become pink around the edges, then flip and cook until shrimp are cooked through, less than a minute.
3. Transfer the shrimp to a plate as they finish cooking. Let them cool while you prepare the other ingredients.
4. Add all other ingredients to a large mixing bowl -- diced avocado, diced tomato, feta cheese, cilantro, lemon juice, olive oil, salt, and pepper -- and toss to mix.
5. Add the shrimp and stir to mix together. Add additional salt and pepper, to taste.

CAPRESE TUNA SALAD STUFFED TOMATOES

Nutrition: Cal 196;Fat 5 g; Carb 5 g;Protein 30 g
Serving 2; Cook time 10 min

Ingredients
- 1 medium tomato
- 1 (5 ounce) can tuna, very well drained
- 2 teaspoons balsamic vinegar
- 1 tablespoon chopped mozzarella (1/4 ounce)
- 1 tablespoon chopped fresh basil
- 1 tablespoon chopped green onion

Instructions

1. Cut the top 1/4-inch off the tomato. Use a spoon to scoop out the insides of the tomato. Set aside while you make the tuna salad.
2. Stir together the drained tuna, balsamic vinegar, mozzarella, basil, and green onion. Put the tuna salad in the hollowed out tomato, and enjoy!

SPICY KIMCHI AHI POKE

Nutrition: Cal 300;Fat 18 g; Carb 5 g;Protein 5 g
Serving 4; Cook time 10 min

Ingredients

- 1 lb sushi-grade ahi tuna, diced to roughly 1 inch
- 1 tablespoon soy sauce (or coconut aminos for paleo)
- 1/2 teaspoon sesame oil
- 1/4 cup mayo
- 2 tablespoons Sriracha
- 1 ripe avocado, diced
- 1/2 cup kimchi
- Chopped green onion
- Sesame seeds

Instructions

1. In a medium mixing bowl, add diced tuna.
2. Add soy sauce, sesame oil, mayo, and Sriracha to the bowl and toss to combine.
3. Add diced avocado and kimchi to the bowl and gently combine.
4. Serve on top of salad greens, cauliflower rice, or traditional rice and top with a sprinkle of chopped green onion and sesame seeds if desired.

PROSCIUTTO BLACKBERRY SHRIMP

Nutrition: Cal 220;Fat 11 g; Carb 6 g;Protein 21 g
Serving 2; Cook time 20 min

Ingredients

- 10 Oz Pre-Cooked Shrimp
- 11 Slices Prosciutto
- 1/3 cup Blackberries, Ground
- 1/3 cup Red Wine
- 2 tbsp. Olive Oil
- 1 tbsp. Mint Leaves, Chopped
- 1-2 Tbsp. Erythritol (to taste)

Instructions

1. Preheat the oven to 425 degrees Fahrenheit (220 degrees Celsius).

2. Slice each piece of prosciutto in half, depending on the size of the shrimp.
3. Wrap a piece of prosciutto around each shrimp, starting from the tail end.
4. Place the wrapped shrimp on a baking sheet and drizzle them with olive oil.
5. Bake the shrimp in the preheated oven for 15 minutes, or until they are cooked through and the prosciutto is crispy.
6. In a pan, add ground blackberries, mint leaves, and erythritol (a sugar substitute).
7. Cook the mixture for 2-3 minutes, allowing the flavors to combine.
8. Mix in red wine and let it reduce while the shrimp cook in the oven.
9. If desired, strain the sauce before serving to remove any solids.
10. Serve the baked prosciutto-wrapped shrimp with the blackberry-mint sauce on the side or drizzled over the top. Enjoy!

SPICY SHRIMP TACO LETTUCE WRAPS

Nutrition: Cal 186;Fat 17 g; Carb 8 g;Protein 2 g
Serving 4; Cook time 20 min

Ingredients

- 20 medium shrimp peeled and deveined (about 1 pound)
- 1 tablespoon oil of choice
- 1 clove garlic minced
- 1/2 teaspoon
- 1/2 teaspoon ground cumin
- 1/4 teaspoon kosher salt
- 1 tablespoon olive oil
- squeeze of lime optional

AVOCADO SALSA

- 1 avocado cut into chunks
- 1 tomato, chopped
- 1/4 cup loosely packed fresh cilantro leaves coarsely chopped
- 1 tablespoon fresh lime juice from half a lime
- 1/2 teaspoon salt
- 1/4 teaspoon black pepper

CILANTRO SAUCE

- 1/4 cup sour cream
- 1/4 cup cilantro
- 1 clove garlic
- 1 tablespoon fresh lime juice
- salt and pepper, to taste

•8-12 lettuce leaves
Instructions
TO COOK THE SHRIMP
1. In a medium bowl whisk together olive oil, garlic, cumin, chili, and salt. Add shrimp and mix until shrimp is covered in seasoning. Heat a large heavy-duty or cast iron skillet on high heat for 2 minutes. Add the olive oil and shrimp. Cook 2-3 minutes per side or until shrimp is cooked through. Turn off heat and finish with a squeeze of lime (optional).

TO MAKE AVOCADO TOMATO SALSA
2. In a medium bowl, gently combine tomato, avocado, cilantro, lime juice and a sprinkle of salt and pepper and mixed through. Set aside.

TO MAKE THE JALAPENO CILANTRO SAUCE
3. Add the sour cream, jalapeno, garlic, cilantro, lime and salt and pepper to a food processor. Blend for 30 seconds or until creamy.

TO ASSEMBLE:
1. Plac two romaine or butter lettuce leaves on top of each-other for each lettuce wraps. Top with 4-5 pieces of shrimp, a few tablespoons of avocado salsa and a genros drizzle of the spicy jalapeno cilantro sauce. Enjoy hot or cold!

SHRIMP AND NORI ROLLS

Nutrition: Cal 340 ;Fat 12 g; Carb 8 g;Protein 25 g
Serving 1 Cook time 10 min

Ingredients
•1 cup shrimp
•1 tbsp. Mayonnaise
•1 thinly sliced green onion
•2 sheets Nori
•¼ cucumber diced and seeded
•1 tbsp. toasted Sesame seeds

Instructions
1. Wash and drain shrimp.
2. Add together shrimp with Mayonnaise and green onions.
3. Place Nori on flat surface and spoon on the shrimp and green onion mixture.
4. Dust with cucumber and sesame seeds.
Roll tightly and cut into bite size pieces.

CRISPY FISH STICKS WITH CAPER DILL SAUCE

Nutrition: Cal 360 ;Fat 14 g; Carb 12 g;Protein 25 g
Serving 1 Cook time 30 min

Ingredients
•1 lb. white fish fillets
•1 cup grated parmesan
•1 cup almond meal/flour
•1/4 tsp. chili powder
•1/2 tsp. dried parsley
•1/4 tsp. salt
•pinch of pepper
•2 tbsp. mayo
•1 egg
•coconut oil for frying

CAPER DILL TARTAR SAUCE
•1/2 cup mayo
•1/2 cup sour cream
•1 1/2 tbsp. capers (including the caper juice)
•2 medium dill/garlic pickles, diced
•2 tbsp. chopped fresh dill
•2 tsp. lemon juice

Instructions
1. Combine the dry ingredients, put in shallow dish and set aside.
2. Whisk together the egg and mayo.
3. Prepare tartar sauce by combining all ingredients cover and refrigerate until the fish is ready.
4. Cut the fillets to desired size. Dip the fish into the egg mixture and dredge in the breading mixture.
5. Heat 1/2-inch oil in a medium skillet and drop 2 fish sticks at a time for consistent cooking.
6. Cook for 1-2 minutes on each side, until golden.
7. Remove and drain on paper-towel.
8. Serve with tartar sauce.

CREAMY SHRIMP AND MUSHROOM SKILLET

Nutrition: Cal 400 ;Fat 12 g; Carb 6 g;Protein 20 g
Serving 2 Cook time 15 min

Ingredients
•4 slices organic uncured bacon
•1 cup sliced mushrooms
•4 oz. smoked salmon

- 4 oz. raw shelled shrimp (I used TJ's Argentinian wild)
- ½ cup heavy whipping cream OR coconut cream for a dairy free option
- 1 pinch Celtic Sea Salt
- freshly ground black pepper

Instructions

1. Cut the bacon into 1-inch pieces and cook them in a skillet over medium heat until they are crispy.
2. Add the sliced mushrooms to the skillet and cook them for about 5 minutes, or until they have softened.
3. Add strips of smoked salmon to the skillet and cook for an additional 2 to 3 minutes, stirring occasionally.
4. Add the shrimp to the skillet and sauté them over high heat for about 2 minutes, or until they are cooked through and pink.
5. Stir in the cream and season with salt to taste.
6. Reduce the heat to low and let the mixture cook for about 1 minute, until it thickens and becomes creamy.
7. Your creamy bacon, mushroom, smoked salmon, and shrimp dish is now ready to be served.

BUTTERED COD IN SKILLET

Nutrition: cal 294;fat 18 g; carb 2 g;protein 30 g
Serving 4; cook time 15 min

Ingredients

- 1 1/2 lbs cod fillets
- 6 tablespoons unsalted butter, sliced

SEASONING

- ¼ teaspoon garlic powder
- ½ teaspoon table salt
- ¼ teaspoon ground pepper
- ¾ teaspoon ground paprika
- Few lemon slices
- Herbs, parsley, or cilantro

Instructions

1. Stir together the ingredients for the seasoning in a small bowl, ensuring they are well combined.
2. If desired, cut the cod into smaller pieces. Season all sides of the cod with the prepared seasoning mixture.
3. Heat 2 tablespoons of butter in a large skillet over medium-high heat until the butter melts and starts to sizzle.

4. Once the butter is melted, add the seasoned cod to the skillet. Cook for about 2 minutes on the first side.
5. Reduce the heat to medium. Carefully turn the cod over and top it with the remaining butter. Cook for an additional 3-4 minutes, or until the cod is cooked through and flakes easily with a fork.
6. The butter will completely melt and coat the cod as it cooks. Be careful not to overcook the cod, as it can become mushy and fall apart.
7. Drizzle the cooked cod with fresh lemon juice for a bright, citrusy flavor. Optionally, you can top it with fresh herbs of your choice.
8. Serve the cod immediately while it's still hot and enjoy its flavorful and tender goodness.

BROCCOLI AND SHRIMP SAUTÉED IN BUTTER

Nutrition: Cal 277;Fat 14 g; Carb 5 g;Protein 30 g
Serving 2; Cook time 15 min

Ingredients

- 1 cup broccoli, cut into small pieces
- 1 clove garlic, crushed
- 300 g shrimp, cleaned
- 2 tbsp butter
- 1 tsp lemon juice
- Salt, to taste

Instructions

1. Begin by chopping the broccoli into small portions, or to your preferred size. Keep in mind that smaller pieces will cook more quickly.
2. Preheat a pan and melt the butter. Once the butter is hot (but not smoking), gently toss in the chopped broccoli and crushed garlic. Stir the ingredients to evenly distribute them in the pan.
3. Allow the broccoli to cook over medium heat for approximately 3-4 minutes. Stir the mixture occasionally to ensure even cooking.
4. Prior to adding the shrimp to the pan, make sure they are cleaned and prepared. Add the shrimp to the pan and let them cook for around 3-4 minutes, or until they turn pink and opaque.
5. Once the shrimp have cooked through, drizzle the lemon juice evenly over the pan, ensuring it is distributed over the broccoli and shrimp.

KETO CALAMARI

Nutrition: Cal 286;Fat 15 g; Carb 11 g;Protein 22 g
Serving 4; Cook time 30 min

Ingredients

- 1 lb fresh squid cleaned
- 1 egg beaten
- 1/2 cup coconut flour
- 1 teaspoon salt
- 1 teaspoon paprika
- 1/2 teaspoon garlic powder
- 1/2 teaspoon onion powder
- Coconut oil for frying (about 1/4 cup)
- Minced cilantro optional
- Sliced Fresno chili optional
- Squeeze of lime optional
- Harissa Mayo
- 1/4 cup mayonnaise
- 1 tablespoon prepared hariss

Instructions

1. Begin by beating the egg in a small bowl. In a separate bowl, combine the coconut flour and spices to create the coating mixture.
2. Make sure the squid is dry, and then dip it into the beaten egg, ensuring it is coated. Next, dredge the squid through the flour mixture, making sure it is evenly coated.
3. Heat the oil in a 10" or larger cast-iron skillet over medium-high heat. Allow the oil to become hot.
4. To fry the squid, work in batches to avoid overcrowding the skillet. Carefully place the coated squid into the hot oil and fry for approximately 2 minutes per side, or until it turns golden and crispy. Once cooked, remove the fried squid from the skillet and drain it on paper towels to remove any excess oil.
5. At this point, you have the option to serve the fried squid as is, or for added flavor, you can toss it with cilantro, chilies, and lime. Additionally, you can serve the squid with harissa mayo as a dipping sauce.

LOW CARB ALMOND CRUSTED COD

Nutrition: Cal 219;Fat 13 g; Carb 4 g;Protein 22 g
Serving 4; Cook time 25 min

Ingredients

- 1 4 filets cod or other white fish
- 1 med lemon zested and juiced
- 1/2 cup crushed almonds can use a food processor or blender to crush
- 1 Tbsp dill either fresh
- 1 Tbsp olive oil
- salt & pepper to taste
- 1 tsp mild to med. chili spice optional
- 4 tsp Dijon mustard more if you like mustard

Instructions

1. Preheat oven to 400 degrees F. Prepare a baking sheet with either parchment paper laid on top or spray with cooking spray
2. Place cod filets on paper towels to drain of water and pat dry. Place on baking sheet.
3. In a small bowl, combine the lemon zest, lemon juice, crushed almonds, dill, oil, salt and pepper and chili spice if using.
4. Spread each cod filet with a tsp or so of Dijon mustard,smoothing it over the entire top of the filet. Divide the almond mixture among the 4 filets, pressing it evely into the mustard with your hands.
5. Bake the fish until opaue at the thickest part, about 7 minutes for most.cod filets (less time for thin filets).
6. Serve with a green vegetable and lemon slices for a great low carb or keto fish dinner.

MEXICAN FISH STEW

Nutrition: Cal 196;Fat 7 g; Carb 8 g;Protein 19 g
Serving 6; Cook time 30 min

Ingredients

- 2 Tbsp olive oil
- 1 med onion chopped
- 1 large carrot sliced thinly
- 3 med celery stalks sliced thinly
- 3-6 cloves garlic smashed or minced
- 1 tsp smoky pepper blend
- 1/2 tsp dried thyme
- 1 cup white wine
- 4 cups chicken broth
- 1/2 cup chopped cilantro
- 2 14 oz cans Rotel diced tomatoes
- 1/2 tsp salt
- 3 leaves bay
- 6 oz scallops
- 7 oz walleye, coarsely chopped
- 1 lb mussels
- 3 oz white fish, coarsely chopped
- 2 med limes, cut into wedges optional
- 1 med lemon, sliced for garnish

Instructions

1.Heat oil over medium-high heat in a Dutch oven or large pot. Sauté onion, carrot, and celery in the oil for 3-5 minutes, or until they become translucent. Add smashed garlic and cook for an additional minute.

2.Stir in the spices, ensuring they coat the onion mixture. Add wine, broth, cilantro, and tomatoes to the pot, and simmer the ingredients together for 15-20 minutes over medium heat. Season with salt to taste.

3.Place all the fish into the pot and cook, covered, for about 5 minutes, or until the mussels open and the white fish becomes opaque.

4.Add sliced lemons to the pot and serve.

6.Optionally, serve the soup with lime wedges that people can squeeze into their individual servings.

CREAMY KETO FISH CASSEROLE

Nutrition: Cal 221;Fat 15 g; Carb 9 g;Protein 27 g
Serving 4; Cook time 30 min

Ingredients
•1 tbsp butter, for greasing baking dish
•3 tbsp olive oil
•1 lb broccoli, small florets
•1 tsp salt
•½ tsp ground black pepper
•4 oz. (1¼ cups) scallions, finely chopped
•2 tbsp small capers (non-pareils)
•1½ lbs white fish (see tip), cut into serving-sized pieces
•1 tbsp dried parsley
•1¼ cups heavy whipping cream
•1 tbsp Dijon mustard
•3 oz. butter, cut into thin, equal slices

Instructions
1.Preheat the oven to 400°F (200°C) and grease a 13" x 9" (33 x 23 cm) baking dish. Set it aside.

2.In a large frying pan, heat the oil over medium-high heat. Add the broccoli and stir-fry for about 5 minutes, or until it becomes lightly browned and tender. Season with salt and pepper.

3.Stir in the scallions and capers, and cook for a couple of minutes. Spoon the broccoli mixture into the prepared baking dish.

4.Arrange the fish among the vegetables in the baking dish.

5.In a medium-sized bowl, whisk together the parsley, whipping cream, and mustard. Pour this mixture over the fish and vegetables. Top with the sliced butter.

6.Bake the dish, uncovered, on the middle rack of the oven for about 20 minutes, or until the fish is cooked through and flakes easily with a fork.

7.Serve the dish as is, or with a side of leafy greens.

GRILLED SALMON WITH AVOCADO SALSA

Nutrition: Cal 528;Fat 43 g; Carb 13 g;Protein 25 g
Serving 2; Cook time 22 min

Ingredients
•2 4-6 oz salmon fillets
•2 tablespoons olive oil
•1 clove garlic minced or crushed
•1/2 teaspoon
•1/2 teaspoon
•1/2 teaspoon onion powder
•1/4 teaspoon black pepper
•1/4 teaspoon salt
•FOR THE AVOCADO SALSA
•1 ripe avocado pitted and diced
•1/2 cup tomato diced (any type of tomato)
•2 tablespoons onion diced
•2 tablespoons cilantro minced
•1 tablespoon olive oil
•1 tablespoon lime juice
•salt and pepper to taste

Instructions
1.In a small bowl, stir together the olive oil, garlic, and spices. Brush or rub the salmon with this spice mixture.

2.Heat a large heavy-duty pan or grill over medium-high heat. Add the salmon to the pan and cook for about 5-6 minutes per side. Once cooked, remove the salmon from the pan and top it with the avocado salsa. Serve immediately.

3.To make the avocado salsa: In a large mixing bowl, add the avocado, tomato, onion, and cilantro. Drizzle with olive oil, fresh lime juice, and a pinch of salt and pepper. Gently mix the ingredients together using a spoon until fully combined. Cover the bowl with plastic wrap until you are ready to serve.

CREAMY CHILE SHRIMP

Nutrition: Cal 103;Fat 6 g; Carb 5 g;Protein 7 g
Serving 4; Cook time 30 min

Ingredients
- 1 lb. shrimp
- 1 chile pepper, cut into thin strips
- ½ cup bell pepper, cut into thin strips
- ½ cup white cabbage
- ½ tsp. cayenne powder
- ½ cup chicken stock
- ½ tsp. black pepper
- ½ cup heavy cream
- ½ tsp. hot sauce
- 1 tbsp. garlic, minced
- ½ tsp. lime juice
- ¼ cup canola oil

Instructions
1. Start by deseeding the green chili and cutting it into thin strips lengthwise.
2. On the Instant Pot, select the sauté function and heat half of the oil. Sauté the bell pepper, cabbage, and green chili for about 3-4 minutes. Once done, remove the sautéed vegetables and keep them warm by covering them with foil.
3. Without cleaning the Instant Pot, add the remaining oil and sauté the ginger and garlic. Then, add the shrimp and turn off the sauté function. Incorporate the spices, hot sauce, and lime juice into the mixture.
4. Pour in the chicken stock and set the Instant Pot to cook on high pressure for 4 minutes. After the cooking time, perform a quick pressure release. Add the sautéed vegetables to the pot and mix everything well.
5. Finally, add the cream and continue sautéing until the sauce thickens slightly. Once ready, serve the dish.

LEMON KALAMATA OLIVE SALMON

Nutrition: Cal 440;Fat 34 g; Carb 3g;Protein 30g
Serving 3; Cook time 25 min

Ingredients
- 4 x 0.3 lb. salmon filets
- 2 tbsps. fresh lemon juice
- ¼ tsp. black pepper
- ½ cup red onion, sliced
- 1 tsp. herbs de Provence
- 1 can pitted kalamata olives
- 1tsp. sea salt
- ½ lemon, thinly sliced
- 1 cup fish broth
- ½ tsp. cumin
- ½ cup essential olive oil

Instructions
1. Start by generously seasoning the salmon fillets with cumin, pepper, and salt. Set your Instant Pot to "Sauté" mode and heat the olive oil. Add the seasoned fish to the pot and brown each side.
2. Stir in the remaining ingredients into the pot and allow them to simmer. Lock the lid of the Instant Pot. Set the pot to manual high pressure for ten minutes. Once the cooking is done, perform a quick release of the pressure.
3. Serve the cooked salmon immediately. Enjoy your flavorful and tender salmon dish prepared using the Instant Pot.

SEAFOOD MEDLEY STEW

Nutrition: Cal 535;Fat 44 g; Carb 8g;Protein 27g
Serving 3; Cook time 25 min

Ingredients
- 2 cups chicken broth
- 2 tbsps. lemon juice
- ½ lb. shrimp
- ½ lb. mussels
- 2 cloves garlic, crushed
- ½ cup coconut cream
- ½ tsp. black pepper
- 100 g. halibut
- 1 dried whole star anise
- 1 bay leaf
- 1 cup light cream
- 3 tbsps. coconut oil

Instructions
1. In the Instant Pot, select the sauté function and heat the coconut oil. Add the bay leaves and star anise to the pot and sauté for approximately 30 seconds.
2. Add the garlic to the pot and continue sautéing.
3. Pour in the broth. Rub fresh lemon juice, salt, and pepper on the fish fillets, and then place them in the pot. Add the shrimp and mussels as well.
4. Close the lid and cook for 10 minutes. Allow the pressure to release naturally.
5. Stir in both creams and let the mixture simmer for a while.

6. Before serving, remember to remove the bay leaves and star anise for a smoother eating experience.

FLAVORED OCTOPUS

Nutrition: Cal 180;Fat 3 g; Carb 1.5 g;Protein 30 g
Serving 4; Соок time 25 min

Ingredients
- 1 tsp chopped cilantro
- 2 tbsps. extra virgin olive oil
- 0.6 pounds octopus
- 2 tsps. garlic powder
- 3 tbsps. lime juice
- salt and pepper, to taste

Instructions
1. Place the octopus in the steaming basket. Season it with garlic powder, salt, and pepper. Drizzle it with olive oil and lime juice.
2. Pour water into the Instant Pot and lower the steaming basket into the pot. Close the lid and cook for 8 minutes on high pressure.
3. Perform a simple pressure release by carefully turning the pressure release valve to the venting position to release the steam.

CRUNCHY ALMOND TUNA

Nutrition: Cal 150;Fat 4 g; Carb 3 g;Protein 21 g
Serving 4; Соок time 15 min

Ingredients
- 2 cans of tuna, drained
- 1 cup shaved almond
- 2 tbsps. butter
- 1 tsp garlic powder
- 1 cup grated cheddar cheese

Instructions
1. Melt the butter in your Instant Pot on "Sauté." Add tuna, almonds, garlic powder, and cheddar. Соок on "Sauté" for 3 minutes.
2. Serve immediately over cauliflower, rice or on its own.

ARUGULA AND SALMON SALAD

Nutrition: Cal 390;Fat 31 g; Carb 6 g;Protein 26 g
Serving 3; Соок time 25 min

Ingredients
- 3 (4-ounce) salmon fillets
- 5 tablespoons extra-virgin olive oil, divided
- 1 teaspoon garlic salt
- Juice of 1 lemon
- 4½ cups arugula

Instructions
1. Preheat your oven to 450°F (230°C) and line a baking sheet with aluminum foil.
2. Rub the salmon fillets with 2 tablespoons of oil and sprinkle them with garlic salt. Place the seasoned fillets on the prepared baking sheet and drizzle lemon juice over the top.
3. Bake the salmon in the preheated oven for 8 to 12 minutes, or until it is cooked through and flakes easily. Once cooked, let the fillets rest for 10 minutes.
4. Divide 1 cup of arugula into each of the 3 storage containers and season with salt and pepper. Place a salmon fillet on top of the arugula in each container.
5. To serve, drizzle each container with 1 tablespoon of oil and toss the arugula to coat it with the dressing.

GRILLED PESTO SALMON WITH ASPARAGUS

Nutrition: Cal 300;Fat 18 g; Carb 2.5 g;Protein 34 g
Serving 4; Соок time 20 min

Ingredients
- 4 (6-ounce) boneless salmon fillets
- Salt and pepper
- 1 bunch asparagus, ends trimmed
- 2 tablespoons olive oil
- ¼ cup basil pesto

Instructions
1. Preheat your grill to high heat and oil the grates to prevent sticking.
2. Season the salmon fillets with salt and pepper. You can also spray them with cooking spray to help prevent sticking to the grill.
3. Place the salmon fillets on the preheated grill and cook for about 4 to 5 minutes on each side, or until the salmon is cooked through and flakes easily with a fork.
4. While the salmon is grilling, toss the asparagus spears with oil to coat them.
5. Place the asparagus on the grill and cook for about 10 minutes, or until the asparagus is tender and slightly charred.
6. Once the salmon and asparagus are cooked, spoon the pesto sauce over the salmon fillets and serve them alongside the grilled asparagus.

GRILLED SALMON AND ZUCCHINI WITH MANGO SAUCE

Nutrition: Cal 485;Fat 32 g; Carb 6,5 g;Protein 43 g
Serving 6; Cook time 6 hours 10 min

Ingredients

- 4 (6-ounce) boneless salmon fillets
- 1 tablespoon olive oil
- Salt and pepper
- 1 large zucchini, sliced in coins
- 2 tablespoons fresh lemon juice
- ½ cup chopped mango
- ¼ cup fresh chopped cilantro
- 1 teaspoon lemon zest
- ½ cup canned coconut milk

Instructions

1. Preheat a grill pan on high heat and spray it liberally with cooking spray to prevent sticking.
2. Brush the salmon fillets with olive oil and season them with salt and pepper. Toss the zucchini with lemon juice and season it with salt and pepper as well.
3. Place the salmon fillets and zucchini on the preheated grill pan.
4. Cook the salmon and zucchini for about 5 minutes on one side, then turn them over and cook for an additional 5 minutes on the other side. The cooking time may vary depending on the thickness of the salmon fillets and the desired level of doneness.
5. While the salmon and zucchini are grilling, combine the remaining ingredients (for the mango sauce) in a blender and blend until smooth. Adjust the consistency and seasoning to your preference.
6. Once the salmon and zucchini are cooked, serve the salmon fillets drizzled with the mango sauce and the grilled zucchini on the side.

FRIED COCONUT SHRIMP WITH ASPARAGUS

Nutrition: Cal 535;Fat 38,5 g; Carb 18 g;Protein 31 g
Serving 6; Cook time 25 min

Ingredients

- 1 ½ cups shredded unsweetened coconut
- 2 large eggs
- Salt and pepper
- 1 ½ pounds large shrimp, peeled and deveined
- ½ cup canned coconut milk
- 1 pound asparagus, cut into 2-inch pieces

Instructions

1. Pour the coconut into a shallow dish, ensuring it forms an even layer.
2. In a bowl, beat the eggs and season them with salt and pepper.
3. Dip each shrimp into the beaten egg mixture, making sure it is coated evenly.
4. Heat the coconut oil in a large skillet over medium-high heat until it is hot and shimmering.
5. Take the coated shrimp and dredge them in the shredded coconut, pressing gently to adhere the coconut to the shrimp.
6. Carefully place the coated shrimp in the hot skillet and fry them for 1 to 2 minutes on each side, or until they turn golden brown and crispy.
7. Once the shrimp are cooked, remove them from the skillet and place them on paper towels to drain any excess oil.
8. Reheat the skillet and add the asparagus spears. Season them with salt and pepper, then sauté them until they are tender-crisp, approximately 3 to 5 minutes.
9. Serve the crispy coconut shrimp alongside the sautéed asparagus for a delicious and satisfying meal.

BALSAMIC SALMON WITH GREEN BEANS

Nutrition: Cal 320;Fat 18 g; Carb 6 g;Protein 35 g
Serving 4; Cook time 25 min

Ingredients

- ½ cup balsamic vinegar
- ¼ cup chicken broth
- 1 tablespoon Dijon mustard
- 2 cloves garlic, minced
- 2 tablespoons coconut oil
- 4 (6-ounce) salmon fillets
- Salt and pepper
- 2 cups trimmed green beans

Instructions

1. In a small saucepan, combine the balsamic vinegar, chicken broth, mustard, and garlic. Place the saucepan over medium-high heat.
2. Bring the mixture to a boil, then reduce the heat to a simmer. Let it simmer for about 15 minutes, or until it has reduced by half, stirring occasionally.

3. Meanwhile, heat the coconut oil in a large skillet over medium-high heat.
4. Season the salmon fillets with salt and pepper on both sides. Carefully add the seasoned salmon to the skillet.
5. Cook the salmon for about 4 minutes, or until it is seared and nicely browned on one side. Flip the salmon fillets and add the green beans to the skillet.
6. Pour the reduced glaze into the skillet with the salmon and green beans. Allow it to simmer for an additional 2 to 3 minutes, or until the salmon is cooked to your desired level of doneness and the green beans are tender.
7. Serve the glazed salmon and green beans hot, with the flavorful glaze drizzled over the top.

SHRIMP AND SAUSAGE "BAKE"

Nutrition: Cal 323;Fat 24 g; Carb 8 g;Protein 20 g
Serving 4; Cook time 35 min

Ingredients
- 2 tablespoons olive oil
- 6 ounces chorizo sausage, diced
- ½ pound (16 to 20 count) shrimp, peeled and deveined
- 1 red bell pepper, chopped
- ½ small sweet onion, chopped
- 2 teaspoons minced garlic
- ¼ cup chicken stock
- Pinch red pepper flakes

Instructions
1. Place a large skillet over medium-high heat and add the olive oil.
2. Sauté the sausage in the skillet until it is warmed through, which should take about 6 minutes.
3. Add the shrimp to the skillet and continue sautéing until the shrimp is opaque and just cooked through, which should take about 4 minutes.
4. Remove the sausage and shrimp from the skillet and transfer them to a bowl. Set aside for now.
5. In the same skillet, add the red pepper, onion, and garlic. Sauté them until they become tender, which should take about 4 minutes.
6. Return the cooked sausage and shrimp to the skillet. Add the chicken stock to the skillet as well.
7. Bring the liquid to a simmer and let it simmer for about 3 minutes.

8. Stir in the red pepper flakes for added spice, if desired. Then, your dish is ready to be served.

HERB BUTTER SCALLOPS

Nutrition: Cal 306;Fat 24 g; Carb 4,5 g;Protein 20 g
Serving 4; Cook time 20 min

Ingredients
- 1 pound sea scallops, cleaned
- Freshly ground black pepper
- 8 tablespoons butter, divided
- 2 teaspoons minced garlic
- Juice of 1 lemon
- 2 teaspoons chopped fresh basil
- 1 teaspoon chopped fresh thyme

Instructions
1. Pat the scallops dry with paper towels to remove any excess moisture. Lightly season them with pepper.
2. Place a large skillet over medium heat and add 2 tablespoons of butter. Allow the butter to melt and heat up.
3. Arrange the scallops in the skillet, making sure they are evenly spaced but not too close together. Sear each side of the scallops until they turn golden brown, which should take about 2½ minutes per side. Be careful not to overcook them, as they can become tough.
4. Once the scallops are cooked, remove them from the skillet and transfer them to a plate. Set them aside while you prepare the sauce.
5. Add the remaining 6 tablespoons of butter to the skillet and allow it to melt. Sauté the garlic in the butter until it becomes translucent, which should take about 3 minutes. Be careful not to burn the garlic.
6. Stir in the lemon juice, basil, and thyme into the skillet with the melted butter and garlic. Return the scallops to the skillet, turning them to coat them evenly in the sauce. Let them heat through for a minute or two.
7. Serve the scallops immediately while they are still hot. They can be enjoyed on their own or paired with a side dish of your choice.

PAN-SEARED HALIBUT WITH CITRUS BUTTER SAUCE

Nutrition: Cal 320;Fat 26 g; Carb 2 g;Protein 22 g
Serving 4; Cook time 25 min

Ingredients
- 4 (5-ounce) halibut fillets, each about 1 inch thick
- Sea salt
- Freshly ground black pepper
- ¼ cup butter
- 2 teaspoons minced garlic
- 1 shallot, minced
- 3 tablespoons dry white wine
- 1 tablespoon freshly squeezed lemon juice
- 1 tablespoon freshly squeezed orange juice
- 2 teaspoons chopped fresh parsley
- 2 tablespoons olive oil

Instructions
1. Begin by patting the fish fillets dry with paper towels. Lightly season them with salt and pepper on both sides. Place the seasoned fillets on a plate lined with paper towels and set them aside.
2. Take a small saucepan and heat it over medium heat. Add the butter to the saucepan and allow it to melt.
3. Sauté the garlic and shallot in the melted butter until they become tender, which should take around 3 minutes. Stir occasionally to prevent burning.
4. Whisk in the white wine, lemon juice, and orange juice into the saucepan with the garlic and shallot. Bring the sauce to a simmer and let it cook for about 2 minutes, or until it slightly thickens.
5. Remove the saucepan from the heat and stir in the parsley. Set the sauce aside.
6. Take a large skillet and heat it over medium-high heat. Add the olive oil to the skillet and let it heat up.
7. Pan-fry the fish fillets in the skillet, cooking them until they are lightly browned and cooked through. This process usually takes around 10 minutes in total, flipping the fillets once during cooking. The cooking time may vary depending on the thickness of the fillets.
8. Once the fish fillets are cooked, serve them immediately. Plate each fillet and spoon a generous amount of the prepared sauce over them.

FISH CURRY

Nutrition: Cal 416;Fat 31 g; Carb 5 g;Protein 26 g
Serving 4; Cook time 35 min

Ingredients
- 2 tablespoons coconut oil
- 1&½ tablespoons grated fresh ginger
- 2 teaspoons minced garlic
- 1 tablespoon curry powder
- ½ teaspoon ground cumin
- 2 cups coconut milk
- 16 ounces firm white fish, cut into 1-inch chunks
- 1 cup shredded kale
- 2 tablespoons chopped cilantro

Instructions
1. Place a large saucepan over medium heat and melt the coconut oil.
2. Sauté the ginger and garlic in the melted coconut oil until they become lightly browned, which should take around 2 minutes.
3. Stir in the curry powder and cumin, and continue sautéing until the mixture becomes very fragrant, about 2 minutes.
4. Add the coconut milk to the saucepan and bring the liquid to a boil.
5. Once it reaches a boil, reduce the heat to low and let it simmer for about 5 minutes. This will allow the coconut milk to infuse with the spices.
6. Add the fish to the simmering liquid. Cook the fish until it is fully cooked through, which usually takes about 10 minutes. The cooking time may vary depending on the thickness of the fish fillets.
7. Stir in the kale and cilantro, allowing them to simmer until the kale wilts, which should take approximately 2 minutes.
8. Once the fish is cooked and the kale is wilted, the dish is ready to be served. You can garnish it with additional cilantro if desired.

ROASTED SALMON WITH AVOCADO SALSA

Nutrition: Cal 320;Fat 26 g; Carb 2 g;Protein 22 g
Serving 4; Cook time 25 min

Ingredients
FOR THE SALSA
- 1 avocado, peeled, pitted,
- and diced
- 1 scallion, white and green parts,
- chopped
- ½ cup halved cherry tomatoes
- Juice of 1 lemon

•Zest of 1 lemon

FOR THE FISH

•1 teaspoon ground cumin

•½ teaspoon ground coriander

•½ teaspoon onion powder

•¼ teaspoon sea salt

•Pinch freshly ground black pepper

•Pinch cayenne pepper

•4 (4-ounce) boneless, skinless

•salmon fillets

•2 tablespoons olive oil

Instructions

TO MAKE THE SALSA

1.In a small bowl, stir together the avocado, scallion, tomatoes, lemon juice, and lemon zest until mixed.

2.Set aside.

TO MAKE THE FISH

1.Preheat the oven to 400°F. Line a baking sheet with aluminum foil and set aside.

2.In a small bowl, stir together the cumin, coriander, onion powder, salt, black pepper, and cayenne until well mixed.

3.Rub the salmon fillets with the spice mix and place them on the baking sheet.

4.Drizzle the fillets with the olive oil and roast the fish until it is just cooked through, about 15 minutes.

5.Serve the salmon topped with the avocado salsa.

SOLE ASIAGO

Nutrition: Cal 300;Fat 24 g; Carb 4 g;Protein 20 g
Serving 4; Cook time 20 min

Ingredients

•4 (4-ounce) sole fillets

•¾ cup ground almonds

•¼ cup Asiago cheese

•2 eggs, beaten

•2&½ tablespoons melted coconut oil

Instructions

1.Preheat the oven to 350°F (175°C). Line a baking sheet with parchment paper and set it aside.

2.Pat the sole fillets dry with paper towels to remove any excess moisture.

3.In a small bowl, stir together the ground almonds and cheese until well combined.

4.Place the beaten eggs in a separate bowl next to the almond mixture.

5.Take one sole fillet and dredge it in the beaten egg, making sure it is fully coated. Then press the fish into the almond mixture, coating it completely with the mixture. Place the breaded fillet onto the prepared baking sheet. Repeat this process with the remaining fillets.

6.Brush both sides of each piece of fish with coconut oil, ensuring they are evenly coated.

7.Bake the sole fillets in the preheated oven for about 8 minutes or until they are cooked through. The cooking time may vary slightly depending on the thickness of the fillets, so keep an eye on them to avoid overcooking.

8.Once the sole is cooked, remove it from the oven and serve it immediately. The breaded almond sole makes a delicious and crispy main dish.

BAKED COCONUT HADDOCK

Nutrition: Cal 406;Fat 31 g; Carb 6 g;Protein 29 g
Serving 4; Cook time 22 min

Ingredients

•4 (5-ounce) boneless haddock fillets

•Sea salt

•Freshly ground black pepper

•1 cup shredded unsweetened coconut

•¼ cup ground hazelnuts

•2 tablespoons coconut oil, melted

Instructions

1.Preheat the oven to 400°F (200°C). Line a baking sheet with parchment paper and set it aside.

2.Pat the haddock fillets very dry with paper towels. Lightly season them with salt and pepper on both sides.

3.In a small bowl, stir together the shredded coconut and hazelnuts until well combined.

4.Dredge each haddock fillet in the coconut mixture, ensuring that both sides of each piece are thickly coated with the mixture.

5.Place the coated fish fillets on the prepared baking sheet. Lightly brush both sides of each piece with coconut oil to help enhance the browning and crispiness.

6.Bake the haddock in the preheated oven for about 12 minutes in total or until the topping is golden and the fish flakes easily with a fork. Cooking times may vary depending on the thickness of the fillets, so keep an eye on them to avoid overcooking.

7.Once the haddock is cooked, remove it from the oven and serve it immediately. The coconut and hazelnut crust will add a delicious crunch to the fish.

CHEESY GARLIC SALMON

Nutrition: Cal 356;Fat 28 g; Carb 2 g;Protein 24 g
Serving 4; Cook time 30 min

Ingredients
- ½ cup Asiago cheese
- 2 tablespoons freshly squeezed
- lemon juice
- 2 tablespoons butter, at room
- temperature
- 2 teaspoons minced garlic
- 1 teaspoon chopped fresh basil
- 1 teaspoon chopped fresh oregano
- 4 (5-ounce) salmon fillets
- 1 tablespoon olive oil

Instructions

1.Preheat the oven to 350°F (175°C). Line a baking sheet with parchment paper and set it aside.

2.In a small bowl, stir together the Asiago cheese, lemon juice, melted butter, garlic, basil, and oregano. Mix until well combined.

3.Pat the salmon fillets dry with paper towels and place them on the prepared baking sheet, skin-side down. Divide the topping mixture evenly between the fillets and spread it across the fish using a knife or the back of a spoon.

4.Drizzle the fish with olive oil to help with browning and moisture.

5.Bake the salmon in the preheated oven for about 12 minutes or until the topping is golden and the fish is just cooked through. Cooking times may vary depending on the thickness of the fillets, so keep an eye on them to avoid overcooking.

6.Once the salmon is cooked, remove it from the oven and serve it immediately. The Asiago cheese and herb topping will create a flavorful crust on top of the fish.

DESSERTS

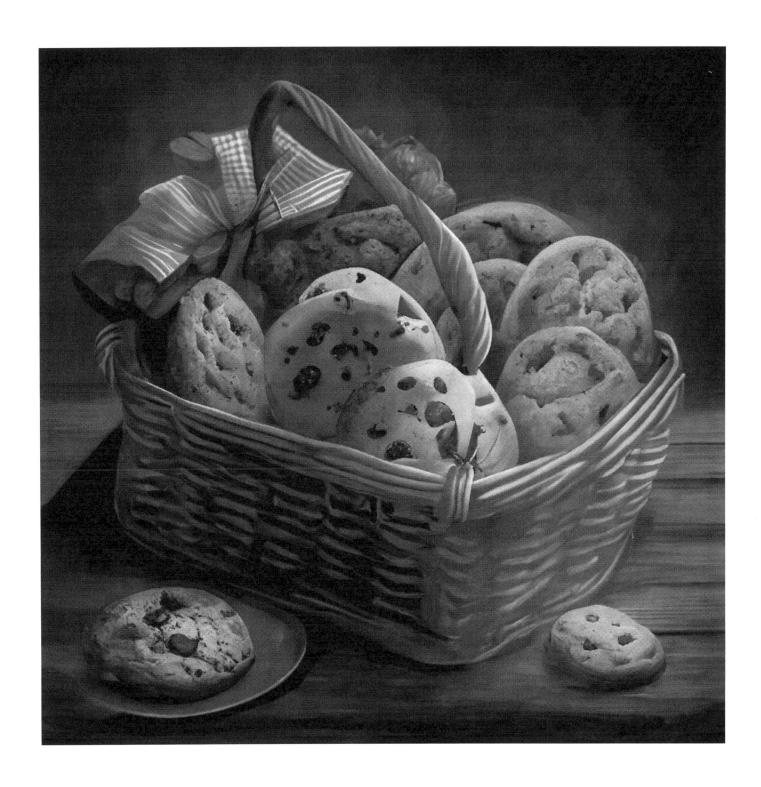

KETO MUFFINS CLASSIC CINNAMON

Nutrition: Cal 190; Fat 13 g; Carb 4.5 g; Protein 5 g
Serving 12; Cook time 30 min

Ingredients

- ½ cup heavy cream
- 5 tablespoon butter, softened
- 2 large eggs
- 1 teaspoon vanilla
- ½ cup powdered sweetener
- 1 ½ cups blanched almond flour
- 2 tablespoons psyllium husk powder
- 2 teaspoon baking powder
- ½ teaspoon nutmeg
- ½ teaspoon ginger
- ¼ teaspoon allspice

FOR THE COVERING:

- 2 tablespoon butter, melted
- 1 teaspoon cinnamon
- ¼ cup granulated sweetener

Instructions

1. Preheat the oven to 350 degrees Fahrenheit (175 degrees Celsius) and line a muffin pan with paper liners.
2. In a medium bowl, use an electric mixer to cream together the butter, sweetener, and vanilla until smooth. Beat in the eggs and cream until well combined.
3. In a separate bowl, whisk together all the dry ingredients except for the topping ingredients. Slowly add the dry mixture to the wet ingredients, continuously mixing with the electric mixer until a smooth batter forms.
4. Spoon even amounts of the batter into each muffin cup, filling them about 3/4 full.
5. Bake for 18-20 minutes or until the edges are golden and set up. You can use a toothpick inserted into the center of a muffin to check if it comes out clean or with a few crumbs.
6. Allow the muffins to cool completely in the pan before removing them. This helps them set and hold their shape.
7. Once the muffins have cooled, brush the tops with melted butter and then roll them in a mixture of cinnamon and sweetener. This will add a delicious cinnamon coating to the muffins.

Serve and enjoy your cinnamon sweetener-coated muffins!

KETO BLUEBERRY MUFFINS

Nutrition: Cal 217; Fat 19 g; Carb 6 g; Protein 7 g
Serving 12; Cook time 30 min

Ingredients

- 2 1/2 cup Wholesome Yum Blanched Almond Flour
- 1/2 cup Besti Monk Fruit Allulose Blend
- 1 1/2 tsp Baking powder
- 1/4 tsp Sea salt (optional, but recommended)
- 1/3 cup Coconut oil (measured solid, then melted; can also use butter)
- 1/3 cup Unsweetened almond milk (at room temperature)
- 3 large Eggs (at room temperature)
- 1/2 tsp Vanilla extract
- 3/4 cup Blueberries

Instructions

1. Preheat the oven to 350 degrees Fahrenheit (177 degrees Celsius) and line a muffin pan with 10 or 12 silicone or parchment paper muffin liners. Use 12 liners for lower calories/carbs or 10 for larger muffin tops.
2. In a large bowl, stir together the almond flour, Besti (sweetener), baking powder, and sea salt.
3. Mix in the melted coconut oil, almond milk, eggs, and vanilla extract. Fold in the blueberries gently.
4. Distribute the batter evenly among the muffin cups, filling each about 2/3 full.
5. Bake for about 20-25 minutes, or until the tops are golden and an inserted toothpick comes out clean.
6. Remove the muffins from the oven and let them cool in the pan for a few minutes. Then transfer them to a wire rack to cool completely.

KETO CHOCOLATE MUFFINS

Nutrition: Cal 246;Fat 16 g;Carb 8 g;Protein 6 g
Serving 12; Cook time 32 min

Ingredients

- 2 cups almond flour (or almond meal)
- ¼ cup unsweetened cocoa
- ¼ teaspoon salt
- ½ teaspoon baking powder
- ¼ cup oil
- ¼ cup sugar-free maple flavored syrup (we use Lakanto)
- 3 large eggs, room temperature
- ½ cup sugar-free, dairy-free dark chocolate chips

Instructions

1. Preheat the oven to 350°F (175°C). Line a cupcake pan with 12 paper liners and set it aside.
2. In a large mixing bowl, whisk together the almond flour, cocoa powder, salt, and baking powder until well combined.
3. Add the oil, maple-flavored syrup, and eggs to the dry ingredients. Mix everything together until well combined and a smooth batter forms.
4. Stir in the chocolate chips, ensuring they are evenly distributed throughout the batter.
5. Spoon the batter evenly into the paper liners, filling each about 2/3 full.
6. Bake in the preheated oven for 18-20 minutes, or until the center of the cupcakes is set. You can test this by inserting a toothpick into the center - if it comes out clean or with a few crumbs, the cupcakes are done.
7. Remove the cupcakes from the oven and allow them to cool in the pan for 5-10 minutes before transferring them to a wire rack to cool completely.
8. Once the cupcakes are completely cooled, store them in an airtight container at room temperature.

KETO LEMON MUFFINS

Nutrition: Cal 209; Fat 25 g; Carb 4.5 g;Protein 8 g
Serving 12; Cook time 40 min

Ingredients

FOR THE MUFFIN:

- 1/2 cup butter, softened
- 3/4 cup granulated erythritol sweetener
- 3 large eggs
- 3 tablespoons lemon juice
- 1 tablespoon lemon zest
- 1 1/2 cup superfine almond flour
- 1/2 cup coconut flour
- 2 teaspoons baking powder
- 1/4 teaspoon xanthan gum or arrowroot powder
- 1/2 teaspoon vanilla extract
- 1 cup full fat sour cream (or 1/2 cup unsweetened almond milk)
- pinch of salt

FOR THE STREUSEL TOPPING:

- 3 tablespoons butter, melted
- 3/4 cup superfine almond flour
- 3 tablespoons granulated erythritol sweetener
- 1 teaspoon grated lemon zest
- 1 tablespoon coconut flour

FOR THE LEMON GLAZE:

- 1/2 cup confectioners style erythritol sweetener
- 3 tablespoons lemon juice

Instructions

FOR THE MUFFIN LAYER:

1. Combine all of the muffin ingredients in a blender and blend for 2-3 minutes or until smooth. The mixture is thick so you'll have to stop a few times and scrape the sides down with a silicone spatula to get it going the first minute or so.
2. Preheat the oven to 350 degrees (F) and then start your streusel topping.

FOR THE STREUSEL TOPPING:

1. Combine the melted butter, almond flour, sweetener, lemon zest and coconut flour in a small bowl and stir well with a fork until a crumbly dough forms.
2. Spoon the muffin batter from the blender into 8 large or 12 regular muffin cups (if you're using foil or thin paper then place inside a muffin tin to support them) – or into a small loaf or cake pan.
3. Crumble the streusel topping in pea sized pieces over the top of the batter.
4. Bake on the middle rack of your oven at 350 degrees for 35 minutes (large muffins) or 25 minutes (average sized muffin) or 50 minutes (loaf or cake pan) OR until a toothpick or knife inserted in the center comes out clean.

FOR THE LEMON GLAZE:

1. Combine the erythritol and lemon juice in a cup or small bowl. Stir with a fork until smooth.

2. If too runny, add another tablespoon of erythritol (or more) until an opaque but still pourable glaze forms.
3. If too stiff to pour, add another teaspoon of lemon juice to loosen.
4. Pour the glaze over the muffins after they are baked and slightly cool. Serve warm or room temperature.
7. Store any leftovers covered in the refrigerator for up to a week.

KETO ALMOND FLOUR MUFFINS

Nutrition: Cal 197; Fat 18 g; Carb 9 g; Protein 8 g
Serving 12; Cook time 30 min

Ingredients
FOR THE MUFFINS
- 2 1/2 cups almond flour blanched almond flour, not almond meal
- 2 teaspoon baking powder
- 1/4 teaspoon salt
- 1/2 cup granulated sweetener of choice erythritol or monk fruit sweetener
- 3 large eggs
- 1/3 cup butter melted (can also use melted coconut oil)
- 6 tablespoon milk of choice I used unsweetened almond milk

FOR THE STREUSEL TOPPING
- 1/2 cup almond flour
- 2 tablespoon coconut flour
- 1/2 cup chopped nuts of choice I used chopped walnuts
- 1 tablespoon cinnamon
- 3 tablespoon granulated sweetener of choice
- 1/4 cup melted butter

ICING DRIZZLE
- 1/4 cup sugar free powdered sugar
- 1-2 tablespoon water

Instructions
1. Preheat the oven to 180°C/350°F. Grease a 12-count muffin tin with muffin liners and set it aside.
2. Prepare the streusel topping by combining all the ingredients in a mixing bowl. Mix until crumbly, and set aside.
3. In a small bowl, whisk together the almond flour, baking powder, and salt. In a separate bowl, add the sweetener, eggs, milk, and melted butter. Whisk together until smooth and glossy.
4. Gently fold the dry ingredients into the wet ingredients until smooth and combined. Distribute the muffin batter evenly among the muffin tin cups. Sprinkle the streusel topping over each muffin.
5. Bake the muffins for 22-25 minutes, or until a skewer inserted into the center comes out clean. Remove from the oven and let them cool in the muffin pan for 10 minutes before transferring them to a wire rack to cool completely.
6. Once cooled, prepare the icing by whisking together the powdered sugar with water. Drizzle the icing over the top of each muffin.

1-MINUTE KETO MUFFINS RECIPE

Nutrition: Cal 113; Fat 6 g; Carb 5 g; Protein 7 g
Serving 1; Cook time 5 min

Ingredients
- 1 eggs - medium
- 2 teaspoon coconut flour or more depending on brand used
- pinch baking powder
- pinch salt

Instructions
1. Grease a ramekin dish or a large coffee mug with coconut oil or butter.
2. In a bowl, mix all the ingredients together with a fork until the mixture is smooth and free of lumps.
3. Microwave the 1-minute keto muffin on HIGH for 45 seconds to 1 minute. Alternatively, you can bake it in an oven at 200°C/400°F for 12 minutes.

KETO PUMPKIN MUFFINS

Nutrition: Cal 204; Fat 13 g; Carb 7 g; Protein 6 g
Serving 12; Cook time 25 min

Ingredients
PUMPKIN SPICE MUFFINS
- 2 cups almond flour
- 1/2 cup Brown Sugar Swerve Sweetener
- 2 tablespoons coconut flour
- 1 tablespoons baking powder
- 2 teaspoons pumpkin pie spice
- 1/2 teaspoon salt

- 1 cup pure pumpkin puree
- 4 large eggs
- 1/2 cup unsweetened almond milk

PECAN CRUMB TOPPING
- 1/3 cup almond flour
- 1/4 cup Brown Sugar Swerve
- 2 tablespoons coconut flour
- 3 tablespoons crushed pecans
- 1 teaspoon cinnamon
- 3 tablespoons butter, cold

Instructions

1. Preheat the oven to 325 degrees F (165 degrees C).
2. In a medium-sized mixing bowl, combine all of the pumpkin muffin ingredients until well combined.
3. Spray a muffin tin or line it with paper liners.
4. Spoon the pumpkin mixture into the muffin tin, filling each cup about 3/4 full. Set aside.
5. In a small bowl, combine the pecan crumb topping ingredients and mash them with a fork until the butter is incorporated and the mixture resembles coarse crumbs.
6. Sprinkle the crumb topping evenly over the muffins.
7. Bake for 20-22 minutes, or until a toothpick inserted into the center of a muffin comes out clean.

KETO STRAWBERRY, ALMOND AND CHOCOLATE MUFFINS

Nutrition: Cal 244; Fat 20 g; Carb 8 g; Protein 6 g
Serving 12; Cook time 35 min

Ingredients

- 25 g (1/4 cup) coconut flour
- 3 tsp baking powder
- 200 g (2 cups) almond meal
- 50 g (1/4 cup) powdered stevia sweetener
- 250 g strawberries, hulled, chopped
- 75 g dark chocolate (85% cocoa), chopped
- 3 eggs, lightly whisked
- 2 tsp vanilla extract
- 60 ml (1/4 cup) almond milk
- 125 g unsalted butter, melted

Instructions

1. Preheat the oven to 170°C (150°C fan forced). Line 12 holes of an 80ml (1/3 cup) capacity muffin pan with paper cases.
2. Sift the coconut flour and baking powder into a large bowl. Add the almond meal, stevia, strawberries, and chocolate, and stir to combine.
3. Whisk the eggs, vanilla, and almond milk together in a jug. Add the egg mixture and butter to the dry ingredients and stir until just combined.
4. Divide the mixture among the prepared muffin holes. Bake for 20-25 minutes or until golden and a skewer inserted into the center comes out clean. Set aside for 5 minutes to cool before transferring to a wire rack to cool completely.

KETO CHOCOLATE CREAM CHEESE MUFFINS

Nutrition: Cal 195; Fat 19 g; Carb 6 g; Protein 6 g
Serving 12; Cook time 30 min

Ingredients

- 1 1/4 cups of finely milled almond flour , measured and sifted
- 1/4 cup cocoa powder
- 1 teaspoon of instant coffee (optional for enhancing chocolate)
- teaspoons of baking powder
- 1/4 teaspoon of sea salt
- 4 tablespoons of unsalted butter, room temperature
- 1 cup plus 2 tablespoons of sugar substitute
- 4 ounces of cream cheese, room temperature
- 1 teaspoon of vanilla extract
- 4 eggs , room temperature
- 1 ounces of baking chocolate (melted)

Instructions

1. Preheat the oven to 400 degrees Fahrenheit and line the muffin pan with your choice of liners.
2. In a medium-sized bowl, combine all the almond flour, cocoa powder, instant coffee, baking powder, and sea salt. Set aside.
3. In a large mixing bowl, beat on high the softened butter, vanilla, and sugar substitute until light and fluffy.
4. Add the cream cheese and combine well until fully incorporated.
5. Add the eggs one at a time, making sure to mix well after each addition.
6. Add all the dry ingredients to the wet ingredients, mixing well until fully combined.

7. Lastly, add the melted baking chocolate in a stream and beat the mixture until fully mixed.
8. Divide the batter evenly into your prepared muffin pan, filling each cup 3/4 full.
9. Bake the muffins for 5 minutes at 400 degrees Fahrenheit. Then, after 5 minutes, reduce your temperature to 350 degrees Fahrenheit and bake for another 10-15 minutes, or until an inserted toothpick comes out clean.
10. Allow the chocolate muffins to cool on a baking rack for at least 10 minutes before enjoying.
11. Store leftovers in the refrigerator for up to 5 days or freeze for up to 3 weeks.

TRIPLE CHOCOLATE ZUCCHINI MUFFINS

Nutrition: Cal 205; Fat 17 g; Carb 4,6 g; Protein 5,5 g
Serving 35; Cook time 35 min

Ingredients

- 6 oz zucchini
- 1 cup classic monk fruit sweetener
- 1 cup coconut flour
- 1/3 cup unsweetened cocoa powder
- 2 1/2 tsp cream of tartar
- 1 tsp baking soda
- 1/2 tsp espresso powder
- 1/4 tsp salt
- 1/4 tsp xanthan gum
- 7 large eggs
- 3/4 tsp pure vanilla extract
- oz 100% Baker's chocolate
- 5 oz unsalted butter or coconut oil for dairy-free
- 3 tbsp 100% cocoa chocolate chips

Instructions

1. Preheat the oven to 350 degrees Fahrenheit and line 2 muffin pans with cupcake liners.
2. Measure and sift the almond flour and set it aside.
3. In a large bowl, using an electric mixer, combine the cream cheese, butter, and beat on high until light and fluffy.
4. Add the sugar substitute and continue to mix well.
5. Add in the eggs one at a time, mixing well between each addition.
6. Next, stir in the sifted almond flour, salt, and baking powder and mix until well combined.
7. Add the lemon extract and lemon zest and mix.
8. Lastly, fold in 1 1/2 cups of the raspberries until fully incorporated.

9. Pour the cake batter into the cupcake-lined muffin pans.
10. Sprinkle a few raspberries on the surface of each muffin.
11. Bake for 20-25 minutes or until an inserted toothpick comes out clean.
12. Muffins can be stored for up to 5 days in the refrigerator or frozen for up to 3 weeks.

KETO PECAN MUFFINS

Nutrition: Cal 270; Fat 30 g; Carb 10 g; Protein 7 g
Serving 6; Cook time 40 min

Ingredients

- 3/4 cup raw pecans, toasted and chopped
- 1/4 cup butter, melted
- 2 large eggs
- 2 tbsp heavy whipping cream
- 1 tsp vanilla extract
- 15-20 drops liquid stevia
- 1/4 tsp Pink Himalayan Salt
- 1 tsp ground cinnamon
- 1 tsp allspice
- 1/4 inch fresh grated ginger
- 2 tsp baking powder
- 1 cup almond flour
- 1/4 cup Low Carb Sugar Substitute
- 1/4 cup Keto Chocolate Chips optional

Instructions

1. Preheat your oven to 350 degrees Fahrenheit. Place the pecans on a sheet pan and toast them for 10-12 minutes until fragrant and lightly browned.
2. In a medium bowl, combine the melted butter, eggs, heavy cream, vanilla extract, and stevia using a hand mixer. Mix until well blended.
3. Add the remaining ingredients, except for the pecans and chocolate chips, to the bowl. Mix again until all ingredients are thoroughly combined.
4. Gently fold in the chocolate chips and toasted, chopped pecans until they are evenly distributed throughout the batter.
5. Grease a muffin tin and evenly distribute the batter among the cups. This recipe should yield 6 large muffins.
6. Bake the muffins in the preheated oven for 20-23 minutes, or until a toothpick inserted into the center comes out clean.

7. Allow the muffins to cool for 5 minutes before serving. For optimal freshness, store the muffins in a zip-top bag in the refrigerator.

KETO PUMPKIN CHIA MUFFINS

Nutrition: Cal 211; Fat 18 g; Carb 3 g; Protein 7 g
Serving 12; Cook time 30 min

Ingredients

DRY INGREDIENTS:
- 1 1/2 cups almond flour
- 1/4 cup ground chia seeds
- 1 tbsp gluten-free baking powder
- 1 tbsp pumpkin pie spice mix
- 1/4 cup Erythritol or Swerve, powdered
- Topping: 6 tbsp pumpkin seeds (pepitas)

WET INGREDIENTS:
- 1 cup pumpkin purée (you can make your own)
- 6 large eggs, separated
- 1/2 cup butter, ghee or virgin coconut oil, melted
- 20-30 drops liquid Stevia extract
- melted coconut oil or ghee for greasing

Instructions

1. Preheat the oven to 175°C (350°F). In a bowl, combine all the dry ingredients, except for the pumpkin seeds, and mix well.
2. Separate the egg whites from the egg yolks. Using a hand beater or electric mixer, whip the egg whites until soft peaks form. In another bowl, combine the egg yolks, melted butter, pumpkin puree, and stevia.
3. Make sure the melted butter is cooled (not hot) and the pumpkin puree and egg yolks are at room temperature. Using a food processor or mixer, process the mixture until well combined. Gradually add the dry mixture, one or two tablespoons at a time, while mixing.
4. Add about a quarter of the whipped egg whites to the mixture and mix gently. Then add the remaining egg whites and fold them into the batter using a slow setting on your mixer or a spatula. Be careful not to deflate the egg whites and keep the batter as fluffy as possible.
5. Line a muffin tray with 12 medium-sized muffin paper cups and lightly grease each cup with a small amount of coconut oil or ghee. Spoon the batter into the paper cups and transfer them to the oven. Alternatively, you can use a silicone muffin tray or silicone muffin cups.
6. Place the tray in the oven and bake for 5 minutes. After 5 minutes, sprinkle the pumpkin seeds over the muffins. Return to the oven and bake for another 30 minutes or until the tops are golden brown.

KETO CARROT MUFFINS

Nutrition: Cal 305; Fat 27 g; Carb 8 g; Protein 7 g
Serving 12; Cook time 40 min

Ingredients

- 300 g / 3 cups grated carrot
- 5 eggs
- 180 g / ¾ cup butter, softened
- 2 very ripe medium bananas
- 150 g / 1 ¼ cup almond flour or ground almonds
- 30 g / scant ¼ cup flaxseed ground
- 50 g / ½ cup walnuts, chopped
- 2 teaspoon baking powder
- 2 teaspoon cinnamon
- 1 teaspoon mixed spice
- 2 teaspoon vanilla essence
- 1 ½ teaspoon granulated stevia
- 100 g / ½ cup cream cheese, full fat

Instructions

1. Preheat your oven to 180 degrees Celsius (356 degrees Fahrenheit).
2. In a blender or mixing bowl, combine the eggs, softened butter, and bananas. Blend or mix until thoroughly combined.
3. Add the ground almonds, flaxseed, spices, vanilla, 1 teaspoon of stevia, and baking powder to the mixture. Mix well to incorporate all the ingredients.
4. Gently stir in the grated carrot and walnuts. Ensure that the carrots are grated and not ground, as grinding them will separate the liquid from the fiber. Avoid this mistake.
5. Grease your muffin tin or line it with paper cups. Pour the dough into the prepared muffin tin, filling each cup.
6. Bake the muffins at 180 degrees Celsius (356 degrees Fahrenheit) for approximately 30 minutes, or until they are nicely browned.
7. For the icing, beat the cream cheese (at room temperature) with 1/2 teaspoon of stevia and a couple of dashes of cinnamon. Once the muffins have cooled, spread the cream cheese mixture onto the muffins.

KETO CRANBERRY ORANGE MUFFINS

Nutrition: Cal 144; Fat 12 g; Carb 8 g; Protein 3.5 g
Serving 12; Соок time 30 min

Ingredients

- •1 oz cream cheese, softened
- •4 eggs
- •2/3 cup (80g) powdered monк fruit sweetener or 2/3 cup (128g) classic monк fruit sweetener
- •2 tbsp (30mL) heavy whipping cream
- •2 tsp orange extract
- •1 tsp cream of tartar
- •1/2 tsp baking soda
- •1/2 tsp pure vanilla extract
- •1/4 tsp salt
- •1/2 cup (4 oz) unsalted butter
- •1/2 cup + 2 tbsp (70g) coconut flour
- •200g fresh cranberries

Instructions

1. Preheat the oven to 350 degrees Fahrenheit (175 degrees Celsius) and line a muffin tin with 12 muffin liners.
2. In a mixing bowl, combine the cream cheese and use an electric mixer to whip it until creamy and fluffy. To the same bowl, add the eggs, monk fruit sweetener, heavy cream, orange extract, cream of tartar, baking soda, vanilla extract, and salt. Mix again with the electric mixer until all the ingredients are well-combined.
3. In a microwave-safe bowl, melt the butter. Add the melted butter and coconut flour to the mixing bowl of eggs and cream cheese mixture. Mix with the electric mixer until everything is fully incorporated. Gently fold in the cranberries.
4. Spoon the dough into the individual muffin liners, flattening it into an even layer using your fingers or the back of a spoon. Transfer the muffin tin to the oven and bake until the tops of the muffins are slightly golden, approximately 23-25 minutes.

KETO CHEESECAKE MUFFINS

Nutrition: Cal 263; Fat 24 g; Carb 6 g; Protein 8 g
Serving 8; Соок time 30 min

Ingredients

- •1 cup almond flour
- •1 tsp baking powder
- •½ cup brown sugar substitute (we use Sukrin Gold)
- •1 tsp ground cinnamon
- •½ cup pecans (chopped)
- •1 tsp vanilla extract
- •4 eggs (large)
- •250 g cream cheese (8oz)
- •salt

Instructions

1. Preheat the oven to 160°C (320°F) and prepare your muffin molds or cases. If using traditional muffin tins, make sure to grease them to prevent sticking. Alternatively, you can use silicone molds, which usually don't require greasing.
2. In a bowl, combine almond flour, baking powder, cinnamon, chopped pecans, sugar substitute, and a pinch of salt. Mix well to ensure all the dry ingredients are evenly distributed.
3. Cut the cream cheese into small cubes. This will add pockets of creamy goodness to the muffins.
4. In a separate jug, whisk together the eggs and vanilla extract using a fork until well blended.
5. Add the egg mixture to the dry ingredients in the bowl and stir until fully combined. Make sure there are no dry spots remaining.
6. Sprinkle the cream cheese cubes into the mixture. Take your time to evenly distribute them throughout the batter, ensuring they are separated and not clumped together.
7. Divide the batter evenly among your prepared muffin molds or cases, filling them about ¾ full.
8. Place the muffin molds in the preheated oven and bake for 20-25 minutes, or until the muffins are golden brown and cooked through. You can check for doneness by inserting a toothpick into the center of a muffin – if it comes out clean or with just a few crumbs, they're ready.

CREAM CHEESE PUMPKIN MUFFINS

Nutrition: Cal 175; Fat 15 g; Carb 10 g; Protein 4 g
Serving 12; Cook time 50 min

Ingredients

- 4 eggs
- 1 egg white
- 1 cup golden monk fruit sweetener
- 1 cup pumpkin puree
- ½ cup unsalted butter, melted
- 2 tbsp coconut oil, melted
- 1 tbsp pumpkin pie spice
- 2 tsp pure vanilla extract
- 1/2 cup + 2 tbsp coconut flour
- 2 tsp cream of tartar
- 1 tsp baking soda
- ¼ tsp salt

FILLING:

- 3 oz cream cheese, softened
- 1 tbsp heavy whipping cream
- 1 tbsp powdered monk fruit sweetener
- ½ tsp pure vanilla extract

Instructions

1. Preheat the oven to 350 degrees Fahrenheit and prepare a muffin tin by lining it with muffin liners.
2. Muffin Batter: In a mixing bowl, combine eggs, egg white, golden monk fruit sweetener, pumpkin puree, melted butter, melted coconut oil, pumpkin pie spice, and vanilla extract. Use an electric mixer to mix the ingredients together. Then, add coconut flour, cream of tartar, baking soda, and salt to the mixture and mix again using an electric mixer. Spoon the batter into the muffin liners.
3. Filling: In a separate bowl, mix the filling ingredients together until well combined. Spoon the filling mixture on top of the pumpkin batter in the muffin liners. Use a toothpick to swirl the filling into the pumpkin mixture.
4. Final Steps: Bake the muffins for about 30-35 minutes or until a toothpick inserted into the center comes out clean.
5. Remove the muffin tin from the oven and allow the muffins to cool almost completely at room temperature before serving.

CHEESY CAULIFLOWER MUFFINS

Nutrition: Cal 77; Fat 5,6 g; Carb 2,7 g; Protein 4,6 g
Serving 11; Cook time 35 min

Ingredients

- 3 cups finely chopped raw cauliflower florets approximately 1/2 a head of cauliflower
- 2 large eggs
- 1 cup shredded cheddar cheese divided
- 1/4 cup almond flour
- 1/2 tsp baking powder
- 1/2 tsp dry Italian seasoning herb blend
- 1/4 tsp onion powder
- 1/4 tsp garlic powder

Instructions

1. Preheat the oven to 375°F and line a cupcake/muffin pan with cupcake liners. Parchment cupcake liners are recommended for easy removal without sticking.
2. In a mixing bowl, combine cauliflower, eggs, 1/2 cup of cheese, almond flour, baking powder, Italian seasoning, onion powder, and garlic powder. Stir the ingredients together using a large spoon or spatula until the mixture is smooth.
3. Using an ice cream scooper, scoop the batter into the muffin cups, filling each cup about 2/3 full. You should be able to fill approximately 11 liners. Sprinkle 1/2 cup of shredded cheese over the muffins.
4. Bake the muffins for 20-25 minutes or until they are completely cooked and are no longer wet to the touch. If desired, garnish with fresh chopped parsley before serving.

DOUBLE CHOCOLATE MUFFINS

Nutrition: Cal 196; Fat 18 g; Carb 6 g; Protein 6 g
Serving 6; Cook time 30 min

Ingredients

- 48 g almond flour
- 30 g golden flaxseed meal finely ground
- 1 teaspoon baking powder
- 70 g unsalted grass-fed butter or 4 TBS coconut oil + 1 TBS coconut cream
- 1/3-1/2 cup allulose xylitol or coconut sugar if paleo (I use 1/2 cup allulose and 1/3 otherwise)
- 40 g cocoa powder
- 1/4 teaspoon kosher salt

- 1/4 teaspoon espresso powder or instant coffee (optional)
- 2 eggs at room temperature

OPTIONAL ADD-INS
- 50-80 g Lily's Sweets dark chocolate bar to taste
- 50-80 g pecans or walnuts
- flakey sea salt to garnish

Instructions
1. Position a rack in the lower third of your oven and preheat it to 350°F/180°C. Line or grease and flour a muffin pan and set it aside.
2. In a medium bowl, add almond flour, flaxseed meal, and baking powder. Whisk the ingredients together until thoroughly combined, and set the bowl aside.
3. In a large heatproof bowl, add butter (or coconut oil and cream), sweetener, cocoa powder, salt, and espresso powder (optional). Melt the mixture over a water bath, whisking constantly. Alternatively, you can melt the mixture in the microwave. Heat it until most of the sweetener has melted and the mixture is well incorporated. Remove from heat and allow the mixture to cool slightly.
4. Add one egg at a time to the mixture, whisking well after each one until fully incorporated. The texture should appear smooth, with all the sweetener dissolving into the mixture. If you used coconut oil, be sure to mix it particularly well. Add the flour mixture to the bowl and whisk vigorously until fully blended, which should take about a minute. Fold in chocolate pieces (or pecans) and spoon the batter into the prepared muffin pan.
5. Bake the muffins for 10-13 minutes if you prefer them extra fudgy (they'll be set but still jiggly), 14-17 minutes for medium fudginess, or 18-20 minutes for a "normal muffin" texture. The baking time may vary slightly from oven to oven, so use these guidelines as a starting point. Keep in mind that the muffins will continue to cook while cooling.
6. Sprinkle the muffins with flaky sea salt (optional) and allow them to cool for at least 15-20 minutes in the muffin pan. They will be particularly fragile right out of the oven if you made them fudgy and with xylitol, so you need to let them set.
7. Store the muffins in an airtight container for 3-4 days. They are best served warm.

KETO CINNAMON EGG LOAF MUFFINS

Nutrition: Cal 152; Fat 15 g; Carb 2,5 g; Protein 4
Serving 12; Cook time 30 min

Ingredients
- 4 eggs, room temperature
- 4 ounces cream cheese, room temperature
- 4 tablespoons butter, room temperature
- 1 teaspoon cinnamon
- 2 tablespoons Steviva Blends Granulated
- 1 teaspoon vanilla extract
- 1/2 cup almond flour
- 2 tablespoons butter, chilled
- 1 teaspoon cinnamon
- 2 tablespoons Steviva Blends
- 1/4 cup chopped pecans
- avocado oil spray

Instructions
1. Preheat the oven to 350°F (175°C).
2. In a blender, combine eggs, cream cheese, butter, 1 teaspoon cinnamon, 2 tablespoons Stevia sweetener, and vanilla extract. Blend until well combined and slightly foamy, which should take about one minute.
3. Grease your muffin cups with avocado oil spray and pour the egg mixture evenly into the muffin cups.
4. Bake for 10 minutes. While the egg loaf muffins are baking, prepare the streusel.
5. In a bowl, add almond flour, cinnamon, Stevia sweetener, 2 tablespoons chilled butter, and pecans. Using your fingertips, combine the ingredients until well mixed but crumbly.
6. After the egg loaf muffins have baked for 10 minutes, top them with the cinnamon streusel. Bake for another 10 minutes.
7. Remove the muffins from the oven and let them cool. They will appear puffy at first, but will sink back down as they cool.

CHOCOLATE CHIP BANANA BREAD MUFFINS

Nutrition: Cal 179; Fat 15 g; Carb 6 g; Protein 4
Serving 12; Cook time 35 min

Ingredients
- 1 oz cream cheese, softened
- 1 tbsp + 2 tsp banana extract
- 1/2 tsp pure vanilla extract

- 1 tsp cream of tartar
- 1/2 tsp baking soda
- 1/4 tsp salt
- 1/2 cup + 2 tbsp coconut flour
- 1/2 cup butter
- 1/3 cup chocolate chips, divided

Instructions

1. Preheat the oven to 350 degrees Fahrenheit (175 degrees Celsius) and line a muffin tin with 12 muffin liners.
2. In a mixing bowl, add eggs, classic monk fruit sweetener, heavy whipping cream, cream cheese, banana extract, vanilla extract, cream of tartar, baking soda, and salt. Use an electric mixer to mix the ingredients until well combined.
3. In a microwave-safe bowl, melt the butter. Add the melted butter and coconut flour to the mixing bowl. Mix again with the electric mixer until the ingredients are fully incorporated. Fold in most of the chocolate chips into the dough, reserving some to top the muffins with. Spoon the dough into the individual muffin liners. Top each muffin dough with the remaining chocolate chips.
4. Bake the muffins in the preheated oven until the tops are slightly golden, which should take about 23-25 minutes.

KETO CHEESY HERB MUFFINS

Nutrition: Cal 216; Fat 20 g; Carb 7,5 g; Protein 5 g
Serving 6; Cook time 40 min

Ingredients

- 6 tablespoons butter
- 1 teaspoon granulated erythritol sweetener
- 1 cup superfine blanched almond flour
- 3 tablespoons coconut flour
- 3/4 teaspoon kosher salt
- 1/4 teaspoon garlic powder
- 2 teaspoons baking powder
- ¼ teaspoon xanthan gum
- 2 eggs
- 1/2 teaspoon fresh thyme leaves
- 1/3 cup unsweetened almond milk
- 1/2 cup shredded sharp cheddar cheese

Instructions

1. Preheat the oven to 375°F (190°C).

2. Grease or line a standard cupcake pan with 8 muffin cups.
3. Place the butter in a medium-sized microwave-safe bowl.
4. Microwave the butter on high, uncovered, for 30 seconds or until melted.
5. Add the sweetener, almond flour, coconut flour, salt, garlic powder, baking powder, xanthan gum, eggs, fresh thyme, almond milk, and cheddar cheese to the bowl. Mix well using a fork until all the ingredients are combined.
6. Spoon the batter into the muffin cups, filling them about 2/3 full.
7. Bake for 22 minutes, or until a toothpick inserted into the center comes out clean.

KETO RICOTTA LEMON POPPYSEED MUFFINS

Nutrition: Cal 142; Fat 13 g; Carb 3 g; Protein 4 g
Serving 12; Cook time 50 min

Ingredients

- 1 cup (112 g) Superfine Almond Flour
- 1/3 cup (0.33 g) Swerve, or alternative sweetener
- 1 teaspoon (1 teaspoon) Baking Powder
- 1/4 cup (61.5 g) full fat ricotta cheese
- 1/4 cup (54.5 g) Coconut Oil
- 3 (3) Eggs
- 2 tablespoons (2 tablespoons) Poppy Seeds, ,
- 4 (4) True lemon packets
- 1/4 cup (59.5 g) Heavy Whipping Cream
- 1 teaspoon (1 teaspoon) Lemon Extract

Instructions

1. In a mixing bowl, combine all the ingredients and beat well until the batter becomes fluffy.
2. Line a muffin pan with silicone cupcake liners.
3. Pour the batter into the muffin pan, dividing it equally into 12 servings.
4. Bake at 350 degrees Fahrenheit (175 degrees Celsius) for 40 minutes or until a knife inserted into the center of a muffin comes out clean.
5. Allow the muffins to cool slightly before removing them from the liners.

CRANBERRY SOUR CREAM MUFFINS

Nutrition: Cal 241; Fat 20 g; Carb 9 g; Protein 9 g
Serving 12; Cook time 40 min

Ingredients

- ½ cup sour cream
- 4 large eggs
- 1 teaspoon vanilla extract
- 3 cups almond flour
- ½ cup Swerve Sweetener
- 2 teaspoon baking powder
- ½ teaspoon cinnamon
- ¼ teaspoon salt
- 1 cup cranberries
- ½ cup chopped pecans optional

Instructions

1. Preheat the oven to 325 degrees Fahrenheit (163 degrees Celsius) and line a muffin tin with parchment or silicone liners.
2. In a large blender jar, combine sour cream, eggs, and vanilla extract. Blend for about 30 seconds until well combined.
3. Add almond flour, sweetener, baking powder, cinnamon, and salt to the blender. Blend again until the batter is smooth, about 30 seconds to a minute. If the batter is too thick, you can add ¼ to ½ cup of water to thin it out, as almond flour brands can vary in consistency.
4. Stir in cranberries by hand, reserving a few for the top of the muffins, and chopped pecans if desired. Divide the mixture evenly among the prepared muffin cups and bake for 25 to 30 minutes, or until the muffins are golden brown and firm to the touch.
5. Remove the muffins from the oven and let them cool completely before serving.

KETO LEMON BLUEBERRY MUFFINS

Nutrition: Cal 130; Fat 10 g; Carb 7 g; Protein 2 g
Serving 12; Cook time 30 min

Ingredients

- ½ cup plain Greek yogurt
- 3 eggs
- juice of 1 lemon
- 2 teaspoons lemon zest
- ¼ cup natural Swerve sweetener
- 1 teaspoon vanilla extract
- 3 cups almond flour
- 1½ teaspoons baking powder
- ½ teaspoon baking soda
- ¼ teaspoon salt
- 1 cup blueberries fresh or frozen

Instructions

1. Preheat the oven to 350°F (175°C).
2. Line a muffin tin with paper liners and set it aside.
3. In a blender, combine Greek yogurt, eggs, lemon juice, lemon zest, Swerve (or your preferred sweetener), and vanilla extract. Blend for about 30 seconds or until the ingredients are well combined.
4. Add almond flour, baking powder, baking soda, and salt to the blender. Blend on high, stopping to scrape down and stir the ingredients once or twice if necessary. Continue blending until the batter is smooth.
5. Gently fold in the blueberries into the batter. Divide the batter evenly among the prepared muffin cups, filling each cup about ¾ full. If desired, sprinkle additional blueberries on top of each muffin.
6. Bake for 25-30 minutes or until the tops of the muffins are set and a toothpick inserted into the center comes out clean.
7. Place the muffin tin on a wire rack and allow the muffins to cool in the tin for 10 minutes. Then, remove the muffins from the tin and let them cool completely on the wire rack.
8. Enjoy your delicious lemon blueberry muffins!

KETO BANANA NUT MUFFINS

Nutrition: Cal 183; Fat 22 g; Carb 7 g; Protein 7 g
Serving 10; Cook time 30 min

Ingredients

- 1 ¼ Cup almond flour
- ½ Cup powdered erythritol
- 2 tablespoons ground flax (feel free to omit if you don't have it...it just adds a bit more depth to the flavors)
- 2 teaspoons baking powder
- ½ teaspoons ground cinnamon
- 5 tablespoon butter, melted

- 2 ½ teaspoons banana extract
- 1 teaspoon vanilla extract
- ¼ cup unsweetened almond milk
- ¼ cup sour cream
- 2 eggs
- ¾ cup chopped walnuts
- 1 tablespoon butter, cold and cut in 4 pieces
- 1 tablespoon almond flour
- 1 tablespoon powdered erythritol

Instructions

1. Preheat oven to 350 Prepare muffin tin with 10 paper liners, and set aside.
2. In a large bowl, mix almond flour, erythritol (or preferred sweetener) flax, baking powder and cinnamon.
3. Stir in butter, banana extract, vanilla extract, almond milk, and sour cream. Add eggs to mixture and gently stir until fully combined.
4. Fill muffin tins about ½-3/4 full with mixture.

CRUMBLE TOPPING

1. Add walnuts, butter, and almond flour to food processor. Pulse a few times until nuts are chopped into small pieces. If mixture seems too dry (sometimes some walnuts are softer than others) feel free to add another tablespoon of butter.
2. Sprinkle bits of the mixture evenly over batter and gently press down. Sprinkle erythritol on top of crumble mixture.
3. Bake for 20 minutes or until golden and toothpick comes out clean. Let cool for at least 30 minutes, an hour or more if possible. This lets them firm up.

KETO SNICKERDOODLE MUFFINS

Nutrition: Cal 287; Fat 26 g; Carb 7 g; Protein 5 g
Serving 12; Cook time 35 min

Ingredients

- 2 cups (220 g) blanched finely ground almond flour
- 2/3 cup (130 g) monk fruit or erythritol
- 4 teaspoons baking powder
- 4 teaspoons ground cinnamon
- 1/2 teaspoon sea salt
- 4 large eggs
- 1/2 cup (120 ml) melted coconut oil
- 1/2 cup (120 ml) non-dairy milk
- 2 teaspoons vanilla extract
- 2/3 cup (100 g) hemp hearts
- Cinnamon Sugar Topping:

- 2 tablespoons melted coconut oil
- 1/4 cup monk fruit or erythritol
- 2 teaspoons ground cinnamon

CINNAMON SUGAR TOPPING:

- 2 tablespoons melted coconut oil
- 1/4 cup monk fruit or erythritol
- 2 teaspoons ground cinnamon

Instructions

1. Preheat the oven to 350°F (177°C) and place 12 muffin liners in a 12-count muffin tin.
2. In a large bowl, combine almond flour, erythritol (or your preferred sweetener), baking powder, cinnamon, and sea salt. Mix until well combined.
3. In a separate smaller bowl, whisk together eggs, melted coconut oil, milk, and vanilla extract. Then, add the egg mixture to the almond flour mixture and stir until fully combined. Fold in the hemp hearts.
4. Divide the batter between the prepared muffin tins and transfer them to the preheated oven. Bake for 15 to 18 minutes, or until the tops are golden.
5. Meanwhile, prepare the cinnamon sugar topping by placing the coconut oil in a small dish and combining erythritol (or your preferred sweetener) and ground cinnamon in a small bowl. Once the muffins are done, one muffin at a time, brush the top with coconut oil before placing it over the cinnamon sugar bowl and sprinkling it with the cinnamon sugar mixture. Lightly shake off any excess and repeat with the remaining muffins.
6. Store the muffins in a sealed container in the fridge for up to a week, or in the freezer for up to a month.

KETO COFFEE CAKE MUFFINS

Nutrition: Cal 222; Fat 18 g; Carb 9 g; Protein 7 g
Serving 12; Cook time 30 min

Ingredients

BATTER:

- 2 tablespoon butter softened
- 2 oz cream cheese softened
- ⅓ cup Joy Filled Eats Sweetener
- 4 eggs
- 2 teaspoon vanilla
- ½ cup unsweetened vanilla almond milk

- 1 cup almond flour
- ½ cup coconut flour
- 1 teaspoon baking powder
- ¼ teaspoon salt

TOPPING:

- 1 cup almond flour
- 2 tablespoon coconut flour
- ¼ cup Joy Filled Eats Sweetener
- ¼ cup butter softened
- 1 teaspoon cinnamon
- ½ teaspoon molasses (optional)

Instructions

1. Preheat the oven to 350°F (177°C) and place 12 muffin liners in a 12-count muffin tin.
2. In a large bowl, combine almond flour, erythritol (or your preferred sweetener), baking powder, cinnamon, and sea salt. Mix until well combined.
3. In a separate smaller bowl, whisk together eggs, melted coconut oil, milk, and vanilla extract. Then, add the egg mixture to the almond flour mixture and stir until fully combined. Fold in the hemp hearts.
4. Divide the batter between the prepared muffin tins and transfer them to the preheated oven. Bake for 15 to 18 minutes, or until the tops are golden.
5. Meanwhile, prepare the cinnamon sugar topping by placing the coconut oil in a small dish and combining erythritol (or your preferred sweetener) and ground cinnamon in a small bowl. Once the muffins are done, one muffin at a time, brush the top with coconut oil before placing it over the cinnamon sugar bowl and sprinkling it with the cinnamon sugar mixture. Lightly shake off any excess and repeat with the remaining muffins.
6. Store the muffins in a sealed container in the fridge for up to a week, or in the freezer for up to a month.

STRAWBERRY VANILLA MUFFIN

Nutrition: Cal 187; Fat 17 g; Carb 4,5 g; Protein 5,5 g
Serving 12; Cook time 30 min

Ingredients

- 2 cups Almond flour
- 2 teaspoons Baking powder
- ¼ teaspoon Salt
- ½ cup Butter melted
- ¼ cup Erythritol or sugar substitute
- 2 teaspoons Vanilla essence
- ⅔ cup Strawberries chopped
- 4 Eggs
- ¼ Cup Water

Instructions

1. Preheat the oven to 180°C (350°F).
2. In a bowl, mix together the almond flour, baking powder, and salt.
3. In another bowl, mix the butter, water, eggs, erythritol, and vanilla essence.
4. Combine the wet and dry ingredients together and stir well. Add the strawberries to the mixture.
5. Pour the batter into muffin liners in a muffin tin.
6. Bake for 15 to 20 minutes, or until the muffins are firm.

FLAXSEED MUFFIN IN A MUG

Nutrition: Cal 283; Fat 22 g; Carb 10 g; Protein 12 g
Serving 1; Cook time 10 min

Ingredients

- 1 Egg
- 1 teaspoon Coconut Oil , melted
- 1 teaspoon Vanilla Extract
- ¼ cup Flaxseed Meal
- ½ teaspoon Baking Powder
- ¼ teaspoon Ground Cinnamon
- 1 tablespoon Erythritol or erythirtol

OPTIONAL INGREDIENTS- RASPBERRY CHOCOLATE CHIP FLAX MUFFIN

- 2 tablespoons Raspberries fresh or frozen
- 1 tablespoon Sugar-free Chocolate Chips

Instructions

1. In a bowl, whisk together the egg, oil, and vanilla. Set aside.
2. Stir in the dry ingredients: flax meal, baking powder, cinnamon, and sugar-free sweetener.
3. Stir in your optional ingredients, such as raspberries and chocolate chips.
4. Transfer the batter into a microwave-safe mug. Make sure the mug is at least 2.5 inches in height to prevent overflowing.
5. Microwave on high for 1 minute and 30 seconds.
6. Allow the muffin to cool for 1 minute before eating to avoid burning yourself.

FLOURLESS PEANUT BUTTER MUFFINS

Nutrition: Cal 208; Fat 13 g; Carb 7,5 g; Protein 15 g
Serving 12; Cook time 35 min

Ingredients

- 1 cup peanut butter (creamy, no sugar added)
- 1 tablespoon coconut oil or butter
- ½ cup Swerve Brown
- 1 teaspoon vanilla extract
- 3 large eggs
- ½ cup collagen protein powder
- 2 teaspoon baking powder
- ¼ teaspoon salt
- ⅓ cup sugar-free chocolate chips

Instructions

1. Preheat the oven to 350°F (175°C) and line a muffin pan with 12 silicone or parchment paper liners.
2. Place the peanut butter and coconut oil in a large microwave-safe bowl. Microwave them until melted and can be stirred together. Alternatively, you can melt them in a pan over low heat.
3. Whisk in the sweetener and vanilla extract until well combined, then whisk in the eggs. Add the collagen, baking powder, and salt, and stir until well combined. Stir in the chocolate chips.
4. Divide the mixture evenly among the prepared muffin cups and bake for 18 to 25 minutes, or until the muffins have risen, are golden brown, and firm to the touch on top.
5. Remove from the oven and let cool in the pan before serving.

KETO GINGERBREAD MUFFINS

Nutrition: Cal 131; Fat 15 g; Carb 6,5 g; Protein 9 g
Serving 12; Cook time 40 min

Ingredients

- ½ cup sour cream
- 3 large eggs
- ¾ teaspoon vanilla extract
- ⅔ cup Swerve Brown lightly packed
- 2 ½ cups almond flour
- ⅓ cup unflavoured whey protein powder or egg white protein
- 1 tablespoon cocoa powder
- 2 teaspoon baking powder
- 2 teaspoon ground ginger
- ½ teaspoon ground cinnamon
- ⅛ teaspoon ground cloves
- ¼ teaspoon salt

VANILLA DRIZZLE

- ⅓ cup powdered Swerve Sweetener
- 1 to 2 tablespoon water
- ½ teaspoon vanilla extract

Instructions

1. Preheat the oven to 350F and line a standard metal muffin pan with 12 silicone or parchment liners.
2. In a large bowl, whisk together the sour cream, eggs, and vanilla extract. Add the sweetener and whisk until well combined, breaking up any clumps with the back of a fork.
3. Add the almond flour, protein powder, cocoa powder, baking powder, ginger, cinnamon, cloves, and salt and stir until well mixed.
4. Divide the batter evenly among the prepared muffins cups, about ¾ full. Bake 18 to 25 minutes, until golden brown and firm to the touch.
5. Remove and let cool in the pan.

VANILLA DRIZZLE

1. In a medium bowl, whisk together the sweetener and just enough water to make a drizzling consistency. Whisk in the vanilla extract.

Drizzle over the cooled muffins.

KETO PEACH MUFFINS

Nutrition: Cal 167; Fat 13 g; Carb 7 g; Protein 7 g
Serving 16; Cook time 50 min

Ingredients

STREUSEL TOPPING

- ½ cup almond flour
- 3 tablespoon Swerve Brown
- ¼ teaspoon salt
- 2 tablespoon melted butter

MUFFINS

- ½ cup sour cream
- 3 large eggs
- 1 teaspoon vanilla extract
- ½ teaspoon peach extract (optional)
- 2 ¼ cups almond flour
- ½ cup Swerve Granular

- ⅓ cup whey protein powder (or egg white protein powder)
- 2 teaspoon baking powder
- ¼ teaspoon salt
- 2 cups finely chopped peaches (about 2 medium peaches)

Instructions

1. In a medium bowl, whisk together the almond flour, Swerve Brown, and salt. Stir in the melted butter and toss until the mixture resembles coarse crumbs. Set aside.

MUFFINS

2. Preheat the oven to 350F and line 16 muffin cups with parchment or silicone liners.
3. In a large bowl, whisk together the sour cream, eggs, and the extracts until smooth. Stir in the almond flour, sweetener, protein powder, baking powder, and salt until well combined.
4. Stir in 1 ½ cups of the peaches and spoon into the prepared muffins cups, filling about ¾ full.
5. Top each muffin with a few additonal pieces of peach, then sprinkle with the streusel mixture. Bake 23 to 28 minutes, until golden brown and just firm to the touch

---

KETO JELLY DONUT MUFFINS

Nutrition: Cal 137; Fat 9 g; Carb 6 g; Protein 7 g

Serving 8; Cook time 50 min

Ingredients

"JELLY" FILLING

- ½ cup raspberries (or chopped strawberries)
- 1 tablespoon water
- ¼ cup powdered Swerve Sweetener
- ¼ teaspoon glucomannan

MINI MUFFINS

- ½ cup coconut flour
- ½ cup Swerve Sweetener
- ¼ cup unflavored whey protein powder
- 1 ½ teaspoon baking powder
- ¼ teaspoon salt
- 4 large eggs
- ¼ cup butter, melted
- ¼ cup water (more if needed)
- ¾ teaspoon vanilla extract
- Powdered sweetener for rolling

Instructions

JELLY FILLING

1. In a small saucepan over medium heat, combine the raspberries and water. Bring to a simmer, then reduce the heat to low and cook until the berries are soft enough to be mashed with a fork.
2. Mash them up, then stir in the sweetener and the glucomannan. Let cool.

MINI MUFFINS

1. Preheat the oven to 350F and grease a metal mini muffin pan well. If yours is not very non-stick, consider using silicone or parchment muffin liners.
2. In a large bowl, combine the coconut flour, sweetener, protein powder, baking powder, and salt. Add the eggs, melted butter, water, and vanilla extract and stir to combine. If the batter is very thick, add another tablespoon or two of water. It should be easily stirred but not really pourable.
3. Divide the mixture among the prepared muffin cups and bake about 15 minutes, or until the tops are firm to the touch. Remove and let cool completely in the pan.

TO ASSEMBLE

1. Once the mini muffins are cool, use a small sharp knife to cut a small cone out of the top of each. Cut off the top of the cone (the part that would be the top of the muffin) and reserve.
2. Fill the holes in the mini muffins with the raspberry filling and replace the tops. Roll the filled mini muffins in powdered sweetener.

KETO CAPPUCCINO MUFFINS

Nutrition: Cal 172; Fat 14 g; Carb 7 g; Protein 7 g

Serving 12; Cook time 45 min

Ingredients

MUFFINS:

- ½ cup sour cream
- 4 large eggs
- 1 teaspoon espresso powder
- ½ teaspoon vanilla extract
- 2 cups almond flour
- ½ cup Swerve Sweetener
- ¼ cup coconut flour
- 2 teaspoon baking powder
- 1 teaspoon cinnamon
- ¼ teaspoon salt

GLAZE:

- ¼ cup powdered Swerve Sweetener
- 2 tablespoon heavy whipping cream
- cinnamon for garnish

Instructions

MUFFINS:

1. Preheat oven to 350F and line a muffin tin with parchment or silicone liners.
2. Combine sour cream, eggs, espresso powder, and vanilla extract in a large blender jar. Blend about 30 seconds.
3. Add the almond flour, sweetener, coconut flour, baking powder, cinnamon, and salt. Blend again until smooth, about 30 seconds to a minute. If your batter is overly thick, add ¼ to ½ cup of water to thin it out (different brands of almond flour can vary).
4. Divide the mixture among the prepared muffin cups and bake 23 to 25 minutes, until just golden brown and firm to the touch. Remove and let cool completely.

GLAZE:

1. In a small bowl, whisk together the powdered sweetener and cream. Drizzle over the cooled muffins. Sprinkle with a little cinnamon.

KETO PANCAKE MUFFINS

Nutrition: Cal 211 Fat 18 g; Carb 8 g; Protein 8 g
Serving 8; Cook time 25 min

Ingredients

- ½ cup plain whole milk yogurt
- 2 tablespoon unsalted butter or coconut oil melted
- 3 tablespoon Swerve Sweetener or equivalent of choice (more if you like sweet muffins)
- 1 teaspoon vanilla extract
- ¼ teaspoon apple cider vinegar
- 1 ¾ cup blanched almond flour
- ½ teaspoon baking soda
- ¼ teaspoon salt
- 3 large eggs
- ½ cup frozen blueberries and raspberries

Instructions

2. Preheat the oven to 350°F (175°C) and line 8 muffin cups with parchment liners or grease the muffin cups very well.
3. In a blender, combine yogurt, butter, sweetener, vanilla, and apple cider vinegar. Place almond flour, baking soda, and salt on top. Blend on low for 10 to 15 seconds until combined.

4. Add eggs to the blender and blend on low for another 15 to 20 seconds, then switch to high speed for 20 to 30 seconds until the eggs are just incorporated into the batter.
5. Stir in all but 2 tablespoons of the frozen berries by hand (do not blend!). Divide the batter among the prepared muffin cups and place a few remaining berries on top of each muffin.
6. Bake for 15 to 18 minutes, until slightly golden brown and a tester inserted in the center comes out clean. Remove from the oven and let cool in the pan for a few minutes, then transfer to a wire rack to cool completely.

KETO MOCHA MUFFINS

Nutrition: Cal 166; Fat 17 g; Carb 9 g; Protein 10 g
Serving 235; Cook time 30 min

Ingredients

- 3 large eggs
- ⅓ cup strong coffee
- 1 teaspoon vanilla extract
- 2 ¼ cups pumpkin seed flour (can sub 2 to 2 ¼ cups almond flour)
- ½ cup Swerve Sweetener
- ¼ cup cocoa powder
- 2 tsp baking powder
- ¼ teaspoon salt
- ¼ cup melted butter
- ⅓ cup sugar-free chocolate chips

Instructions

1. Preheat the oven to 325°F (163°C) and line a mini muffin pan with silicone or parchment liners.
2. In a blender or food processor, combine the eggs, coffee, and vanilla extract. Blend for a few seconds to combine.
3. Add the pumpkin seed flour, sweetener, cocoa powder, baking powder, and salt. Blend on high until well combined. Add the melted butter and blend again until smooth.
4. If your batter is overly thick, add a little more liquid (coffee or water) 1 tablespoon at a time. The batter should be scoopable but not pourable.
5. Stir in most of the chocolate chips by hand, reserving a few for the tops of the muffins. Fill the mini muffin cups almost to the top. You will get about 30 mini muffins, so you may need to work in batches.

6. Add a few of the reserved chips to the top of each muffin. Bake for 15 to 20 minutes, until the tops are set and firm to the touch. Remove from the oven and let cool in the pan.

BROWN BUTTER PECAN MUFFINS

Nutrition: Cal 250; Fat 22 g; Carb 9 g; Protein 8 g
Serving 12; Cook time 30 min

Ingredients
- 1/2 cup unsalted butter
- 2 1/2 cups almond flour
- 1/2 cup Brown Swerve
- 1/3 cup whey protein powder
- 2 1/2 tsp baking powder
- 1/2 tsp salt
- 3 large eggs
- 1/2 cup water
- 1/2 tsp caramel or vanilla extract
- 1/2 cup chopped, toasted pecans

Instructions
1. In a medium saucepan over medium heat, melt the butter. Continue to cook until the butter becomes a deep amber color, about 4 minutes. Let cool for 15 minutes.
2. Preheat the oven to 350°F (177°C) and line a muffin pan with parchment or silicone liners.
3. In a large bowl, whisk together the almond flour, Swerve, protein powder, baking powder, and salt. Stir in the eggs, browned butter, water, and extract until well combined. Stir in the chopped pecans, reserving a few for the top of the muffins.
4. Divide the batter among the prepared muffin cups and add a few chopped pecans to the top of each. Bake for 18 to 25 minutes, until golden brown and firm to the touch.
5. Remove from the oven and let cool completely.

MAPLE WALNUT MUFFINS

Nutrition: Cal 260; Fat 23 g; Carb 7 g; Protein 8 g
Serving 12; Cook time 30 min

Ingredients
MUFFINS
- 2 cups almond flour
- 1/2 cup granulated Swerve Sweetener (more if you like things sweeter)
- 1/3 cup unflavored whey protein powder
- 1/4 cup coconut flour (or an additional cup almond flour)
- 2 tsp baking powder
- 1/4 tsp salt
- 3 large eggs
- 1/2 cup butter, melted
- 3/4 cup unsweetened almond milk
- 1 tsp maple extract
- 3/4 cup chopped walnuts, divided

GLAZE
- 1/4 cup confectioner's Swerve Sweetener
- 2 tbsp heavy cream
- 1/2 tsp maple extract
- 1 to 2 tbsp water to thin glaze

Instructions
MUFFINS
1. Preheat oven to 325F and grease 12 muffin tins well or line with paper liners.
2. In a large bowl, combine almond flour, Swerve Sweetener, protein powder, coconut flour, baking powder and salt. Stir in eggs, melted butter, almond milk and maple extract until well mixed. Stir in 1/2 cup of the walnuts.
3. Divide batter between prepared muffin cups. Sprinkle with remaining chopped nuts, pressing lightly to adhere. Bake 25 to 30 minutes, until set and golden brown. Remove and let cool.

GLAZE
1. In a small bowl, combine confectioner's Swerve, cream and maple extract. Add just enough water to thin it out to a drizzling consistency. Drizzle over cooled muffins.

PECAN CHEESECAKE MUFFINS

Nutrition: Cal 263; Fat 3 g; Carb 4 g; Protein 8 g
Serving 8; Cook time 30 min

Ingredients
- 1 cup almond flour
- 1 tsp baking powder
- ½ cup brown sugar substitute (we use Sukrin Gold)
- 1 tsp ground cinnamon
- ½ cup pecans (chopped)
- 1 tsp vanilla extract
- 4 eggs (large)
- 250 g cream cheese (8oz)

- Salt

Instructions

1. Preheat the oven to 160°C (320°F) and prepare your muffin molds or cases. Grease the tin, preferably using a silicone mold for easy removal without the need for additional greasing.
2. In a bowl, combine almond flour, baking powder, cinnamon, pecans, sugar substitute, and a pinch of salt.
3. Chop the cream cheese into small cubes.
4. In a jug, whisk together the eggs and vanilla using a fork.
5. Add the egg mixture to the dry ingredients and stir until well combined.
6. Sprinkle the cream cheese cubes into the mixture, ensuring they are evenly distributed and not clumped together.
7. Divide the mixture among your muffin molds.
8. Bake in the oven for 20-25 minutes or until the muffins are golden brown and fully cooked.

BLUEBERRY LEMON MUFFINS

Nutrition: Cal 180; Fat 15 g; Carb 7 g; Protein 6 g
Serving 10; Cook time 25 min

Ingredients

- 1 ¾ cups super fine almond flour
- ¼ cup Oat Fiber , see notes
- ¾ cup of fresh blueberries
- eggs
- ⅓ cup sour cream
- ⅓ cup heavy cream
- ½ cup monk fruit/allulose
- teaspoons baking powder
- Zest and juice of 1 lemon
- 1 teaspoon vanilla extract
- Pinch of salt

Instructions

1. Preheat the oven to 350°F. In a bowl, combine the flour, baking powder, oat fiber, and salt. Whisk them together and set aside.
2. In a separate bowl, add the wet ingredients, including the sweetener, and mix using a hand mixer or whisk.
3. Gradually add the dry ingredients into the wet mixture and mix just until combined. Be careful not to overmix. Gently fold in the blueberries. Scoop the batter into silicone cupcake liners or paper liners.
4. Bake for 18-20 minutes or until a toothpick inserted into the center comes out clean. Allow the muffins to cool before serving.

BUTTER PECAN COOKIES

Nutrition: Cal 146; Fat 14 g; Carb 3 g; Protein 2 g
Serving 16; Cook time 30 min

Ingredients

- 4 oz cold salted butter cut into pieces
- 1 cup almond flour
- ⅓ cup coconut flour
- ⅔ cup Joy Filled Eats Sweetener
- 2 teaspoon gelatin
- 1 teaspoon vanilla
- 1 cup pecans

Instructions

1. Preheat the oven to 350°F and line a large cookie sheet with parchment paper.
2. In a food processor, combine the butter, almond flour, coconut flour, 1/3 cup of the sweetener, gelatin, and vanilla. Pulse until the mixture forms wet crumbs. Add the pecans and pulse until they are chopped, and the dough comes together into a ball.
3. Divide the dough into 16 pieces. Place the remaining 1/3 cup sweetener in a shallow bowl. Roll each piece of dough into a ball, then coat it in the sweetener by pressing it into a disc. Flip it over and press again so that both sides are dusted with sweetener. Place the coated dough on the prepared baking sheet. Repeat with the remaining dough.
4. Bake for 15-17 minutes or until the edges are golden. Begin checking them around the 8-10 minute mark, as they may bake quickly in some ovens.

KETO JAM COOKIES

Nutrition: Cal 65; Fat 6 g; Carb 2 g; Protein 1 g
Serving 28; Cook time 30 min

Ingredients

- 4 oz cold salted butter cut into pieces (1 stick)
- 1 cup almond flour
- ⅓ cup coconut flour
- ⅓ cup Joy Filled Eats Sweetener
- 2 teaspoon gelatin
- 1 teaspoon vanilla
- ⅓ cup finely shredded unsweetened coconut
- about ¼ cup no sugar added or reduced carb jam

Instructions

1. Preheat the oven to 350°F.
2. In a food processor, combine the butter, almond flour, coconut flour, sweetener, gelatin, and vanilla. Pulse the mixture until it forms a ball of dough. Divide the dough into 28 balls and roll each ball in shredded coconut. Place the coated balls on a parchment-lined baking sheet and press them down to create a small well in the center using your thumbs.
3. Bake the cookies for 14-17 minutes or until they are lightly browned around the edges. Use a small upside-down measuring spoon to press down the center of each cookie. Place 1/2 teaspoon of jam into the well of each cookie. Allow the cookies to cool completely and store them in the refrigerator.

ENGLISH TOFFEE CAPPUCCINO COOKIES

Nutrition: Cal 253; Fat 25 g; Carb 5 g; Protein 4 g
Serving 8; Cook time 45 min

Ingredients

DOUGH INGREDIENTS:

- 4 oz cold salted butter cut into pieces
- 1 cup almond flour
- 2 tablespoon cocoa powder
- 1 tablespoon instant coffee
- ⅓ cup Joy Filled Eats Sweetener
- 2 teaspoon gelatin
- 1 teaspoon vanilla

TOFFEE:

- ½ cup Joy Filled Eats Sweetener
- ⅛ cup heavy cream
- ⅛ cup salted butter

CHOCOLATE:

- ¼ cup sugar free chocolate chips
- 1 teaspoon butter

Instructions

1. Preheat the oven to 350°F and line 8 holes of a cupcake tin with foil liners.
2. In a food processor, combine all the dough ingredients and pulse until a uniform dough forms.
3. Divide the dough into 8 balls and place each ball in a foil-lined cupcake tin.
4. Bake for 18 minutes or until the dough is slightly firm to the touch. Allow them to cool completely.
5. Meanwhile, in a medium saucepan, combine the sweetener, cream, and butter. Cook over medium heat, stirring frequently, until the mixture turns a deep golden brown and thickens. This process can take around 10-15 minutes, so monitor it carefully. Let it cool for ten minutes.
6. Use a tart tamper or the back of a tablespoon to make an indent in each cookie cup. Fill the indent with the caramel.
7. Melt the chocolate in the microwave or using a double boiler. If using the microwave, stir the chocolate every thirty seconds until fully melted. Spread the tops of the cookies with the melted chocolate.
8. It's important to note that the toffee center will become hard when refrigerated for more than a few hours, so it is recommended to store these cookies at room temperature. They should remain fresh for 2-3 days.

CRUNCHY PEANUT COOKIES

Nutrition: Cal 139; Fat 3 g; Carb 4 g; Protein 4 g
Serving 18; Cook time 27 min

Ingredients

- 1 cup unsweetened almond milk or 1% milk
- 1/2 cup fat free plain Greek yogurt
- 2 cups (9 oz) frozen strawberries
- 1 1/2 ripe medium bananas
- 1/2 cup quick oats or old fashioned oats
- 1 Tbsp honey
- 1/2 tsp vanilla extract

Instructions

1. Preheat the oven to 350°F and line a large cookie sheet with parchment paper.
2. In a food processor, combine the butter, almond flour, 1/3 cup of sweetener, coconut flour, gelatin, vanilla, and salt. Pulse until the mixture forms wet crumbs. Add the peanuts and pulse until the nuts are chopped.
3. Divide the dough into 18 pieces. Place the remaining 1/3 cup of sweetener in a shallow bowl. Roll each piece of dough into a ball, then roll it in the sweetener and press it into a disc. Flip it over and press again so that both sides are coated with sweetener. Place the dough discs on the prepared baking sheet. Repeat with the remaining dough.
4. Bake for 17-19 minutes or until the edges are golden. Allow them to cool completely. These cookies will firm up even more when refrigerated.

KETO VANILLA COOKIES

Nutrition: Cal 89; Fat 8 g; Carb 2 g; Protein 1 g
Serving 20; Cook time 30 min

Ingredients
- 1 stick cold salted butter cut into pieces
- 1 cup almond flour
- ⅓ cup coconut flour
- ⅓ cup Joy Filled Eats Sweetener
- 2 teaspoon gelatin
- 2 teaspoon vanilla

ICING INGREDIENTS:
- ½ cup xylitol ground into a powder (or ⅔ cup of another powdered sweetener)
- 2 teaspoon vanilla
- 1 tablespoon almond milk
- 1 tablespoon butter melted

Instructions
1. Preheat the oven to 350°F.
2. In a food processor, combine all the dough ingredients and pulse until they are well combined.
3. To make round cookies: Divide the dough into 20 balls and place them on a parchment-lined baking sheet. Press them down with your fingers to flatten.
4. To make cut-out cookies: Roll the dough out between two sheets of parchment paper on top of a cookie sheet. Remove the top sheet and make shapes in the dough, keeping them 1-2 inches apart. Remove the excess dough

between the shapes. Repeat with the remaining dough.
5. Bake for 14-18 minutes or until the edges are lightly browned. Allow the cookies to cool completely.
6. Stir together the ingredients for the icing. Spread the icing on the cooled cookies. Place them on waxed paper and refrigerate to allow the icing to harden, making them stackable.

MAPLE CREAM SANDWICH COOKIES

Nutrition: Cal 161; Fat 16 g; Carb 2 g; Protein 2 g
Serving 8; Cook time 27 min

Ingredients
- ¾ cup almond flour
- 3 tablespoon Joy Filled Eats Sweetener
- 3 tablespoon butter softened
- 1 teaspoon maple extract
- ½ teaspoon gelatin

MAPLE BUTTERCREAM:
- 5 tablespoon butter
- ½ cup Joy Filled Eats Sweetener
- ½ teaspoon maple extract

Instructions
1. Preheat the oven to 350°F and line a cookie sheet with parchment paper.
2. In a bowl, combine the cookie ingredients and mix using a wooden spoon until the dough comes together easily. Divide the dough into 16 pieces and roll each into a ball. Place the balls on the prepared cookie sheet, or shape the dough into a log and slice it into 16 pieces.
3. Using the bottom of a measuring cup or drinking glass, flatten the cookies to a thickness of ¼ inch. If the dough sticks to the bottom, gently slide it off and place it back on the parchment paper.
4. Bake for 10-12 minutes, or until the edges are golden. If your oven runs hot, start checking after 8 minutes. Allow the cookies to cool completely.
5. While the cookies are cooling, use an electric mixer to mix the butter for the icing. Gradually add the sugar and mix until smooth. Add the maple extract.
6. Once the cookies are completely cooled, flip half of them upside down and divide the icing between them. Top each with a second cookie. Refrigerate for at least an hour to allow the

icing to set. Otherwise, the icing may ooze out when you bite into them.

'APPLE' PIE COOKIES

Nutrition: Cal 192; Fat 18 g; Carb 8 g; Protein 4 g
Serving 16; Cook time 60 min

Ingredients

- 1 medium zucchini peeled and diced
- 1 tablespoon coconut oil
- 3 tablespoon Joy Filled Eats Sweetener
- 1 tablespoon cinnamon
- 1 teaspoon gluccomannan

CRUST INGREDIENTS:

- 1 ⅓ cup almond flour
- teaspoon coconut flour
- 4 tablespoon butter
- 3 tablespoon Joy Filled Eats Sweetener
- 1 tablespoon cold water
- 1 tablespoon gelatin

Instructions

1. Heat coconut oil in a large frying pan over medium heat. Sauté zucchini until softened. Add the sweetener and cinnamon and cook for a couple more minutes. Sprinkle glucomannan on top and mix well. Set aside.
2. Preheat the oven to 350°F.
3. In a food processor, combine the crust ingredients and pulse until a dough forms. Roll it out into a large rectangle, about ¼ inch thick, and cut out 16 circles with a diameter of 1.5-2 inches (you can use an upside-down cup).
4. Divide the filling between the cookies. Re-roll the scraps of dough and cut thin strips to create a criss-cross pattern on top of the cookies. You can gently press or crimp the strips around the edges.
5. Bake for 20-30 minutes or until golden brown.

LOW CARB LEMON COOKIES

Nutrition: Cal 70; Fat 7 g; Carb 3 g; Protein 2 g
Serving 24; Cook time 25 min

Ingredients

- 4 oz cold salted butter (1 stick) cut into pieces
- 1 cup almond flour
- ⅓ cup coconut flour
- ⅓ cup Joy Filled Eats Sweetener

- 2 teaspoon gelatin
- 1 teaspoon lemon extract or zest

ICING INGREDIENTS:

- 1 cup powdered erythritol
- 1-2 tablespoon lemon juice
- lemon zest optional

Instructions

1. Preheat the oven to 350°F.
2. In a food processor, combine all the dough ingredients and pulse until a uniform dough forms. Divide the dough into 24 balls and place them on a parchment-lined baking sheet. Press down on each ball with your fingers. Sprinkle a little more sweetener on top.
3. Bake for 12-15 minutes or until lightly browned around the edges. Allow the cookies to cool for at least 10 minutes.
4. In a small bowl, combine the powdered sweetener with 1 tablespoon of lemon juice. Stir until smooth. Add additional lemon juice if needed. Spread the mixture on the cooled cookies.
5. Garnish the cookies with lemon zest.

KETO FRUIT PIZZA COOKIES

Nutrition: Cal 115; Fat 9 g; Carb 5 g; Protein 4 g
Serving 10; Cook time 25 min

Ingredients

- 4 oz cold salted butter cut into pieces
- 1 cup almond flour
- ⅓ cup coconut flour
- ⅓ cup Joy Filled Eats Sweetener
- 2 teaspoon gelatin
- 1 teaspoon vanilla

TOPPING INGREDIENTS:

- 3 oz cream cheese softened
- 2 tablespoon Joy Filled Eats Sweetener
- 1-2 teaspoon half and half
- ½ teaspoon vanilla
- fresh berries

Instructions

1. Preheat the oven to 350°F.
2. In a food processor, combine the dough ingredients and pulse until a uniform dough forms.
3. Divide the dough into 10 balls and place them on a parchment-lined baking sheet. Use the bottom of a glass coated with additional

sweetener to press each ball into 2.5-inch circles. Press down further with your fingers if necessary.

4. Bake for 14-16 minutes or until lightly browned around the edges. Allow the cookies to cool completely.

5. Use an electric mixer to whip the cream cheese until fluffy. Add the powdered sweetener and mix well. Gradually add the half and half, 1 teaspoon at a time, until the mixture reaches a spreadable consistency. Add the vanilla extract and mix well. Use this mixture to top the cooled cookies. Garnish with fresh berries. Store the cookies in the refrigerator.

GLAZED MAPLE WALNUT COOKIES

Nutrition: Cal 132; Fat 12 g; Carb 3 g; Protein 2 g
Serving 16; Cook time 35 min

Ingredients
- 1 cup walnuts
- 4 oz cold salted butter (1 stick) cut into pieces
- ½ cup almond flour
- ⅓ cup coconut flour
- ⅓ cup Joy Filled Eats Sweetener
- teaspoon gelatin
- 1 teaspoon maple extract
- 1 teaspoon cinnamon

GLAZE INGREDIENTS:
- ½ cup powdered erythritol
- 1 tablespoon half and half
- 1 teaspoon cinnamon
- ½ teaspoon maple extract

Instructions
1. Preheat the oven to 350°F. Line a large cookie sheet with parchment paper.
2. Place the walnuts in a food processor and pulse until finely chopped. Add the butter, almond flour, coconut flour, sweetener, gelatin, maple extract, and cinnamon. Pulse until the mixture forms wet crumbs.
3. Divide the dough into 16 pieces. Roll each piece into a ball and place them on the prepared baking sheet. Gently press down on each ball to flatten slightly.
4. Bake for 18-22 minutes or until the edges are golden. Allow the cookies to cool completely.
5. In a small bowl, stir together the ingredients for the glaze. Use a pastry brush to brush the

glaze on top of the cookies. Place the cookies in the refrigerator to chill. The glaze will harden in the refrigerator, allowing you to stack the cookies.

CHOCOLATE CHIP SHORTBREAD COOKIES

Nutrition: Cal 107; Fat 9 g; Carb 6 g; Protein 3 g
Serving 16; Cook time 30 min

Ingredients
- 4 oz cold salted butter cut into pieces
- 1 cup almond flour
- ⅓ cup coconut flour
- ⅓ cup Joy Filled Eats Sweetener
- 2 teaspoon gelatin
- 1 teaspoon vanilla
- ⅔ cup sugar-free chocolate chips

CHOCOLATE COATING:
- 3 oz sugar-free chocolate chips

Instructions
1. Preheat the oven to 350°F.
2. In a food processor, combine the first 6 dough ingredients and pulse until a uniform dough forms. Stir in the chocolate chips.
3. Divide the dough into 16 balls and place them on a parchment-lined baking sheet. Press down on each ball with your fingers to flatten them slightly.
4. Bake for 16-18 minutes or until lightly browned around the edges. Allow the cookies to cool completely.
6. Melt the chocolate in the microwave or using a double boiler. If using the microwave, stir the chocolate every thirty seconds until fully melted. Dip each cookie halfway into the melted chocolate, allowing any excess to drip off. Place the dipped cookies on waxed paper to harden.

CRANBERRY COOKIES

Nutrition: Cal 110; Fat 9 g; Carb 4 g; Protein 2 g
Serving 16; Cook time 35 min

Ingredients
- 4 oz cold salted butter, cut into pieces
- 1 cup almond flour
- ⅓ cup coconut flour
- ⅓ cup Joy Filled Eats Sweetener

- 2 teaspoon gelatin
- 1 teaspoon vanilla
- ½ cup sugar-free dried cranberries divided

LEMON GLAZE:

- 3 tablespoon powdered erythritol such as Swerve
- 1 teaspoon lemon extract
- 1 teaspoon water
- 1 tablespoon sugar-free dried cranberries chopped

Instructions

1. Preheat the oven to 350°F. Line a baking sheet with parchment paper.
2. Add the butter, flours, sweetener, gelatin, vanilla, and 2 tablespoons of the dried cranberries to the food processor. Pulse until the cranberries are chopped and the dough comes together in a ball. Add the remaining cranberries and pulse just until they are mixed in.
3. Divide the dough into 2 balls. Press each ball into a circle on the parchment-lined baking sheet. Cut each circle into 8 wedges using a pizza slicer or knife.
4. Bake for 15 minutes. Cool for 10 minutes, then separate the wedges so that there is an inch or so of space between each wedge. Bake for an additional 10 minutes, or until golden. Allow the cookies to cool completely.
5. Stir together the powdered sweetener, lemon extract, and water until smooth to make the glaze. Drizzle the glaze over the cooled cookies. Optionally, sprinkle chopped cranberries on top for garnish.

KETO MAGIC COOKIES

Nutrition: Cal 150; Fat 14 g; Carb 6g; Protein 3 g
Serving 12; Cook time 25 min

Ingredients

- 2 tablespoon coconut cream
- 2 tablespoon butter softened, not melted
- ¼ cup Joy Filled Eats Sweetener
- 2 egg yolks
- ½ cup sugar-free chocolate chips
- ½ cup walnuts (or other nuts of your choice)
- ½ cup unsweetened flaked coconut
- 1 teaspoon coconut flour optional

Instructions

1. Preheat oven to 350.
2. Stir together the butter and coconut cream until smooth. Add the sweetener and egg yolks. Mix

well. Add the rest of the ingredients. Scoop onto a parchment lined baking sheet to form 12 cookies. Press down to flatten the tops.
3. Bake for 20 minutes or until golden.

SUGAR FREE LEMON BARS

Nutrition: Cal 69; Fat 4 g; Carb 7 g; Protein 4 g
Serving 24; Cook time 25 min

Ingredients

- 4 oz cold salted butter (1 stick) cut into pieces
- 1 cup almond flour
- ⅓ cup coconut flour
- ⅓ cup Joy Filled Eats Sweetener
- 2 teaspoon gelatin
- 1 teaspoon lemon extract or zest

ICING INGREDIENTS:

- 1 cup powdered erythritol
- 1-2 tablespoon lemon juice
- lemon zest optional

Instructions

1. Preheat the oven to 350°F.
2. Combine all the dough ingredients in a food processor and pulse until a uniform dough forms. Divide the dough into 24 balls and place them on a parchment-lined baking sheet. Press down on each ball with your fingers. Sprinkle a little more sweetener on top.
3. Bake for 12-15 minutes or until lightly browned around the edges. Allow the cookies to cool for at least 10 minutes.
4. In a small bowl, combine the powdered sweetener and 1 tablespoon of lemon juice. Stir until smooth. If needed, add additional lemon juice to achieve the desired consistency. Spread the glaze on the cooled cookies.
5. Garnish the cookies with lemon zest.

LOW CARB OATMEAL COOKIES

Nutrition: Cal 117; Fat 10 g; Carb 7 g; Protein 2 g
Serving 24; Cook time 22 min

Ingredients

- 4 oz butter softened
- ½ cup Joy Filled Eats Sweetener
- 1 teaspoon molasses
- 1 egg
- 1 teaspoon vanilla
- 1 cup almond flour

- 1 teaspoon baking soda
- 1 cup gluten-free oats
- 1 cup sugar-free butterscotch chips
- ½ cup unsweetened coconut flakes
- ½ teaspoon cinnamon

Instructions

1. Preheat the oven to 350°F.
2. In a large bowl, cream together the butter and sweetener until well combined. Add in the molasses, eggs, and vanilla, and mix well.
3. Stir in the almond flour, baking soda, and cinnamon until the dry ingredients are fully incorporated.
4. Fold in the oats, butterscotch chips, and coconut, ensuring they are evenly distributed throughout the dough.
5. Form 24 cookies and place them on 2 parchment-lined cookie sheets. Bake for 12 minutes until they are soft but golden around the edges. Allow the cookies to cool completely on the trays before transferring them to a storage container.

KETO VANILLA COOKIES

Nutrition: Cal 89; Fat 8 g; Carb 2 g; Protein 1 g
Serving 20; Cook time 30 min

Ingredients

- 1 stick cold salted butter cut into pieces
- 1 cup almond flour
- ⅓ cup coconut flour
- ⅓ cup Joy Filled Eats Sweetener
- 2 teaspoon gelatin
- 2 teaspoon vanilla

ICING INGREDIENTS:

- ½ cup xylitol ground into a powder (or ⅔ cup of another powdered sweetener)
- 1 teaspoon vanilla
- 1 tablespoon almond milk
- 1 tablespoon butter melted

Instructions

1. Preheat the oven to 350°F.
2. Combine all the dough ingredients in the food processor and pulse until well combined.
3. To make round cookies: Divide the dough into 20 balls and place them on a parchment-lined baking sheet. Press them down gently with your fingers.
4. To make cut-out cookies: Roll out the dough between two sheets of parchment paper on top of a cookie sheet. Remove the top sheet and make shapes in the dough, keeping them 1-2 inches apart. Remove the dough in between the shapes. Repeat with the remaining dough.
5. Bake for 14-18 minutes or until lightly browned around the edges. Allow the cookies to cool completely.
6. Stir together the ingredients for the icing. Spread the icing on the cooled cookies. Place them on waxed paper and refrigerate to harden the icing so that they can be stacked.

KETO MOLASSES COOKIES

Nutrition: Cal 167; Fat 14 g; Carb 9 g; Protein 4 g
Serving 25; Cook time 22 min

Ingredients

- 4 oz cold salted butter, cut into pieces
- 1 cup almond flour
- ⅓ cup coconut flour
- ⅓ cup Joy Filled Eats Sweetener
- 2 teaspoon gelatin
- 1 teaspoon vanilla
- 2 teaspoon molasses
- 1 tsp fresh ginger finely grated

Instructions

1. Preheat the oven to 350°F.
2. Combine the dough ingredients in the food processor and process until the dough comes together in a ball. This should take about a minute.
3. Divide the dough into 25 balls and place them on a parchment-lined baking sheet. Press them down gently with your fingers, flipping them over so the flat side is up.
4. Bake for 10-12 minutes or until lightly browned around the edges. Allow the cookies to cool completely.

KETO BROWNIE COOKIES

Nutrition: Cal 218; Fat 20 g; Carb 9 g; Protein 7 g
Serving 8; Cook time 22 min

Ingredients

- 1 cup raw sunflower seed kernels
- ½ cup xylitol (or ¼ cup of my sweetener)
- 4 tablespoon butter, softened
- 2 eggs
- ½ cup cocoa powder
- ½ cup sugar-free chocolate chips

Instructions

1. Preheat the oven to 350°F.
2. Finely chop the sunflower seed kernels in a food processor. Add the xylitol, butter, eggs, and cocoa powder. Pulse until a dough forms. Stir in the chocolate chips.
3. Drop 8 scoops of dough onto a parchment-lined baking sheet. Bake for 12 minutes or until firm to the touch in the center. Allow the cookies to cool for 10 minutes.

KETO COOKIE DOUGH ICE CREAM SANDWICHES

Nutrition: Cal 257; Fat 29 g; Carb 8 g; Protein 5 g
Serving 16; Cook time 30 min

Ingredients

- 4 tablespoon butter
- 4 tablespoon cream cheese
- 2 cups almond flour
- ½ cup Joy Filled Eats Sweetener
- 1 teaspoon molasses
- 1 teaspoon vanilla
- 1 cup sugar free chocolate chips or chopped sugar free or dark chocolate

ICE CREAM INGREDIENTS:

- 2 cups heavy cream
- 1 cup half and half
- 1 cup almond milk
- 1 egg yolks
- ½ cup Joy Filled Eats Sweetener
- 1 tablespoon vanilla
- 1 tablespoon glycerin
- 1 cup sugar free chocolate chips optional

Instructions

1. Line an 8x8 square baking pan with parchment paper or foil.
2. In a large bowl, beat the butter, cream cheese, and sweetener using an electric mixer. Add almond flour, vanilla, molasses, and chocolate chips. Mix well. Spread half of the cookie dough in the bottom of the pan and smooth it gently. Cover with another layer of parchment paper or foil. Spread the remaining dough onto the second layer. Place the pan in the freezer.
3. Meanwhile, prepare the ice cream. Combine all the ice cream ingredients in a blender and blend until smooth. Pour the mixture into an ice cream machine and churn according to the manufacturer's instructions. If desired, add additional chocolate chips during the last minute of churning. Once the ice cream has firmed up, remove the cookie dough from the freezer and remove the top layer. Pour ¾ of the ice cream onto the bottom layer of cookie dough. Save the remaining ice cream in a separate container.
4. It's best not to top it with the top cookie dough layer just yet. Allow it to firm up a little more. Place both the top layer of dough and the ice cream in the freezer separately. After an hour or two, remove them from the freezer and top the ice cream with the top layer of cookie dough.
5. Freeze for an additional 3-4 hours. If you have any extra ice cream left, you can enjoy it while you wait for the ice cream cake to freeze.
6. Remove from the freezer and cut into squares using a sharp knife. Individually wrap each square with plastic wrap for storage.

KETO COOKIE DOUGH BROWNIE FAT BOMBS

Nutrition: Cal 240; Fat 20 g; Carb 8 g; Protein 13 g
Serving 18; Cook time 40 min

Ingredients

- 1 cups almond flour
- ¼ cup Joy Filled Eats Sweetener
- 4 tablespoon butter softened
- 1 oz cream cheese softened
- 1 teaspoon vanilla
- ½ teaspoon molasses optional
- ¼ cup sugar-free chocolate chips

BROWNIE DOUGH:

- ¾ cup almond flour
- ¼ cup Joy Filled Eats Sweetener
- ¼ cup cocoa powder
- 4 tablespoon butter softened
- 1 oz cream cheese softened
- 1 teaspoon vanilla

COATING:

- 1 cups sugar-free chocolate chips
- 2 teaspoon refined coconut oil

Instructions

1. In a medium bowl, combine all the ingredients for the cookie dough and mix until smooth.

2. In another medium bowl, combine all the ingredients for the brownie dough and mix until smooth.
3. Scoop small balls of each dough onto a waxed paper-lined cookie sheet. You will get between 15-20 balls from each dough.
4. Take one ball of each dough and press them together. Roll the mixture between your hands to form a ball. Repeat with the remaining dough.
5. Melt the chocolate chips and coconut oil in the microwave, stirring every 30 seconds. Once it is 75% melted, stir until the chips are completely melted.
4. Cover each cookie/brownie dough ball with the melted chocolate. Place them back on the lined cookie sheet. Refrigerate to set the chocolate. Store in the fridge.

KETO PUMPKIN COOKIES

Nutrition: Cal 196; Fat 14 g; Carb 6 g; Protein 3 g
Serving 12; Cook time 35 min

Ingredients

- 4 oz butter
- ½ cup Joy Filled Eats Sweetener
- 1 cup almond flour
- ½ cup coconut flour
- 1 egg
- 1 cup pumpkin
- 1 teaspoon vanilla
- 1 teaspoon baking powder
- 1 teaspoon baking soda
- ½ teaspoon pumpkin spice

CREAM CHEESE FILLING:

- 4 oz cream cheese
- 1.5 tablespoon salted butter
- ½ cup powdered erythritol

Instructions

1. Preheat oven to 350. Line two cookie sheets with parchment paper.
2. Cream together the butter and sweetener in a stand mixer until light and fluffy. Add the remaining cookie ingredients. Mix well, scraping the sides as needed.
3. Scoop 24 cookies onto the prepared baking sheets. Press and smooth into a circle about ¾ inch thick.
4. Bake for 20-25 minutes. Cool completely.

CREAM CHEESE FILLING:

1. Whip the cream cheese and butter in a stand mixer until light and fluffy, scraping down the sides as needed.
2. Add the powdered erythritol. Mix for 2-3 minutes until fluffy. Scrape down the sides and mix for another minute.
3. Spread or pipe the filling between a pair of cookies. Repeat.

RASPBERRY CHEESECAKE COOKIES

Nutrition: Cal 190; Fat 18 g; Carb 5.6 g; Protein 4 g
Serving 12; Cook time 30 min

Ingredients
SHORTBREAD COOKIE

- 4 oz cold salted butter cut into pieces (1 stick)
- 1 cup almond flour
- ⅓ cup coconut flour
- ⅓ cup Joy Filled Eats Sweetener
- 2 teaspoon gelatin
- 1 teaspoon vanilla

RASPBERRY CHEESECAKE FILLING

- 4 oz cream cheese
- ¼ cup sugar free raspberry jam
- 2 tablespoon Joy Filled Eats Sweetener

TOPPING

- ¼ cup sugar free white chocolate chips
- 1 teaspoon coconut oil

Instructions

1. Preheat oven to 350.
2. Combine the butter, almond flour, coconut flour, sweetener, gelatin, and vanilla in the food processor and pulse until it comes together in a ball of dough. Divide into 12 balls. Put on a parchment-lined lined baking sheet and press down making a little well with your thumbs.
3. Combine the filling ingredients and divide between the wells.
4. Bake for 16-18 minutes or until lightly browned around the edges. Cool completely.
5. Optional: Melt the white chocolate chips and coconut oil in a small bowl in the microwave stirring every 30 seconds. Drizzle the cookies with melted white chocolate.
6. Store in the fridge in an airtight container for up to 1 week or freezer for up to 3 months.

KETO FUNFETTI COOKIE BITES

Nutrition: Cal 225; Fat 22 g; Carb 5 g; Protein 5 g
Serving 8; Cook time 20 min

Ingredients

- cups almond flour
- 4 oz butter
- ¼ cup Joy Filled Eats Sweetener
- 2 teaspoon gelatin
- ½ teaspoon vanilla
- ½ teaspoon almond extract
- ½ teaspoon butter extract
- 3 tablespoon sugar-free sprinkles

Instructions

1. Preheat the oven to 350°F (175°C).
2. Combine all the dough ingredients (except the sprinkles) in the food processor and process until a ball of dough forms. This should take about 2-3 minutes at high speed. Add the sprinkles and pulse just until they are evenly distributed throughout the dough.
3. Press the dough into an 8x10-inch rectangle, about 1/2 inch thick, on a parchment-lined baking sheet. Cut the dough into 1/2-inch squares and separate them.
4. Bake for 8-10 minutes or until the edges are lightly browned. Allow the cookies to cool completely.

KETO COOKIE DOUGH BROWNIES

Nutrition: Cal 260; Fat 26 g; Carb 7 g; Protein 5 g
Serving 16; Cook time 50 min

Ingredients

- 4 oz dark 85% or unsweetened chocolate
- ¾ cup of butter 1.5 sticks
- ¾ cup Joy Filled Eats Sweetener
- 3 eggs
- 1 teaspoon vanilla
- ½ cup Trim Healthy Mama Baking Blend OR 2 tablespoon each coconut flour, almond flour, & golden flax meal
- ½ cup sugar-free chocolate chips

COOKIE DOUGH INGREDIENTS:

- 1 cup almond flour
- 4 tablespoon butter softened
- 1 oz cream cheese softened
- ¼ cup Joy Filled Eats Sweetener
- 1 teaspoon molasses
- 1 teaspoon vanilla
- 1 teaspoon coconut flour
- ½ cup sugar-free chocolate chips

Instructions

1. Preheat the oven to 350°F (175°C). Spray an 8x8 baking dish liberally with cooking spray.
2. In a glass bowl, melt the chocolate and butter in the microwave. Add the next four ingredients and stir until smooth. Stir in the chocolate chips.
3. Pour the mixture into the prepared baking pan and spread it evenly. Bake for 30-35 minutes or until the center is no longer jiggly. Allow it to cool completely.
4. To make the cookie dough, stir together all the ingredients (except the chocolate chips) until smooth. Stir in the chocolate chips. Spread the cookie dough on top of the cooled brownies.

PIGNOLI COOKIES

Nutrition: Cal 107; Fat 10 g; Carb 2 g; Protein 3 g
Serving 26; Cook time 35 min

Ingredients

- 2 cups slivered almonds
- ½ cup Joy Filled Eats Sweetener
- ¼ cup egg whites
- 8 oz pine nuts
- powdered erythritol optional

Instructions

1. Preheat the oven to 350°F (175°C).
2. Process the almonds and sweetener in a food processor for 5 minutes, scraping down the sides occasionally. Add the egg whites and process until the mixture comes together and reaches a peanut butter-like consistency.
3. Place the pine nuts in a shallow bowl. Drop tablespoons of the dough into the pine nuts. Roll the dough balls around, covering them with nuts. Place them on a parchment-lined baking sheet.
4. Bake for 20-25 minutes or until slightly golden. Allow them to cool completely, and if desired, dust with powdered sweetener.

PEANUT BUTTER CUP COOKIES

Nutrition: Cal 109; Fat 10 g; Carb 4 g; Protein 4 g
Serving 30; Cook time 30 min

Ingredients

- 2 large eggs
- ½ cup coconut oil
- ½ cup peanut butter
- 1 teaspoon vanilla
- ⅓ cup peanut flour
- ¾ cup Joy Filled Eats Sweetener
- 1 teaspoon salt
- ½ cup almond flour
- ¼ cup coconut flour
- 1 teaspoon aluminum-free baking powder

TOPPING INGREDIENTS:

- 3 oz sugar free chocolate chips or chopped chocolate
- 2 oz heavy cream
- ¼ cup peanuts (roasted salted)

Instructions

1. Preheat the oven to 350°F (175°C).
2. In a mixing bowl, whisk together the eggs, melted coconut oil, peanut butter, and vanilla extract.
3. Add the peanut butter powder, sweetener, salt, almond flour, coconut flour, and baking powder to the bowl. Mix until well combined.
4. Divide the batter evenly among 30 mini muffin cups lined with aluminum liners.
5. Bake for 14-16 minutes or until the edges turn golden. While the cookies are still warm and in the pan, use a tart tamper or the rounded back of a teaspoon to create a well in the center of each cookie. Allow them to cool completely.
6. To make the ganache, heat the cream until it is just below boiling point. Pour the hot cream over the chocolate and stir until the mixture is smooth.
7. Fill the cooled cookies with the prepared ganache. Top each cookie with a few peanuts.

CHOCOLATE THUMBPRINT COOKIES

Nutrition: Cal 73; Fat 6 g; Carb 3 g; Protein 2 g
Serving 24; Cook time 30 min

Ingredients

- 4 oz cold salted butter cut into pieces
- 1 cup almond flour
- ⅓ cup coconut flour
- ⅓ cup Joy Filled Eats Sweetener
- 2 teaspoon gelatin
- 1 teaspoon vanilla

NUT TOPPING:

- ⅔ cup sliced almonds
- 2 teaspoon Joy Filled Eats Sweetener

CHOCOLATE GANACHE:

- ⅓ cup sugar free chocolate chips
- 3 tablespoon heavy cream

Instructions

1. Preheat the oven to 350°F (175°C).
2. In a food processor, combine the 2/3 cup sliced almonds and 2 teaspoons sweetener. Pulse until the almonds are chopped. Transfer to a small bowl and set aside.
3. In the same food processor, combine all the dough ingredients. Pulse until a uniform dough forms. Divide the dough into 24 balls and roll each ball in the almond topping. Place them on a parchment-lined baking sheet and press them down with your thumbs, creating a small well in the center. Sprinkle a little more almond topping on each cookie.
4. Bake for 12-15 minutes or until lightly browned around the edges. Allow them to cool for at least 10 minutes.
5. Meanwhile, put the chocolate chips and heavy cream in a microwave-safe bowl. Heat for 30 seconds, then stir. Heat for another 30 seconds, then stir again. Repeat this process until the chocolate has melted. Stir until smooth.
6. Divide the chocolate ganache between the thumbprint cookies, filling each well. Sprinkle a little more of the chopped almonds on top of each cookie.

EGGLESS CHOCOLATE CHIP COOKIES

Nutrition: Cal 180; Fat 18 g; Carb 5 g; Protein 4 g
Serving 18; Cook time 25 min

Ingredients

- 4 oz cold salted butter, cut into pieces (1 stick)
- 1 cup almond flour
- ⅓ cup coconut flour
- ⅓ cup Joy Filled Eats Sweetener
- 2 teaspoon gelatin
- 1 teaspoon vanilla
- 1 tsp molasses
- ¾ cup sugar-free chocolate chips

Instructions

1. Preheat the oven to 350°F (175°C). Line a baking sheet with parchment paper.
2. In a food processor, combine the dough ingredients (excluding the chocolate chips). Process until the dough comes together in a ball, which should take about a minute.
3. Transfer the dough to a mixing bowl and stir in the chocolate chips.
4. Divide the dough into 18 balls and place them on the parchment-lined baking sheet. Press down on each ball with your fingers to flatten them slightly.
5. Bake for 15 minutes or until the cookies are firm to the touch and golden around the edges.

RASPBERRY AND CHOCOLATE COOKIES

Nutrition: Cal 140; Fat 13 g; Carb 5 g; Protein 3 g
Serving 15; Cook time 30 min

Ingredients

- 4 oz cold salted butter cut into pieces
- 1 cup almond flour
- ⅓ cup coconut flour
- ⅓ cup Joy Filled Eats Sweetener
- 2 teaspoon gelatin
- 1 teaspoon vanilla
- ½ cup sugar-free white chocolate chips
- ½ cup freeze-dried raspberries chopped

Instructions

1. Preheat the oven to 350 degrees Fahrenheit (175 degrees Celsius).
2. In a food processor, combine the first 6 dough ingredients (as specified in your recipe) and pulse until a uniform dough forms. Then, stir in the white chocolate chips and dried raspberries until they are evenly distributed.
3. Divide the dough into 15 equal-sized balls and place them on a parchment-lined baking sheet. Use your fingers to gently press down on each ball to flatten them slightly.
4. Bake the cookies in the preheated oven for 14 to 16 minutes, or until they are lightly browned around the edges. Allow the cookies to cool completely before serving.

KETO NO-BAKE COOKIES

Nutrition: Cal 170; Fat 18 g; Carb 5 g; Protein 4 g
Serving 12; Cook time 25 min

Ingredients

- 2 tbsp butter
- 2/3 cup natural chunky peanut butter (or any nut butter)
- 1 cup unsweetened shredded coconut
- 1 tbsp cocoa powder
- 4 drops liquid vanilla stevia (or liquid sweetener of choice)

Instructions

1. In a microwave-safe bowl, place the butter and melt it in the microwave.
2. Stir in the peanut butter and cocoa powder until the mixture is smooth and well combined.
3. Add the shredded coconut and stevia to the bowl, and mix everything together until fully incorporated.
4. Use a tablespoon to scoop spoonfuls of the mixture onto a small sheet pan or any dish that will fit in your freezer, such as a cutting board or plate. Make sure to line the pan or dish with parchment paper to prevent sticking.
5. Place the pan or dish in the freezer and let the cookies freeze for about 15 minutes, or until they become firm.
6. Once the cookies are frozen, you can cut and separate the parchment paper, ensuring that each cookie still has a piece of paper underneath to prevent them from sticking together. Store the cookies in a sealed container or bag in your refrigerator.

KETO COOKIE DOUGH FAT BOMBS

Nutrition: Cal 332; Fat 30 g; Carb 7 g; Protein 4 g
Serving 20; Cook time 20 min

Ingredients

- 1 (8oz) package cream cheese (softened)
- 6 tbsp peanut butter (no sugar added)
- 3 tbsp butter (softened)
- 1 tsp vanilla
- 1/3 cup swerve
- 1/3 cup sugar-free chocolate chips

Instructions

1. In a mixing bowl, combine all the ingredients except for the chocolate chips. Use a mixer to cream everything together until well combined.
2. Gently fold in the chocolate chips into the dough until they are evenly distributed.
3. Use a small cookie scoop or spoon to portion out the dough onto a parchment paper-lined cookie sheet or a container that can fit into your freezer. Alternatively, you can use silicone molds for shaping the cookies.
4. Place the cookie sheet or container in the freezer and let the cookies freeze for about 1 hour or until they are firm.
5. Once frozen, transfer the cookies to ziplock bags or airtight containers and store them in your freezer for future enjoyment.

NO BAKE PEANUT BUTTER COOKIES

Nutrition: Cal 159; Fat 15 g; Carb 5 g; Protein 5 g
Serving 12; Cook time 20 min

Ingredients

- 1 Cup Flaked Almonds (or chopped nuts of choice)
- 1/2 Cup Shredded Coconut
- 1/2 Cup Peanut Butter
- 1/2 Cup Stevia
- 50g/1.76 ounces Unsalted Butter or 1/4 Cup Coconut Oil For Dairy Free

Instructions

1. Line a baking tray with well-greased baking paper to prevent the cookies from sticking.
2. In a bowl, combine the almonds and coconut, mixing them together.
3. In a small saucepan over medium heat, place the peanut butter, stevia, and butter or coconut oil.
4. Heat the mixture until the butter has melted and you have a smooth, creamy, buttery sauce.
5. Pour the peanut butter mixture over the almond mixture and stir until well combined, ensuring that all the dry ingredients are coated.
6. Using a tablespoon, drop spoonfuls of the mixture onto the prepared baking tray, spacing them apart to allow for spreading.
7. Place the tray in the fridge for a few hours to allow the cookies to set and harden. This will help them become crispy.
8. Once the cookies have hardened, remove them from the fridge and enjoy them crisp and chilled.

KETO CRACKERS

Nutrition: Cal 121; Fat 10 g; Carb 3 g; Protein 6 g
Serving 8; Cook time 25 min

Ingredients

- 1 cup almond flour
- 1 cup shredded cheese cheddar cheese
- 1/4 teaspoon salt
- 1-2 tablespoon water

Instructions

1. Preheat the oven to 180°C/350°F. Line a large baking sheet with parchment paper to prevent the crackers from sticking.
2. In a high-speed blender or food processor, add almond flour, shredded cheese, and salt. Blend the ingredients well until a dough-like consistency forms. If the dough is too crumbly, you can add a tablespoon or two of water to help bind it together.
3. Place a large sheet of parchment paper on a flat kitchen surface. Transfer the dough onto the parchment paper and place another sheet of parchment paper on top. Press down on the dough to flatten it and then use a rolling pin to roll it out to a thickness of about 1/4 inch. You can adjust the thickness to your preference.
4. Using a pizza cutter or a sharp knife, slice the rolled-out dough into squares or rectangles to form crackers. Transfer the crackers onto the lined baking sheet, spacing them apart to allow for even baking.
5. Bake the crackers in the preheated oven for approximately 12 minutes, flipping them halfway through the baking time to ensure

even browning. Keep an eye on them to prevent over-browning or burning.

6. Once the crackers are golden and crispy, remove them from the oven and allow them to cool completely on a wire rack or the baking sheet. Cooling will help the crackers become even more crisp.

7. Once cooled, you can store the crackers in an airtight container at room temperature for a few days. Enjoy them as a tasty and crunchy snack on their own or pair them with your favorite dips or spreads.

CRANBERRY ALMOND BISCOTTI COOKIES

Nutrition: Cal 112; Fat 9 g; Carb 6 g; Protein 5 g
Serving 14; Cook time 45 min

Ingredients

- 2 eggs
- 1 teaspoon vanilla
- ⅓ cup low carb sugar substitute
- ¼ teaspoon lemon stevia drops or plain stevia and a half teaspoon lemon extract
- 1 ½ cups almond flour
- ¼ cup coconut flour
- ½ teaspoon baking soda
- ¼ teaspoon sea salt
- ½ cup sugar free dried cranberries
- ½ cup sliced almonds
- low carb dark chocolate melted, optional

Instructions

1. In a mixing bowl, beat together the eggs, vanilla extract, Swerve, and stevia using an electric mixer until the mixture becomes frothy.

2. In a separate bowl, combine the almond flour, coconut flour, baking soda, and salt.

3. Add the flour mixture to the wet mixture and stir until a dough forms.

4. Stir in the cranberries and almonds.

5. Line a cookie sheet with parchment paper and shape the dough into a long rectangle on the prepared sheet.

6. Bake in a preheated oven at 350°F (175°C) for approximately 20 minutes or until the top has browned.

7. Remove from the oven and allow the cookie rectangle to cool completely.

8. Slice the cooled cookie rectangle into thin pieces on a slight diagonal. Lay each slice on its side in a baking pan.

9. Bake the slices for about 15-20 minutes at 350°F (175°C) until toasted.

10. Allow the slices to cool, and if desired, drizzle melted chocolate over them as a finishing touch.

KETO SNOWBALL COOKIES

Nutrition: Cal 108; Fat 11 g; Carb 2 g; Protein 2 g
Serving 24; Cook time 27 min

Ingredients

- 2 cups Almond flour
- ½ cup Butter unsalted and softened
- ⅓ cup Swerve confectioner sugar substitute
- 1 teaspoon Vanilla extract
- ⅔ cup Chopped pecans
- pinch of salt
- ½ cup Swerve confectioners sugar substitute for coating the cookies once baked

Instructions

1. In a mixing bowl, add the butter and 1/3 cup of sugar substitute. Beat the mixture until it becomes creamy and smooth.

2. Add the almond flour, salt, and vanilla extract to the bowl. Mix everything together until well combined.

3. Fold in the pecans into the dough, ensuring they are evenly distributed.

4. Take the dough and shape it into 24 evenly sized balls. Place the balls on a tray or baking sheet and transfer them to the freezer. Allow them to freeze for approximately 30 minutes.

5. Preheat your oven to 350 degrees Fahrenheit (175 degrees Celsius).

6. Once the dough balls are frozen, remove them from the freezer and place them on a lined baking sheet. Bake the cookies in the preheated oven for 10-12 minutes, or until the bottoms are lightly browned.

7. After removing the cookies from the oven, let them cool for several minutes.

8. While the cookies are still warm, roll them in the remaining sugar substitute to coat them.

SOUR CREAM CAKE

Nutrition: Cal 310; Fat 27 g; Carb 10 g; Protein 10 g
Serving 12; Cook time 70 min

Ingredients
CAKE

- 2 cups almond flour
- 1/3 cup coconut flour
- 1/3 cup unflavored whey protein powder
- 1 tbsp baking powder
- 1/4 tsp salt
- 1/2 cup butter, softened
- 1/2 cup full fat sour cream
- 3/4 cup Swerve Sweetener
- 4 large eggs, room temperature
- 1 tsp vanilla extract

PECAN STREUSEL

- 1/2 cup almond flour
- 3 tbsp Swerve Sweetener
- 1 1/2 tsp ground cinnamon
- 2 tbsp butter, melted
- 1/2 cup chopped pecans

Instructions
STREUSEL:

1. In a small bowl, whisk together almond flour, Swerve Sweetener, and cinnamon. Add the melted butter and mix until the texture resembles coarse crumbs. Fold in pecans.

CAKE:

2. Preheat the oven to 325°F (163°C) and thoroughly grease a 9x5-inch loaf pan.
3. In a medium bowl, whisk together almond flour, coconut flour, whey protein, baking powder, and salt.
4. In a large bowl, cream the butter and sour cream until smooth. Gradually add Swerve Sweetener, mixing until well combined. Add the eggs one at a time, followed by the vanilla extract, mixing thoroughly after each addition.
5. Gently fold in the almond flour mixture until the dough is well combined.
6. Spread half of the batter into the prepared loaf pan and sprinkle with half of the streusel mixture. Spread the remaining batter on top, and finish with the remaining streusel.
7. Cover the cake with aluminum foil, and bake for 50 minutes. Remove the foil and continue baking for an additional 15 to 20 minutes, or until the cake is golden brown and a toothpick inserted into the edges comes out clean.
8. Remove the cake from the oven and allow it to cool completely before serving.

CRANBERRY ORANGE CAKE

Nutrition: Cal 227; Fat 18 g; Carb 9 g; Protein 8 g
Serving 16; Cook time 70 min

Ingredients
CAKE:

- 3 cups cranberries
- Sweetener equivalent to 1/3 cup sugar
- 1/4 cup water
- 2 1/2 cups almond flour
- 1/2 cup coconut flour
- 1/4 cup unflavored whey protein powder
- 1 tbsp baking powder
- 1/4 tsp salt
- 1/2 cup butter, softened
- Sweetener equivalent to 3/4 cup sugar
- 4 large eggs, room temperature
- 1 tbsp orange zest
- 1/2 tsp orange extract
- 2/3 cup almond milk, room temperature
- 1/2 cup chopped pecans (optional)

OPTIONAL GLAZE:

- 3 tbsp powdered sweetener (erythritol or xylitol)
- 1 tbsp water

Instructions

1. In a large saucepan, combine cranberries, sweetener, and water. Bring to a boil, then reduce heat and simmer until cranberries have burst. Mash with a fork or wooden spoon.
2. Preheat the oven to 325°F (163°C) and grease a 9-inch springform pan (using other pans is possible, but it may be more challenging to remove the cake neatly, and baking time may vary).
3. In a large bowl, whisk together almond flour, coconut flour, whey protein powder, baking powder, and salt.
4. In another large bowl, cream the butter and sweetener until smooth and well combined. Mix in eggs, orange zest, and orange extract. Add half of the almond flour mixture, followed by the almond milk, mixing well after each addition. Stir

in the remaining almond flour mixture until well combined.

5.Spread about two-thirds of the batter in the prepared baking pan. Layer the cranberry sauce evenly over the batter. Mix pecans into the remaining batter and spread it over the cranberry sauce.

6.Bake for 40 to 50 minutes, or until the top is golden brown and firm to the touch, and a toothpick inserted in the center comes out clean with no raw batter attached. Remove the cake from the oven and let it cool for at least 30 minutes. Carefully run a sharp knife around the inside edges of the pan and remove the sides.

OPTIONAL GLAZE:

7.Stir together powdered sweetener and water and drizzle over cooled cake.

BLACKBERRY CAKE RECIPE

Nutrition: Cal 204; Fat 18 g; Carb 7 g; Protein 5 g
Serving 16; Cook time 70 min

Ingredients
CAKE

- 1 ¼ cups almond flour
- ¼ cup coconut flour
- 1 teaspoon baking powder
- ½ cup Joy Filled Eats Sweetener
- ⅓ cup melted coconut oil
- ½ cup canned coconut milk
- 1 teaspoon vanilla
- 4 eggs

TOPPING

- 2 cups blackberries
- 1 cup almonds
- 2 tablespoon Joy Filled Eats Sweetener
- 2 tablespoon coconut oil

Instructions
1.Preheat oven to 350.
2.Stir together the dry cake ingredients in a medium bowl. Add all the other cake ingredients and mix well with a wooden spoon. Spread in a greased 8 x 8-inch baking dish. Sprinkle the blackberries on top of the cake batter.
3.Bake for 15 minutes.
4.Meanwhile, combine the ingredients for the topping in a food processor. Process until the

nuts are chopped and wet crumbs form. Sprinkle evenly over the partially baked cake.

5.Bake for an additional 40-55 minutes until the cake is firm to the touch, golden, and doesn't jiggle when lightly shaken. The center should feel as firm as the edge when lightly pressed with your fingertip.

CINNAMON CARROT CAKE

Nutrition: Cal 282; Fat 27 g; Carb 6 g; Protein 6 g
Serving 8; Cook time 10 min

Ingredients

- 1 large carrot
- 1/4 cup Low Carb Sugar Substitute
- 1/2 tsp liquid stevia
- 1/2 cup butter, melted
- 2 large eggs, room temperature
- 2/3 cup almond flour
- 2 tbsp coconut flour
- 1 tsp cinnamon
- 1 tsp baking soda
- pinch of salt

TOPPING

- 4 tbsp butter, room temperature
- 1/2 cup almond flour
- 1 tbsp coconut flour
- 3 tbsp Low Carb Sugar Substitute
- 1/4 tsp liquid stevia
- 1 tsp cinnamon
- pinch of salt

Instructions

1.Preheat the oven to 350°F and prepare an 8-inch round cake pan by greasing it with coconut oil spray or lining it with parchment paper.
2.Grate the carrot and set it aside.
3.In a large bowl, combine erythritol, stevia, melted butter, and eggs using a whisk.
4.Add the shredded carrot, almond flour, coconut flour, cinnamon, baking soda, and salt to the bowl. Mix until well combined.
5.Spoon the batter into the prepared round cake pan and set it aside while you prepare the topping.
6.To make the topping, combine all the ingredients in a mixing bowl using a spoon or your hands.
7.Sprinkle the topping over the batter and bake for 30-35 minutes.

8.Use a toothpick to test for doneness. Allow the cake to cool for 15-20 minutes before transferring and slicing.

9.For optimal freshness, store the cake in an airtight container in the refrigerator for up to 10 days.

ALMOND CAKE

Nutrition: Cal 231; Fat 22 g; Carb 5 g; Protein 6 g
Serving 1; Cook time 60 min

Ingredients

- 2 cups almond flour
- 1 cup granular sweetener (monk fruit is what I use)
- 1/2 cup plus 2 tablespoons olive oil
- 4 eggs
- 2 teaspoons baking powder
- 2 teaspoons cinnamon
- 1 teaspoon almond extract
- coconut oil for greasing

Instructions

1.Preheat the oven to 350 degrees Fahrenheit and lightly grease an 8x8 baking dish.

In a small bowl, combine almond flour, sweetener, and olive oil. Mix together until the mixture becomes crumbly.

2.Set aside just under 1 cup of the crumble mixture. **3.**Please note that you should lightly measure the mixture without packing it tightly.

4.In a large bowl, add the remaining crumble mixture, eggs, baking powder, cinnamon, and almond extract. Mix well using hand beaters.

5.Pour the mixture into the prepared baking dish.

6.Sprinkle the reserved crumble mixture evenly over the top of the batter.

7.Bake for approximately 50 minutes or until the center is fully cooked.

SKILLET CHOCOLATE CHIP COFFEE CAKE

Nutrition: Cal 275; Fat 25 g; Carb 8 g; Protein 9 g
Serving 10; Cook time 65 min

Ingredients

CRUMB TOPPING:
- ¼ cup almond flour
- 1 tablespoon Swerve Sweetener

- 1 & ½ tsp cinnamon
- 1 tablespoon butter softened

CAKE:
- 2 cups almond flour
- ¼ cup unflavoured whey protein powder
- 2 teaspoon baking powder
- ¼ teaspoon salt
- 6 tablespoon butter softened
- ½ cup Swerve Sweetener
- 2 large eggs room temperature
- 1 teaspoon vanilla extract
- ½ cup almond milk
- ½ cup dark chocolate chips, sugar-free

Instructions

1.In a small bowl, whisk together almond flour, sweetener, and cinnamon. Cut in butter until mixture resembles coarse crumbs. Set aside.

2.For the cake, preheat oven to 325F and grease a 10 inch oven-proof skillet (does not need to be cast iron, but it's great if it is!)

3.In a medium bowl, whisk together the almond flour, whey protein powder, baking powder and salt.

4.In a large bowl, beat butter with sweetener until well combined. Beat in eggs and vanilla, then beat in half the almond flour mixture. Beat in almond milk and remaining almond flour until well combined.

5.Stir in chocolate chips and spread batter in prepared skillet. Bake 25 minutes, then remove from oven and sprinkle with topping. Return to oven and bake another 15 to 20 minutes, until sides are beginning to brown and center is just firm to the touch.

6.Remove and let cool at least 20 minutes before serving (cake will fall apart easily if you remove it while it's still very warm).

CINNAMON ROLL CAKE

Nutrition: Cal 222; Fat 20 g; Carb 5,5 g; Protein 7 g
Serving 16; Cook time 50 min

Ingredients

CINNAMON FILLING:
- 3 tablespoon Swerve Sweetener
- 2 teaspoon ground cinnamon

CAKE:
- 3 cups almond flour
- ¾ cup Swerve Sweetener
- ¼ cup unflavoured whey protein powder
- 2 teaspoon baking powder

- ½ teaspoon salt
- 3 large eggs
- ½ cup butter melted
- ½ teaspoon vanilla extract
- ½ cup almond milk

1 tablespoon melted butter

CREAM CHEESE FROSTING:

- 3 tablespoon cream cheese softened
- 2 tablespoon powdered Swerve Sweetener
- 1 tablespoon heavy whipping cream
- ½ teaspoon vanilla extract

Instructions

1. Preheat oven to 325F and grease an 8x8 inch baking pan.
2. For the filling, combine the Swerve and cinnamon in a small bowl and mix well. Set aside.
3. For the cake, whisk together almond flour, sweetener, protein powder, baking powder, and salt in a medium bowl.
4. Stir in the eggs, melted butter and vanilla extract. Add the almond milk and continue to stir until well combined.
5. Spread half of the batter in the prepared pan, then sprinkle with about two thirds of the cinnamon filling mixture. Spread the remaining batter over top and smooth with a knife or an offset spatula.
6. Bake 35 minutes, or until top is golden brown and a tester inserted in the center comes out with a few crumbs attached.
7. Brush with melted butter and sprinkle with remaining cinnamon filling mixture. Let cool in pan.
8. For the frosting, beat cream cheese, powdered erythritol, cream and vanilla extract together in a small bowl until smooth. Pipe or drizzle over cooled cake.

KETO PUMPKIN CRUNCH CAKE

Nutrition: Cal 215; Fat 19 g; Carb 7 g; Protein 5 g
Serving 18; Cook time 75 min

Ingredients

- 1 ½ cups pumpkin puree
- 3 large eggs room temperature
- ⅔ cup Swerve Granular
- ½ cup heavy whipping cream
- 2 teaspoon pumpkin pie spice

- ¼ teaspoon salt
- 1 box Swerve Yellow Cake Mix divided
- 1 cup chopped pecans
- ⅓ cup Swerve Brown
- ½ cup butter melted

Instructions

1. Preheat the oven to 350°F and grease a 9×13 inch glass or ceramic baking pan.
2. In a large bowl, whisk together the pumpkin, eggs, sweetener, whipping cream, pumpkin spice, and salt. Measure out ½ cup of the cake mix and whisk into the pumpkin mixture until smooth.
3. Pour into the prepared baking pan, then sprinkle the remaining cake mix evenly overtop.
4. In a small bowl, whisk the pecans with the Swerve Brown. Sprinkle this evenly over the cake mix, then drizzle the melted butter evenly over the pecans.
5. Bake 45 to 55 minutes, until the top is just firm to the touch and a rich, deep brown. It will still be very soft underneath.
6. Remove and let cool to room temperature. You can also eat it warm, or chill it in the refrigerator to firm it up.

MACADAMIA NUT KETO CAKE

Nutrition: Cal 138; Fat 13 g; Carb 5 g; Protein 2 g
Serving 12; Cook time 45 min

Ingredients

- 2 whole eggs
- 1/4 cup butter
- 1/2 cup sour cream coconut cream
- 1/4 cup ground flax meal
- 1/4 cup coconut flour
- 1/4 cup almond flour
- 1/2 cup keto brown sugar
- 1 tbsp ground cinnamon
- 1 teaspoon baking powder
- 1 teaspoon vanilla extract
- 1 teaspoon star anise seed
- 1/2 teaspoon salt
- 1/4 teaspoon allspice powder
- 1/2 cup macadamia nuts chopped

Instructions

1. Preheat the oven to 350° F.
2. Whisk eggs in a small bowl. Add butter and cream.

3. In a second bowl, mix all dry ingredients together. Reserve the nuts to be either blended into the batter or sprinkled on top.
4. Combine the dry ingredients with the egg mixture. If desired, blend the nuts in now. Pour batter into greased 8 by 8-inch glass baking dish. If the nuts are not blended in to the dough, sprinkle them on top now.
5. Bake for 30 minutes. Test the center with a knife. If it is ready, remove from the oven and let cool. Serve warm, room temperature or cold.

RHUBARB CAKE

Nutrition: Cal 330; Fat 29 g; Carb 14 g; Protein 12 g
Serving 10; Cook time 10 min

Ingredients
- 3 cups (425g) rhubarb, sliced
- 1/2 cup (100g) plus 2 tablespoons granulated erythritol sweetener, divided
- 3 cups (288g) almond flour
- 1/3 cup (25g) unflavored whey protein powder
- 2 teaspoons baking powder
- 1/4 teaspoon salt
- 1/2 cup (113g) unsalted butter, melted
- 3 large (150g) eggs
- 1/2 cup (113g) unsweetened almond milk
- 1/2 teaspoon vanilla extract

FOR THE CRUMB TOPPING:
- 1/4 cup (24g) almond flour
- 2 tablespoons pecans, finely chopped
- 1 tablespoon granulated erythritol sweetener
- 1 tablespoon unsalted butter, room temperature

Instructions
1. In a medium bowl, toss together the sliced rhubarb and 2 tablespoons of the sweetener. Set aside.
2. Preheat the oven to 350F and grease a 9-inch springform pan very well.
3. In a medium bowl, whisk together the almond flour, remaining 1/2 cup of sweetener, whey protein powder, baking powder, and salt.
4. Stir in the melted butter, eggs, almond milk, and vanilla extract until well combined. Spread 2/3 of the batter in prepared pan. Sprinkle with the rhubarb and dot the remaining batter over in small spoonfuls. Bake 30 minutes.

TO MAKE THE CRUMB TOPPING

1. While the cake is baking, combine the crumb topping ingredients in a small bowl, cutting in the room temperature butter until it resembles coarse crumbs. Sprinkle the crumb topping over the cake and cover with foil.
2. Bake another 20 to 30 minutes, until the edges are golden brown and the center is firm to the touch. Remove and let cool, then run a sharp knife around the inside of the pan to loosen. Remove the sides.

KETO LEMON BLUEBERRY MUG CAKE

Nutrition: Cal 210; Fat 23 g; Carb 8g; Protein 6 g
Serving 1; Cook time 18 min

Ingredients
- ⅓ cup coconut flour
- ⅓ cup Swerve Sweetener
- Zest from one lemon
- 1 teaspoon baking powder
- ¼ teaspoon salt
- 3 large eggs
- ⅓ cup coconut oil melted
- ⅓ cup water
- ½ teaspoon lemon extract
- ⅓ cup blueberries

Instructions
1. In a medium bowl, whisk together the coconut flour, sweetener, lemon zest, baking powder, and salt.
2. Stir in the eggs, coconut oil, water, and lemon extract. Stir in the blueberries and divide the batter between 4 mugs.
3. Cook each mug in the microwave on high for about 1 minute 30 seconds. Cook longer if desired.

KETO PUMPKIN CARAMEL LAVA CAKES

Nutrition: Cal 259; Fat 29 g; Carb 5 g; Protein 6 g
Serving 4; Cook time 45 min

Ingredients
- ½ recipe Sugar-Free Caramel Sauce
- ⅓ cup pumpkin puree
- ¼ cup butter, melted
- 2 large eggs, room temperature
- ½ teaspoon vanilla extract

- 6 tablespoon powdered Swerve Sweetener
- 6 tablespoon almond flour
- 1 teaspoon pumpkin pie spice

Instructions

1. Make the caramel sauce according to the directions, but leave out the additional water in Step 4. Let it cool completely before proceeding.
2. Preheat the oven to 350F and lightly grease 4 small (4 ounce) ramekins.
3. In a large bowl, whisk together the pumpkin puree, melted butter, eggs, and vanilla extract. Stir in the sweetener, almond flour, and pumpkin pie spice until well combined.
4. Divide about ⅔ of the batter between the ramekins to cover the bottom of each. Use a spoon to make a well in the batter (you want some batter to cover the bottom of the ramekin but raised on the sides).
5. Spoon 1 tablespoon of caramel sauce into each well. Use the remaining batter to cover the caramel in each ramekin.
6. Bake 20 to 25 minutes, until the cakes are golden brown and the tops are just barely firm to the touch. The caramel sauce may be bubbling up a bit through the top.
7. Remove and let cool 10 minutes before serving in the ramekins (these will not stand up to be flipped out of the ramekins).
8. Top with keto vanilla ice cream, if desired, and the remaining caramel sauce. If the sauce has thickened considerably, add a tablespoon of water and re-warm gently in the pan.

SLOW COOKER KETO CHOCOLATE CAKE

Nutrition: Cal 205; Fat 17 g; Carb 9 g; Protein 8 g
Serving 10; Cook time 3 hours

Ingredients

- 1 cup plus 2 tablespoon almond flour
- ½ cup Swerve Granular
- ½ cup cocoa powder
- 3 tablespoon unflavoured whey protein powder can sub egg white protein powder
- 1 ½ teaspoon baking powder
- ¼ teaspoon salt
- 6 tablespoon butter melted
- 3 large eggs
- ⅔ cup unsweetened almond milk
- ¾ teaspoon vanilla extract
- ⅓ cup sugar-free chocolate chips optional

Instructions

1. Grease the insert of a 6 quart slow cooker well.
2. In a medium bowl, whisk together almond flour, sweetener, cocoa powder, whey protein powder, baking powder and salt.
3. Stir in butter, eggs, almond milk and vanilla extract until well combined, then stir in chocolate chips, if using.
4. Pour into prepared insert and cook on low for 2 to 2 ½ hours. It will be gooey and like a pudding cake at 2 hours, and more cakey at 2 ½ hours.
5. Turn slow cooker off and let cool 20 to 30 minutes, then cut into pieces and serve warm. Serve with lightly sweetened whipped cream.

KETO SMOOTHITES AND DRINKS

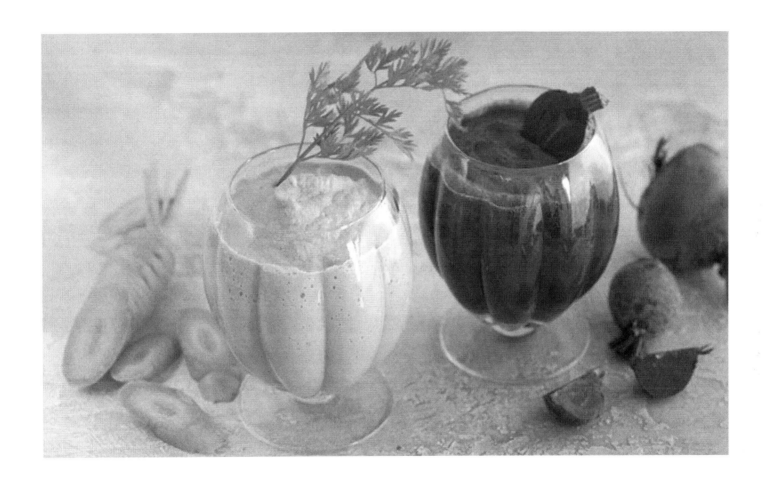

CREAMY CHOCOLATE MILKSHAKE

Nutrition: Cal 292; Fat 25 g; Carb 4 g; Protein 15 g
Serving 2; Cook time 10 min

Ingredients

- 16 oz. unsweetened almond milk, vanilla
- 1 packet stevia
- 4 oz. heavy cream
- 1 scoop Whey Isolate Chocolate protein powder
- ½ cup crushed ice

Instructions

Place all of the ingredients in your blender, and blend until you get a creamy smoothie.

FAT BURNING ESPRESSO SMOOTHIE

Nutrition: Cal 270; Fat 16 g; Carb 2 g; Protein 30 g
Serving 1; Cook time 10 min

Ingredients

- 1 scoop Isopure Zero Carb protein powder
- 1 espresso shot
- ¼ c Greek yogurt, full fat
- Liquid stevia, to sweeten
- Pinch of cinnamon
- 5 ice cubes

Instructions

Place all of the ingredients in your blender, and blend until you get a creamy smoothie.

ALMOND BUTTER & BANANA PROTEIN SMOOTHIE

Nutrition: Cal 402; Fat 3 g; Carb 37 g; Protein 19 g
Serving 1; Cook time 10 min

Ingredients

- 1 small frozen banana
- 1 cup unsweetened almond milk
- tablespoons almond butter
- tablespoons unflavored protein powder
- 1 tablespoon sweetener of your choice (optional)
- ½ teaspoon ground cinnamon

Instructions

Place all of the ingredients in your blender, and blend until you get a creamy smoothie.

BLUEBERRY BLISS

Nutrition: Cal 302; Fat 25 g; Carb 4 g; Protein 15 g
Serving 2; Cook time 10 min

Ingredients

- 16 oz. unsweetened almond milk, vanilla
- 1 packet stevia
- 4 oz. heavy cream
- 1 scoop Whey Isolate Vanilla protein powder
- ¼ cup frozen blueberries, unsweetened

Instructions

Place all of the ingredients in your blender, and blend until you get a creamy smoothie.

CINNAMON ROLL SMOOTHIE

Nutrition: Cal 165; Fat 3 g; Carb 1,6 g; Protein 15 g
Serving 1; Cook time 10 min

Ingredients

- 1 cup unsweetened almond milk
- 2 tbsp. vanilla protein powder
- ½ tsp cinnamon
- ¼ tsp vanilla extract
- 1 packet stevia
- 1 tbsp. chia seeds 1 cup ice cubes

Instructions

Place all of the ingredients in your blender, and blend until you get a creamy smoothie.

BLUEBERRY AVOCADO SMOOTHIE

Nutrition: Cal 377; Fat 22 g; Carb 4 g; Protein 32 g
Serving 1; Cook time 10 min

Ingredients

- 1 cup unsweetened almond milk, vanilla
- 1 tbsp. heavy cream
- ½ avocado, peeled, pitted, sliced
- 1 scoop Isopure Coconut Zero Carb protein powder
- ¼ cup frozen blueberries, unsweetened
- Liquid stevia, to sweeten

Instructions

Place all of the ingredients in your blender, and blend until you get a creamy smoothie.

BLACKBERRY CHOCOLATE SHAKE

Nutrition: Cal 338; Fat 34 g; Carb 4 g; Protein 4 g
Serving 2; Cook time 10 min

Ingredients

- 1 cup unsweetened coconut milk
- ¼ cup fresh blackberries
- 2 tbsp. cacao powder
- Liquid stevia, to sweeten
- 6 ice cubes
- ¼ tsp xanthan gum
- 1-2 tbsp. MCT oil

Instructions

Place all of the ingredients in your blender, and blend until you get a creamy smoothie.

PUMPKIN PIE BUTTERED COFFEE

Nutrition: Cal 125; Fat 12 g; Carb 2 g; Protein 4 g
Serving 1; Cook time 10 min

Ingredients

- 12 oz. hot coffee
- 2 tbsp. canned pumpkin
- 1 tbsp. regular butter, unsalted
- ¼ tsp pumpkin pie spice
- Liquid stevia, to sweeten

Instructions

Place all of the ingredients in your blender, and blend until you get a creamy smoothie.

CUCUMBER SPINACH SMOOTHIE

Nutrition: Cal 335; Fat 33 g; Carb 4 g; Protein 3 g
Serving 1; Cook time 10 min

Ingredients

- 2 large handfuls spinach
- ½ cucumber, peeled and cubed
- 6 ice cubes
- 1 cup coconut milk
- Liquid stevia, to sweeten
- ¼ tsp xanthan gum
- 1-2 tbsp. MCT oil

Instructions

Place all of the ingredients in your blender, and blend until you get a creamy smoothie.

ORANGE CREAMSICLE

Nutrition: Cal 290; Fat 25 g; Carb 4 g; Protein 15 g
Serving 2; Cook time 10 min

Ingredients

- 16 oz. unsweetened almond milk, vanilla
- 1 packet stevia
- 4 oz. heavy cream
- 1 scoop Whey Isolate Tropical Dreamsicle protein powder
- ½ cup crushed ice

Instructions

Place all of the ingredients in your blender, and blend until you get a creamy smoothie.

CAYENNE CHOCOLATE SHAKE

Nutrition: Cal 258; Fat 26 g; Carb 3 g; Protein 3 g
Serving 2; Cook time 10 min

Ingredients

- ¼ cup coconut cream
- 2 tbsp. unrefined coconut oil
- 1 tbsp. whole chia seeds, spectrum
- 2 tbsp. cacao
- Dash of vanilla extract
- Pinch of ground cinnamon
- ½ pinch cayenne powder
- ½ - 1 cup water
- Ice cubes, if desired

Instructions

Place all of the ingredients in your blender, and blend until you get a creamy smoothie.

SHAMROCK SHAKE

Nutrition: Cal 200; Fat 19 g; Carb 4,5 g; Protein 2 g
Serving 1; Cook time 10 min

Ingredients

- 1 cup coconut milk, unsweetened
- 1 avocado, peeled, pitted, sliced
- Liquid stevia, to sweeten
- 1 cup ice
- 1 tbsp. pure vanilla extract
- 1 tsp pure peppermint extract

Instructions

Place all of the ingredients in your blender, and blend until you get a creamy smoothie.

CHAI COCONUT SHAKE

Nutrition: Cal 233; Fat 20 g; Carb 5 g; Protein 4 g
Serving 2; Cook time 10 min

Ingredients

- 1 cup unsweetened coconut milk
- 1 tbsp. pure vanilla extract
- 2 tbsp. almond butter
- ¼ cup unsweetened shredded coconut
- 1 tsp ground ginger
- 1 tsp ground cinnamon
- Pinch of allspice
- 1 tbsp. ground flaxseed
- 5 ice cubes

Instructions

Place all of the ingredients in your blender, and blend until you get a creamy smoothie.

AVOCADO ALMOND SMOOTHIE

Nutrition: Cal 252; Fat 18 g; Carb 5 g; Protein 17 g
Serving 2; Cook time 10 min

Ingredients

- ½ cup unsweetened almond milk, vanilla
- ½ cup half and half
- ½ avocado, peeled, pitted, sliced
- 1 tbsp. almond butter
- 1 scoop Isopure Zero Carb protein powder
- Pinch of cinnamon
- ½ tsp vanilla extract
- 2-4 ice cubes
- Liquid stevia, to sweeten

Instructions

Place all of the ingredients in your blender, and blend until you get a creamy smoothie.

STRAWBERRY ALMOND DELIGHT

Nutrition: Cal 305; Fat 25 g; Carb 7 g; Protein 15 g
Serving 2; Cook time 10 min

Ingredients

16 oz. unsweetened almond milk, vanilla
1 packet stevia
4 oz. heavy cream
1 scoop Whey Isolate Vanilla protein powder
¼ cup frozen strawberries, unsweetened

Instructions

Place all of the ingredients in your blender, and blend until you get a creamy smoothie.

CREAMY BLACKBERRY

Nutrition: Cal 237; Fat 22 g; Carb 6 g; Protein 2 g
Serving 2; Cook time 10 min

Ingredients

- 1 cup fresh blackberries
- 1 cup ice cubes
- Liquid stevia, to sweeten
- ¾ cup heavy whipping cream

Instructions

Place all of the ingredients in your blender, and blend until you get a creamy smoothie.

PEANUT BUTTER MILKSHAKE

Nutrition: Cal 253; Fat 23 g; Carb 7 g; Protein 5 g
Serving 2; Cook time 10 min

Ingredients

- ½ cup coconut milk, regular
- 1 cup unsweetened almond milk, vanilla
- 2 tbsp. all natural peanut butter
- 1 tsp vanilla extract
- 1 cup ice cubes
- 1 packet stevia

Instructions

Place all of the ingredients in your blender, and blend until you get a creamy smoothie.

RASPBERRY SMOOTHIE

Nutrition: Cal 285; Fat 22 g; Carb 7 g; Protein 14 g
Serving 2; Cook time 10 min

Ingredients

- ½ cup fresh raspberries
- 1 cup unsweetened almond milk, vanilla
- 1 scoop prebiotic fibre (Pinnaclife Prebiotic Fibre)
- 1 scoop Vanilla Whey Isolate protein powder
- 2 tbsp. coconut oil
- ¼ cup coconut flakes, unsweetened
- 3-4 ice cubes

Instructions

Place all of the ingredients in your blender, and blend until you get a creamy smoothie.

LEPRECHAUN SHAKE

Nutrition: Cal 217; Fat 13 g; Carb 7 g; Protein 13 g
Serving 2; Cook time 10 min

Ingredients

- ½ avocado, peeled, pitted, sliced
- ¼ cup unsweetened coconut milk
- Small bunch of baby spinach
- ¼ cup fresh mint
- 1 scoop Isopure Zero Carb Whey Protein Isolate
- 1 tsp vanilla extract
- Liquid stevia, to sweeten
- Water, if desired
- 2-3 ice cubes, if desired

Instructions

Place all of the ingredients in your blender, and blend until you get a creamy smoothie.

BREAKFAST EGG SMOOTHIE

Nutrition: Cal 266; Fat 17 g; Carb 6 g; Protein 22 g
Serving 2; Cook time 10 min

Ingredients

- ½ cup coconut milk, unsweetened
- ½ cup Lifeway Organic Whole Milk Kefir, plain
- 4 tbsp. chia seeds
- 1 oz. egg substitute dry powder

Instructions

Place all of the ingredients in your blender, and blend until you get a creamy smoothie.

PEANUT BUTTER CARAMEL SHAKE

Nutrition: Cal 366; Fat 35 g; Carb 6 g; Protein 7 g
Serving 1; Cook time 10 min

Ingredients

- 1 cup ice cubes
- 1 cup coconut milk, unsweetened
- 2 tbsp. natural peanut butter
- 2 tbsp. Sugar-free Torani Salted Caramel
- ¼ tsp. xanthan gum, to thicken smoothie
- 1 tbsp. MCT oil

Instructions

Place all of the ingredients in your blender, and blend until you get a creamy smoothie.

CREAMY GREEN MACHINE

Nutrition: Cal 279; Fat 18 g; Carb 9 g; Protein 18 g
Serving 2; Cook time 10 min

Ingredients

½ cup unsweetened almond milk, vanilla
½ cup half and half
½ avocado, peeled, pitted, sliced
½ cup frozen blueberries, unsweetened
1 cup spinach
1 tbsp. almond butter
1 scoop Isopure Zero Carb protein powder
2-4 ice cubes
1 packet stevia

Instructions

Place all of the ingredients in your blender, and blend until you get a creamy smoothie.

COCONUT SUPERFOOD SMOOTHIE

Nutrition: Cal 272; Fat 22 g; Carb 8 g; Protein 15 g
Serving 2; Cook time 10 min

Ingredients

- ½ cup unsweetened almond milk, vanilla
- ½ cup coconut cream
- 1 scoop Isopure Zero Carb protein powder
- ½ cup frozen blueberries, unsweetened
- 2-4 ice cubes

Instructions

Place all of the ingredients in your blender, and blend until you get a creamy smoothie.

CREAMY STRAWBERRY

Nutrition: Cal 140; Fat 39 g; Carb 9 g; Protein 27 g
Serving 2; Cook time 10 min

Ingredients

- 1 cup ice cubes
- ½ cup water
- 1 scoop Isopure Zero Carb Strawberry protein powder
- 3 slices avocado, peeled, pitted
- 1 oz. MCT oil
- 1/2 cup frozen strawberries, unsweetened

Instructions

Place all of the ingredients in your blender, and blend until you get a creamy smoothie.

SPRING SMOOTHIE

Nutrition: Cal 263; Fat 19 g; Carb 8 g; Protein 12 g
Serving 2; Cook time 10 min

Ingredients
- 2 large handfuls mixed greens (spinach and kale)
- 1 oz. almonds, unsalted
- ¼ cup frozen blueberries, unsweetened
- 1 tbsp. chia seeds
- 1 cup raspberry tea, unsweetened

Instructions
Place all of the ingredients in your blender, and blend until you get a creamy smoothie.

VANILLA HEMP

Nutrition: Cal 250; Fat 20 g; Carb 9 g; Protein 7 g
Serving 2; Cook time 10 min

Ingredients
- 1 cup water
- 1 cup unsweetened hemp milk, vanilla
- 1 ½ tbsp. coconut oil, unrefined
- ½ cup frozen berries, mixed
- 4 cup leafy greens (kale and spinach)
- 1 tbsp. flaxseeds or chia seeds
- 1 tbsp. almond butter

Instructions
Place all of the ingredients in your blender, and blend until you get a creamy smoothie.

CACAO SUPER SMOOTHIE

Nutrition: Cal 445; Fat 14 g; Carb 9 g; Protein 16 g
Serving 2; Cook time 10 min

Ingredients
- ½ cup unsweetened almond milk, vanilla
- ½ cup half and half
- ½ avocado, peeled, pitted, sliced
- ½ cup frozen blueberries, unsweetened
- 1 tbsp. cacao powder
- 1 scoop Whey Isolate Vanilla protein powder
- Liquid stevia, to sweeten

Instructions
Place all of the ingredients in your blender, and blend until you get a creamy smoothie.

PEPPERMINT MOCHA

Nutrition: Cal 198; Fat 16 g; Carb 9 g; Protein 3 g
Serving 2; Cook time 10 min

Ingredients
- 1 cup cold coffee
- 1/3 Organic Chocolove Dark Chocolate, 73%
- 2 tbsp. avocado, peeled, pitted, sliced
- ½ cup half and half
- 2 tbsp. fresh mint (about 20 leaves) or 1 tsp mint extract
- 2 tsp cacao powder ¼ cup water
- Liquid stevia, to sweetener
- ¼ cup ice cubes

Instructions
Place all of the ingredients in your blender, and blend until you get a creamy smoothie.

HAPPY GUT SMOOTHIE

Nutrition: Cal 410; Fat 33 g; Carb 8 g; Protein 12 g
Serving 1; Cook time 10 min

Ingredients
- 2-3 cup spinach leaves
- 1 ½ tbsp. coconut oil, unrefined
- ½ cup plain full fat yogurt
- 1 tbsp. chia seeds 1 serving aloe vera leaves
- ½ cup frozen blueberries, unsweetened
- 1 tbsp. hemp hearts
- 1 cup water
- 1 scoop Pinnaclife Prebiotic Fibre

Instructions
Place all of the ingredients in your blender, and blend until you get a creamy smoothie.

STRAWBERRY CHEESECAKE SMOOTHIE

Nutrition: Cal 247; Fat 19 g; Carb 8 g; Protein 3 g
Serving 1; Cook time 10 min

Ingredients
- ½ cup frozen strawberries, unsweetened
- ½ cup unsweetened vanilla almond milk
- Liquid stevia, to sweeten
- ½ tsp vanilla extract
- 2 oz. cream cheese, regular
- 3-4 ice cubes

•Water, optional

Instructions

Place all of the ingredients in your blender, and blend until you get a creamy smoothie.

SILKEN TOFU SMOOTHIE

Nutrition: Cal 208; Fat 12 g; Carb 10 g; Protein 18 g
Serving 2; Cook time 10 min

Ingredients

•½ cup strawberries, unfrozen

•Silken tofu

•1 cup unsweetened almond milk, vanilla

•Pinch of cinnamon

•Liquid Stevia, to sweeten

Instructions

Place all of the ingredients in your blender, and blend until you get a creamy smoothie.

MANGO GREEN TEA & CARROT SMOOTHIE

Nutrition: Cal 133; Fat 9 g; Carb 10 g; Protein 6 g
Serving 2; Cook time 10 min

Ingredients

•2 cup water

•½ cup baby carrots

•Pinch of fresh ginger

•½ cup frozen mango

•Liquid stevia, to sweeten

•1 tbsp. chia seed

Instructions

Place all of the ingredients in your blender, and blend until you get a creamy smoothie.

PUMPKIN PARADISE

Nutrition: Cal270; Fat 10 g; Carb 10 g; Protein 30 g
Serving 1; Cook time 10 min

Ingredients

•½ cup unsweetened almond milk, vanilla

•½ cup water

•½ cup canned pumpkin

•½ tsp pumpkin pie spice

•Stevia packet

•1 scoop Isopure Zero Carb protein powder

•1 oz. cream cheese

•2-3 ice cubes

•Ground cinnamon, to taste

Instructions

Place all of the ingredients in your blender, and blend until you get a creamy smoothie.

CREAMY GREEN SMOOTHIE

Nutrition: Cal 315; Fat 25 g; Carb 10 g; Protein 13 g
Serving 2; Cook time 10 min

Ingredients

•¼ avocado, peeled, pitted, sliced

•4 broccoli florets, if desired

•1 bunch of kale and spinach

•1 slice honeydew

•½ cup coconut milk

•2 tbsp. plain Greek yogurt, full fat

•1 tbsp. almond butter

•½ cup unsweetened almond milk, vanilla

•¼ cup water, optional

•½ scoop Isopure Zero Carb Protein powder

Instructions

Place all of the ingredients in your blender, and blend until you get a creamy smoothie.

RED VELVET SMOOTHIE

Nutrition: Cal 228; Fat 16 g; Carb 13 g; Protein 7 g
Serving 2; Cook time 10 min

Ingredients

•2 cup unsweetened almond milk, vanilla

•2 cup ice cubes

•2-3 slices avocado, peeled, pitted, sliced

•1 beet, small, cooked

•2 tbsp. cacao

•¼ tsp pure vanilla extract

•Liquid stevia, to sweeten

Instructions

Place all of the ingredients in your blender, and blend until you get a creamy smoothie.

WHIPPED SHAKE

Nutrition: Cal 238; Fat 22 g; Carb 13 g; Protein 7 g
Serving 1; Cook time 10 min

Ingredients

•1 cup unsweetened almond milk

•1/3 cup heavy whipping cream

•2-4 drops liquid stevia

- ½ tsp vanilla extract
- 2 tbsp. cacao (use 1 tbsp. for lower carbohydrate)
- 3 ice cubes

Instructions

Place all of the ingredients in your blender, and blend until you get a creamy smoothie.

GREEN AND BLUE SMOOTHIE

Nutrition: Cal 230; Fat 4 g; Carb 12 g; Protein 38 g
Serving 1; Cook time 10 min

Ingredients

- 1/4 cup frozen blueberries
- 1/3 cup unsweetened almond milk •
- 1/2 cup Greek or Fage yogurt (plain or full-fat)
- 1 scoop vanilla isolate protein
- or 2 tablespoons gelatin plus
- 1 teaspoon vanilla extract
- 1 cup spinach, loosely packed
- 1/3 cup ice

Instructions

Place all of the ingredients in your blender, and blend until you get a creamy smoothie.

BERRY POLKA DOT DANCE

Nutrition: Cal 268; Fat 4 g; Carb 9 g; Protein 14 g
Serving 2; Cook time 10 min

Ingredients

- 1 1/2 cup unsweetened almond milk
- 1 cup spinach
- 2 tablespoons flax seeds
- 1/3 cup frozen blackberries
- 1/3 cup frozen blueberries
- 1 scoop vanilla isolate protein or 2 tablespoons gelatin plus
- 1 teaspoon vanilla extract

Instructions

Place all of the ingredients in your blender, and blend until you get a creamy smoothie.

ALMOND STRAWBERRY DELIGHT

Nutrition: Cal 352; Fat 24 g; Carb 9 g; Protein 26 g
Serving 2; Cook time 10 min

Ingredients

- 16 ounces unsweetened almond milk, vanilla
- 1 packet stevia or 2 teaspoons Splenda

- 4 ounce heavy cream
- 2 scoops vanilla isolate protein or 4 tablespoons gelatin plus 1 teaspoon vanilla extract
- 1/4 cup frozen strawberries, unsweetened

Instructions

Place all of the ingredients in your blender, and blend until you get a creamy smoothie.

CREAMY BLACKBERRY

Nutrition: Cal 300; Fat 17 g; Carb 12 g; Protein 25 g
Serving 1; Cook time 10 min

Ingredients

- 1 cup fresh blackberries
- 1 packet stevia or 2 teaspoons Splenda
- 3/4 cup heavy whipping cream
- 2 scoops vanilla isolate protein or 4 tablespoons gelatin plus
- 2 teaspoon vanilla extract
- 1 cup ice cubes

Instructions

Place all of the ingredients in your blender, and blend until you get a creamy smoothie.

SPICY GREEN SALAD SMOOTHIE

Nutrition: Cal 267; Fat 2 g; Carb 10 g; Protein 3 g
Serving 2; Cook time 10 min

Ingredients

- 1 cup fresh white cabbage
- 1 handful fresh baby kale
- 1 handful fresh parsley
- 1 lemon juice, squeezed into the blender
- 1 medium Roma or Heirloom tomato
- 1/2 cup water
- 1/2 habanero pepper, remove seeds
- 1/2 Italian cucumber
- 5–6 ice cubes

Instructions

Place all of the ingredients in your blender, and blend until you get a creamy smoothie.

SUPERFOOD COCONUT SMOOTHIE

Nutrition: Cal 216; Fat 15 g; Carb 9 g; Protein 13 g
Serving 2; Cook time 10 min

Ingredients

- 1/2 cup coconut cream

- 1/2 cup frozen blueberries
- 1/2 cup unsweetened almond milk, vanilla
- 1 scoop vanilla isolate protein or 2 tablespoons gelatin plus
- 1 teaspoon vanilla extract
- 2-4 ice cubes

Instructions

Place all of the ingredients in your blender, and blend until you get a creamy smoothie.

DAIRY-FREE GREEN SMOOTHIE

Nutrition: Cal 230; Fat 4 g; Carb 9 g; Protein 2 g
Serving 2; Cook time 10 min

Ingredients

- 1 cup raw cucumber, peeled and sliced
- 1 cup romaine lettuce
- 1 tablespoon fresh ginger, peeled and chopped
- 1/2 cup kiwi fruit, peeled and chopped
- 1/2 Half avocado (remove pit and scoop flesh out of shell)
- 1/3 cup chopped fresh pineapple
- 2 tablespoons fresh parsley
- 3 teaspoons Splenda
- 4 cups water

Instructions

Place all of the ingredients in your blender, and blend until you get a creamy smoothie.

COCONUT CHAI SMOOTHIE

Nutrition: Cal 420; Fat 38 g; Carb 13 g; Protein 7 g
Serving 2; Cook time 10 min

Ingredients

- 1/4 cup unsweetened shredded coconut
- 1 cup unsweetened coconut milk
- 1 tablespoon ground flaxseed
- 1 tablespoon pure vanilla extract
- 1 teaspoon ground cinnamon
- 1 teaspoon ground ginger
- 2 tablespoons almond butter
- Pinch of allspice
- 5 ice cubes

Instructions

Place all of the ingredients in your blender, and blend until you get a creamy smoothie.

SPICY GREEN SALAD SMOOTHIE

Nutrition: Cal 154; Fat 3 g; Carb 10 g; Protein 2 g
Serving 1; Cook time 10 min

Ingredients

- 1 cup fresh white cabbage
- 1 handful fresh baby kale
- 1 handful fresh parsley
- 1 lemon juice, squeezed into the blender
- 1 medium Roma or Heirloom tomato
- 1/2 cup water
- 1/2 habanero pepper, remove seeds
- 1/2 Italian cucumber
- 5–6 ice cubes

Instructions

Place all of the ingredients in your blender, and blend until you get a creamy smoothie.

GREEN MINTY PROTEIN SHAKE

Nutrition: Cal 184; Fat 10 g; Carb 9 g; Protein 13 g
Serving 2; Cook time 10 min

Ingredients

- 1 packet stevia or 2 teaspoons Splenda
- 1/4 teaspoon peppermint extract
- 1/2 cup almond milk, unsweetened
- 1/2 avocado
- 1 scoop vanilla or
- chocolate isolate protein
- 1 cup spinach, fresh
- 1 cup ice

Instructions

Place all of the ingredients in your blender, and blend until you get a creamy smoothie.

PEPPERMINT PATTY

Nutrition: Cal 166; Fat 5 g; Carb 9 g; Protein 28 g
Serving 2; Cook time 10 min

Ingredients

- 1/4 teaspoon mint extract
- 1 scoop chocolate isolate protein
- 1 cup unsweetened almond milk
- 1 cup spinach
- 2 tbsp. unsweetened cocoa powder
- Ice cubes

Instructions

Place all of the ingredients in your blender, and blend until you get a creamy smoothie.

BLUE-RASPBERRY SMOOTHIE

Nutrition: Cal 191; Fat 6 g; Carb 12 g; Protein 26 g
Serving 1; Cook time 10 min

Ingredients

- 1/4 cup blueberries, frozen
- 1/4 cup raspberries, frozen
- 1 ½ cups unsweetened almond milk
- 1 pack gelatin or 1 scoop isolate protein

Instructions

Place all of the ingredients in your blender, and blend until you get a creamy smoothie

BLUEBERRY CHIA SMOOTHIE

Nutrition: Cal 160; Fat 3 g; Carb 9 g; Protein 4 g
Serving 1; Cook time 10 min

Ingredients

- ½ cup blueberries
- 1/2 banana
- 1/2 cup nonfat milk
- 1/2 cup plain nonfat Greek Yogurt
- 1 tablespoon chia seeds
- 1/2 cup ice

Instructions

Place all of the ingredients in your blender, and blend until you get a creamy smoothie.

STRAWBERRY-ALMOND CRUNCH SMOOTHIE

Nutrition: Cal 135; Fat 10 g; Carb 11 g; Protein 4 g
Serving 1; Cook time 10 min

Ingredients

- 2 tablespoons almonds
- 1/2 teaspoon cinnamon
- 1/2 cup organic
- strawberries, frozen
- 1 cup unsweetened almond milk, vanilla
- 2 iced cubes

Instructions

Place all of the ingredients in your blender, and blend until you get a creamy smoothie.

PEACH PIE SHAKE

Nutrition: Cal 209; Fat 4 g; Carb 11 g; Protein 28 g
Serving 1; Cook time 10 min

Ingredients

- 1 peach, pitted
- 1 scoop vanilla protein powder or 2 tablespoons gelatin plus
- 1 teaspoon vanilla extract
- 1/4 cup plain Greek yogurt
- 2 pinches of cinnamon
- 2/3 cup unsweetened almond milk
- 8-10 ice cubes

Instructions

Place all of the ingredients in your blender, and blend until you get a creamy smoothie.

BUTTERED PUMPKIN PIE COFFEE

Nutrition: Cal 12; Fat 3 g; Carb 10 g; Protein 1 g
Serving 1; Cook time 10 min

Ingredients

- 1/4 teaspoon pumpkin pie spice
- 1 tablespoon regular butter, unsalted
- 12 ounces hot coffee
- 2 tablespoons canned pumpkin
- 1 packet stevia or 2 teaspoons Splenda

Instructions

Place all of the ingredients in your blender, and blend until you get a creamy smoothie.

PEANUT BUTTER CRUNCH CHOCOLATE SMOOTHIE

Nutrition: Cal 236; Fat 19 g; Carb 11 g; Protein 3 g
Serving 2; Cook time 10 min

Ingredients

- 1 cup unsweetened almond milk
- 1/3 cup heavy whipping cream
- 1 packet stevia or 2 teaspoons Splenda
- 1/2 teaspoon vanilla extract
- 1 tablespoon unsweetened cocoa powder
- 3 ice cubes

Instructions

Place all of the ingredients in your blender, and blend until you get a creamy smoothie.

MANGO ALMOND SMOOTHIE

Nutrition: Cal 130; Fat 3 g; Carb 12 g; Protein 25 g
Serving 2; Cook time 10 min

Ingredients

- 125 g mango, frozen
- 3/4 cup unsweetened almond milk
- 1 pack gelatin or 1 scoop isolate protein
- 1 tablespoon flax seeds
- 1/2 cup ice cubes

Instructions

Place all of the ingredients in your blender, and blend until you get a creamy smoothie.

ALMOND STRAWBERRY SMOOTHIE

Nutrition: Cal 162; Fat 6 g; Carb 4 g; Protein 26g
Serving 2; Cook time 10 min

Ingredients

- 16 ounces unsweetened Almond milk
- 8 almonds
- 2 large strawberry, frozen
- 1 1/2 scoop whey protein powder or 3 tablespoon gelatin
- 6 ice cubes

Instructions

Place all of the ingredients in your blender, and blend until you get a creamy smoothie.

CHOCOLATE AVOCADO CREAM SMOOTHIE

Nutrition: Cal 433; Fat 32 g; Carb 15 g; Protein 25 g
Serving 2; Cook time 10 min

Ingredients

- 1 avocado, frozen
- 1/2 cup heavy cream
- 1 tablespoons dark chocolate
- 1 teaspoon Splenda
- 1 pack gelatin or 1 scoop chocolate isolate protein
- 1 cup water

Instructions

Place all of the ingredients in your blender, and blend until you get a creamy smoothie.

BERRIES & CREAM KETO PROTEIN SMOOTHIE

Nutrition: Cal 540; Fat 50 g; Carb 7 g; Protein 10 g
Serving 1; Cook time 10 min

Ingredients

- 1 cup coconut milk
- ⅓ cup frozen raspberries
- 1 Tbsp coconut oil or MCT oil
- 1 scoop collagen
- sweetener of choice, to taste

Instructions

Place all of the ingredients in your blender, and blend until you get a creamy smoothie.

CUCUMBER CELERY MATCHA KETO SMOOTHIE

Nutrition: Cal 280; Fat 27 g; Carb 10 g; Protein 3 g
Serving 1; Cook time 10 min

Ingredients

- ½ cup cashew milk
- 1 baby cucumber
- 1 stalk celery
- ½ avocado
- 1 Tbsp coconut oil or MCT oil
- 1 tsp matcha powder
- sweetener of choice, to taste

Instructions

Place all of the ingredients in your blender, and blend until you get a creamy smoothie.

GOLDEN MILK KETO SMOOTHIE

Nutrition: Cal 420; Fat 50 g; Carb 4 g; Protein 6 g
Serving 1; Cook time 10 min

Ingredients

8 coconut milk ice cubes, thawed slightly (or ~1 cup coconut milk)
2 Tbsp additional coconut milk or water
½ tsp vanilla
1 Tbsp coconut oil or MCT oil
½ tsp turmeric
¼ tsp cinnamon
pinch of ground ginger
pinch of salt
sweetener of choice, to taste

Instructions

Place all of the ingredients in your blender, and blend until you get a creamy smoothie.

CINNAMON ALMOND BULLETPROOF SMOOTHIE

Nutrition: Cal 500; Fat 48 g; Carb 11 g; Protein 9 g
Serving 1; Cook time 10 min

Ingredients

- 1 cup coffee
- 4 coconut milk ice cubes, or ~⅓-½ cup coconut milk
- 1 Tbsp coconut oil or MCT oil
- 2 Tbsp almond butter
- 1 Tbsp flax meal
- ½ tsp cinnamon
- sweetener of choice, to taste
- pinch of salt

Instructions

Place all of the ingredients in your blender, and blend until you get a creamy smoothie.

BLACKBERRY CHEESECAKE KETO SMOOTHIE

Nutrition: Cal 450; Fat 41 g; Carb 14 g; Protein 5 g
Serving 1; Cook time 10 min

Ingredients

- ½ cup blackberries, frozen
- ¼ cup 2 oz cream cheese (or full-fat coconut milk, for dairy-free)
- 1 Tbsp coconut oil or MCT oil
- ¼ tsp vanilla extract
- sweetener of choice, to taste
- pinch of salt
- ¼ cup coconut milk
- ½ cup water

Instructions

Place all of the ingredients in your blender, and blend until you get a creamy smoothie.

MOCHA KETO COFFEE SHAKE

Nutrition: Cal 142; Fat 3 g; Carb 28 g; Protein 4 g
Serving 1; Cook time 10 min

Ingredients

- ¾ cup coconut milk, frozen into ice cubes (~6-8 cubes)
- ½ cup cold brew coffee, or leftover cold coffee
- scoop chocolate keto meal shake, or chocolate protein powder of choice
- 1 Tbsp cashew butter

Instructions

1. Pour coconut milk into ice cube tray and freeze overnight, until set.
2. When ready to drink, add all ingredients to a blender and blend until smooth.

KETO CHOCOLATE SHAKE

Nutrition: Cal 409; Fat 39 g; Carb 10 g; Protein 6 g
Serving 1; Cook time 10 min

Ingredients

- ¾ cup unsweetened almond milk, or milk of choice
- 3 Tbsp heavy cream, or coconut cream
- 1½ tsp cocoa powder
- 10g 90%+ dark chocolate, (or keto chocolate chips)
- 1 Tbsp nut butter of choice
- 1-2 Tbsp low carb sweetener of choice, to taste, (i.e., erythritol or monk fruit)
- ⅓ cup ice
- 1-3 tsp coconut or MCT oil, (for additional fat, optional)

OPTIONAL ADDITION:

- ½-1 scoop protein powder or collagen powder

Instructions

Place all of the ingredients in your blender, and blend until you get a creamy smoothie.

VEGAN KETO PUMPKIN CREAM COLD BREW

Nutrition: Cal 53; Fat 3 g; Carb 5 g; Protein 3 g
Serving 1; Cook time 10 min

Ingredients

¾ cup cold brew or cold brew concentrate
½ cup water, use less water for a stronger brew

KETO PUMPKIN CREAM COLD BREW FOAM

- 1 cup milk of choice
- 1 tsp canned pumpkin puree
- ½ tsp pumpkin pie spice
- ⅛ tsp glucomannan powder
- pinch of salt

Instructions

1. Combine cold brew and water as desired. Serve over ice.
2. Separately, combine milk of choice, pumpkin puree, pumpkin pie spice, glucomannan powder, and salt. If desired, add stevia drops or sweetener of choice to taste.
3. Use a frother or immersion blender to mix ingredients together until frothy! Froth/blend for 2-3 minutes, let it sit for a minute, then continue blending for another minute until thickened and holding form.
4. Pour foam on top of cold brew, sprinkle with pumpkin pie spice, and serve.

CINNAMON DOLCE LATTE

Nutrition: Cal 235; Fat 22 g; Carb 5 g; Protein 13 g
Serving 1; Cook time 10 min

Ingredients
- 1/2 cup unsweetened milk of choice
- 6 ounces cold brewed coffee
- 1/2 tablespoon chia seeds
- 1/2 teaspoon ceylon cinnamon
- 1 scoop Perfect Keto Collagen Powder
- 1 tablespoon Perfect Keto MCT Oil

OPTIONAL
1 handful ice
keto friendly sweetener of choice to taste

Instructions
Place all of the ingredients in your blender, and blend un-til you get a creamy smoothie.

ENERGIZING KETO SMOOTHIE

Nutrition: Cal 250; Fat 26 g; Carb 4 g; Protein 4 g
Serving 1; Cook time 10 min

Ingredients
- 1 cup unsweetened cashew milk
- 1 tablespoon Perfect Keto MCT Oil
- 1 tablespoon Perfect Keto Nut Butter
- 2 teaspoons maca powder
- 1 handful ice

Instructions
Place all of the ingredients in your blender, and blend un-til you get a creamy smoothie.

CHOCOLATE SEA SALT SMOOTHIE

Nutrition: Cal 235; Fat 20 g; Carb 11,5 g; Protein 5,5 g
Serving 1; Cook time 10 min

Ingredients

- 1 avocado (frozen or not)
- 2 cups almond milk
- 1 tablespoon tahini
- 1/4 cup cocoa powder
- 1 scoop Perfect Keto 'Chocolate' Base
- Stevia or monk fruit to taste

Instructions
Place all of the ingredients in your blender, and blend un-til you get a creamy smoothie.

ACAI ALMOND BUTTER SMOOTHIE

Nutrition: Cal 235; Fat 20 g; Carb 11,5 g; Protein 5,5 g
Serving 1; Cook time 10 min

Ingredients
- 1 100g Pack Unsweetened Acai Puree
- 3/4 cup Unsweetened Almond Milk
- 1/4 of an Avocado
- 3 tbsp Collagen or Protein Powder
- 1 tbsp Coconut Oil or MCT Oil Powder
- 1 tbsp Almond Butter
- 1/2 tsp Vanilla Extract
- 2 drops Liquid Stevia

Instructions
If you are using individualized 100 gram packs of acai puree, run the pack under lukewarm water for a few seconds until you are able to break up the puree into smaller pieces. Open the pack and put the contents into the blender.

Place the remaining ingredients in the blender and blend until smooth. Add more water or ice cubes as needed.

Drizzle the almond butter along the side of the glass to make it look cool.

STRAWBERRY AVOCADO KETO SMOOTHIE

Nutrition: Cal 106; Fat 7 g; Carb 10 g; Protein 1 g
Serving 1; Cook time 10 min

Ingredients
- 1 lb Frozen strawberries
- 1 1/2 cups Unsweetened almond milk
- 1 large Avocado
- 1/4 cup Besti Powdered Monk Fruit Allulose Blend

Instructions

Place all of the ingredients in your blender, and blend un-til you get a creamy smoothie.

KETO SMOOTHIE – BLUEBERRY

Nutrition: Cal 215; Fat 10 g; Carb 7 g; Protein 23 g
Serving 1; Cook time 10 min

Ingredients

- 1 cup Coconut Milk or almond milk
- 1/4 cup Blueberries
- 1 tsp Vanilla Extract
- 1 tsp MCT Oil or coconut oil
- 30 g Protein Powder

Instructions

Place all of the ingredients in your blender, and blend until you get a creamy smoothie.

CHOCOLATE FAT BOMB SMOOTHIE

Nutrition: Cal 240; Fat 11 g; Carb 4 g; Protein 13 g
Serving 1; Cook time 10 min

Ingredients

- 70 g avocado, frozen pieces 1/2 a cup
- 1 scoop perfect keto chocolate collagen
- 1 tbsp cacao powder
- 1 cup almond milk
- ½ – 1 cup ice

Instructions

Place all of the ingredients in your blender, and blend until you get a creamy smoothie.

KETO CREAMY HOT CHOCOLATE

Nutrition: Cal 183; Fat 15 g; Carb 1 g; Protein 10 g
Serving 1; Cook time 10 min

Ingredients

- 1 scoop Perfect Keto chocolate collagen
- 2 tbsp pure cream (heavy whipping cream)
- 1 cup boiling water

Instructions

Add chocolate collagen and cream to a cup of boiling water

Blend to combine. You could do this in your blender, with a milk frother or stick blender

KETO DAIRY FREE SHAMROCK SHAKE

Nutrition: Cal 137; Fat 3 g; Carb 3 g; Protein 4 g
Serving 1; Cook time 10 min

Ingredients

- ½ medium avocado
- 1 scoop dairy free vanilla protein powder (about 30g)
- ½ cup almond or coconut milk
- 8 ice cubes
- ⅛ teaspoon peppermint extract
- 5 drops natural green food coloring (optional for color)
- 2 tablespoon coconut milk whipped cream (optional)
- 1 tablespoon sugar-free dark chocolate chips

Instructions

Place all of the ingredients in your blender, and blend until you get a creamy smoothie.

KETO BLUEBERRY CHEESECAKE SMOOTHIE

Nutrition: Cal 311; Fat 27 g; Carb 9 g; Protein 6 g
Serving 1; Cook time 10 min

Ingredients

- ½ medium avocado
- 1 scoop dairy free vanilla protein powder (about 30g)
- ½ cup almond or coconut milk
- 8 ice cubes
- ⅛ teaspoon peppermint extract
- 5 drops natural green food coloring (optional for color)
- 2 tablespoon coconut milk whipped cream (optional)
- 1 tablespoon sugar-free dark chocolate chips

Instructions

Place all of the ingredients in your blender, and blend until you get a creamy smoothie.

HIGH PROTEIN KETO STRAWBERRY SMOOTHIE

Nutrition: Cal 205; Fat 14 g; Carb 8 g; Protein 13 g
Serving 2; Cook time 10 min

Ingredients

- ½ medium avocado
- 1 scoop dairy free vanilla protein powder (about 30g)
- ½ cup almond or coconut milk
- 8 ice cubes
- ⅛ teaspoon peppermint extract
- 5 drops natural green food coloring (optional for color
- 2 tablespoon coconut milk whipped cream (optional)
- 1 tablespoon sugar-free dark chocolate chips

Instructions

Place all of the ingredients in your blender, and blend until you get a creamy smoothie.

Conclusion

We hope that by the time you've reached the last pages of "Keto for Women Over 60: 500 Great Recipes for Weight Loss and a Healthy Life," you've gained the knowledge, confidence, and enthusiasm to begin a ketogenic journey that's perfect for you. You can now take control of your life and health by knowing the incredible benefits of the ketogenic diet for women over 60, learning how to stick to it, and discovering how to optimize ketosis.

In this book, we delved into the health benefits of the ketogenic diet and offered concrete advice on how to enter and remain in a state of nutritional ketosis for women over the age of 60. You can ease into a ketogenic diet with the help of the accompanying meal plan and exhaustive list of permitted products.

Keep in mind that persistence and commitment are crucial as you go forward on your trip. Recognize and enjoy your progress, and use setbacks as opportunities to grow. The ketogenic diet may aid in healthy aging and provide a lively sense of well-being and vitality.

Finally, we hope that you find success in your efforts to improve your health, happiness, and overall quality of life. The 500 tasty and healthy recipes in this book are a testament to the efficacy of the ketogenic diet and are meant to inspire you to cook delicious and healthy food that will help you achieve your health and fitness goals. Here's to a beautiful, fruitful, and long life for all women over 60!

JASMINE PATEL

Made in the USA
Columbia, SC
09 July 2023

20200213R00124